HUMAN REPRODUCTIVE SYSTEM - ANATOMY, ROLES AND DISORDERS

TESTIS

ANATOMY, PHYSIOLOGY AND PATHOLOGY

Human Reproductive System - Anatomy, Roles and Disorders

Additional books in this series can be found on Nova's website
under the Series tab.

Additional E-books in this series can be found on Nova's website
under the E-book tab.

Human Anatomy and Physiology

Additional books in this series can be found on Nova's website
under the Series tab.

Additional E-books in this series can be found on Nova's website
under the E-book tab.

HUMAN REPRODUCTIVE SYSTEM - ANATOMY, ROLES AND DISORDERS

TESTIS

ANATOMY, PHYSIOLOGY AND PATHOLOGY

YOICHI NEMOTO
AND
NORIO INABA
EDITORS

Nova Science Publishers, Inc.
New York

For permission to use material from this book please contact us:
Telephone 631-231-7269; Fax 631-231-8175
Web Site: http://www.novapublishers.com

LIBRARY OF CONGRESS CATALOGING-IN-PUBLICATION DATA

ISBN 978-1-61942-739-6

Published by Nova Science Publishers, Inc. † New York

CONTENTS

PREFACE

In this book, the authors present current research in the study of the anatomy, physiology and pathology of the testes. Topics discussed in this compilation include the roles and regulatory mechanism of proton pumping V-ATPase in spermatozoa and epididymis physiology; oxidative stress as a converging mechanism of testicular damage; the pathophysiology of the testis after ischemia reperfusion injury; beta-actin implications in the seminiferous tubule; heat stress damage in mammalian testis; and the effect of plasticizers on testis and Sertoli cell functions.

Chapter 1 - Mammalian spermatogenesis is a complex physiological process that takes place inside seminiferous tubules in the testis. This process involves a fine balance between cell proliferation, differentiation and apoptosis, ending up with a motile spermatozoon. In most mammals the testes are kept 4-5 °C below body core temperature in the scrotum and the spermatogenic process proceeds with a blood and oxygen supply that appears to be fairly independent of changes in other vascular beds in the body. Despite this well-controlled environment, special circumstances (i.e. genetics), lifestyle, occupational work, pathologies (e.g. diabetes, cryptorchidism and varicocele) and environmental exposure to low oxygen (hypoxia) can result in a decrease of blood flow, nutrients and oxygen supply along with increased temperature. All of these conditions, besides those that cause some pathological conditions, may lead to subfertility or infertility. However, they also represent unique conditions that help us to address some crucial questions about the cell biology and physiology of spermatogenesis: what advantage is there for the spermatogenic cell processes mentioned above taking place under mild hypothermia? What are the molecular and physiological processes that make spermatocytes especially vulnerable to high temperatures? What mechanisms of adaptation take place in the seminiferous tubules cells under hypoxia? What mechanisms lead to a decreased sperm output from spermatogenesis under hypoxia? Do these conditions have similar physiological and molecular pathways? In this chapter, we will review the available literature on human and animal models concerning "extreme" conditions for spermatogenesis, such as: heat stress, hypoxia and pathological conditions like varicocele, cryptorchidism and diabetes. Our analyses suggest that germ cell apoptosis, oxidative stress and DNA damage are common features in all of these "extreme" conditions. Furthermore, oxidative damage seems to be present in all of these conditions during the initiation step of cellular damage. This oxidative stress in the testicle is critical when it poses an imminent risk to the viability and quality of the reproductive cells of animals and humans subjected to extreme conditions. Thus, about 25% of infertile patients are diagnosed with elevated levels of reactive oxygen species (ROS) in semen samples. It is well documented that oxidative damage and elevated ROS levels in germ cells lead to apoptosis, a likely cause of hypospermatogenesis and low sperm production in these patients.

Chapter 2 - Recent developments in immunology and cell biology highlighted the importance of inflammation in the pathogenesis of post-ischemic organ dysfunction due to ischemia-reperfusion injury (IRI). IRI is often observed in the testis after testicular torsion – detorsion of the spermatic cord. The inflammatory aspect of IRI includes both the cellular and humoral components. A growing body of evidence, primarily from animal models of IRI and preliminary human studies are unveiling the potential role of leukocytes and leukocyte adhesion molecules in IRI. Multiple mechanisms have been postulated for the leukocyte-mediated testicular injury following ischemia-reperfusion. Reperfusion of ischemic testis is often associated with microvascular dysfunction that is evidenced as diminished endothelium-dependent dilation in arterioles, enhanced fluid filtration and leukocyte plugging in capillaries, and the trafficking of leukocytes and plasma protein extravasation in postcapillary venules. Activated endothelial cells in all segments of the microcirculation produce more oxygen free radicals, but less nitric oxide, in the early phase of reperfusion. This imbalance leads to production and release of inflammatory mediators such as platelet-activating factor and tumor necrosis factor, which activate endothelial cells in remote organs that are not exposed to the initial ischemic insult such as the contralateral testis. The cellular and molecular mechanisms resulting to IRI are still eluding, and adjuncts to surgical intervention have received little attention. Adaptational responses to IRI including ischemic preconditioning, have been demonstrated that allow for protection of briefly ischemic tissues against the harmful effects of subsequent prolonged ischemia. Likewise, rapid intermittent interruptions of blood flow at the early phase of reperfusion, a phenomenon called postconditioning, mechanically alter reperfusion hydrodynamics in a more beneficial fashion. Moreover, pharmaceutical agents emerging from preclinical research of the basic cellular and molecular events responsible for the post-torsion testicular changes and pathology may also be usefulness as potential treatment on testes injury after ischemia and reperfusion. Understanding the cellular and molecular effects is important in order to offer better prognosis to the adult infertility that may experience males with a history of torsion. The following chapter emphasizes current knowledge of basic science outcomes of testicular torsion and addresses the pathophysiology of testicular ischemia-reperfusion, the role of leukocytes in the post-ischemic inflammatory cascade, and the potential therapeutic alternatives and preventive manoeuvres that may diminish the post-torsion testicular damage.

Chapter 3 - The regulation of pH is critical for a wide variety of biological processes, including fertilization and spermatogenesis. Acrosomes in spermatozoa are acidic inside and contain hydrolytic enzymes essential for penetrating the *zona pellucida* around the eggs. The lumen of epididymis and vas deferens is also acidic, which is required for the maturation and storage of spermatozoa in a quiescent state. The proton pumping vacuolar-type ATPase (V-ATPase) is responsible for acidification of organelles and tissues. V-ATPase is a large multi-subunit enzyme with structural variations: six out of 12 subunits of the mammalian enzyme have more than two isoforms that are specific for cell and/or organelle. We found that the E subunit has two isoforms E1 and E2, which are expressed specifically in testis and ubiquitously in all cells, respectively. V-ATPase with E1 isoform is localized in the acrosome of spermatozoa and is necessary for assembly of the entire enzyme. In the epididymis and vas deferens, V-ATPase is localized in the plasma membrane of narrow and clear cells. In these cells, proton secretion is regulated via recycling of this enzyme: alkaline luminal pH triggers the accumulation of V-ATPase molecules in the apical membrane, whereas lower pH reduces their accumulation. In this review, we summarize and discuss possible roles and regulatory mechanism(s) of V-ATPase in fertilization and spermatogenesis.

Chapter 4 - The mammalian testis exerts two main functions in two different compartments: synthesis of steroids and production of spermatozoa. These specific functions are controlled by gonadotropins and numerous locally synthesized factors, among them testosterone, growth factors and more recently estrogens. Indeed since 1993, we know that germ cells in male gonad synthesize estrogens. As a matter of fact aromatase has been demonstrated in numerous mammalian species (review Carreau and Hess, 2010). Aromatase is localized in immature Sertoli cells then in Leydig cells and germ cells in mature rat and it is clear that aromatase transcripts are more expressed in pachytene spermatocytes than in round spermatids but conversely the aromatase activity is reversed. What is interesting is that germ cells not only express aromatase but are also equipped of estrogen receptors (both genomic and non genomic effects). In addition from numerous models of mice (either ArKO, or ERαKo or ERβKO) and from men deficient in aromatase we know that estrogens are necessary for a full achievement of spermatogenesis (otherwise the number and motility of spermatozoa are decreased; Carreau et al 2010). In addition looking on the putative effects of endocrine disruptors, it is now clear that they are deleterious since estrogen receptors are everywhere in the male genital tract. Therefore estrogens which are also demonstrated in ejaculated spermatozoa of man are necessary not only on the germ cells renewal, spermatogenesis but also for the final maturation of that sperm cell.

Chapter 5 - Junctional devices in Sertoli cells play a key role in maturation and differentiation of germ cells. However, the cellular and subcellular organization of these specializations are still not totally understood. By combining light and electron microscopic techniques using β-actin immunolabeling and prosaposin and glutaredoxin antibodies to label Sertoli cytoplasm, we observed the structural (by confocal microscopy) and fine structural (by electron microscopy) organization of tight and adherent junctions, which are the morphological substrate of the blood testis barrier (BTB). The association to the beta actin also characterizes ectoplasmic specializations (ES) found at two different level of the seminiferous epithelium. We also used freeze fracture to analyze the characteristics of tubular bulbar complexes (TBC), a known component of apical ectoplasmic specializations. These different approaches also allowed us to study the complex arrangement of the actin cytoskeleton of Sertoli cells branches, which surround germ cells in different stages of the spermatogenic cycle. Our results show a consistent labelling for β-actin before, during and after the release of spermatozoa in the tubular lumen (spermiation) suggesting a significant role of the actin network in spermatic cell differentiation. In conclusion, significant interrelations among the β-actin network, the junctional complexes of the BTB and the ectoplasmic specializations were detected at different stages of the seminiferous cycle.

Chapter 6 - Testes in anurans are a structure that posses distinct morphology and coloration. Spermatogenesis in these groups is a complex and organized process that involves spermatogenic cysts progression through in the seminiferous epithelium. The germ cells are grouped with Sertoli cells and constitute spermatogenic cyst. Germ cells are distinct in species of different families.

Chapter 7 - Germ cell apoptosis have been recognized as an important event in order to regulate daily sperm production in humans and in animal models as well. Several studies in rat, mouse and monkeys have shown that testicular mild heat stress (43°C for 15 min) induces a massive increase in germ cell apoptosis along with oxidative damage and activation of diverse signaling pathways. In addition, heat stress produces a decrease in sperm viability, increase sperm damage and decrease embryo quality. In human, testis exposure to heat stress may result from occupational exposure, life style or clinical disorders including cryptorchidism or varicocele. Thus, in the past years researchers have focused on two major areas; the first is to find the molecular signaling pathway trigger by heat stress, and 2) to seek for new molecules with antioxidant abilities which may prevent germ cell apoptosis and/or to improve sperm performance. However, the link between heat stress and male infertility in humans still remains controversial. Here we critically review the available literature in human and animal models, and we propose a new model which explain the elevate apoptosis rate and sperm damage observed after heat stress. Finally we review the available data in pharmacological therapies to protect testicular damage from heat stress.

Chapter 8 - Over the past five decades there have been reports of progressive decline in male reproductive health, which has been correlated with increase in the amount of chemical pollutants in the environment. Plastics are one of the major environmental pollutants today and have become an integral part of urban lifestyle. Polyvinyl chlorides (PVC) and polycarbonates (PC) make up most of household plasticware. During manufacture of PVC and PC, polymers are treated with phenolic additives called "plasticizers" that enhance their flexibility and toughness. Some of these phenolic compounds have estrogenic and anti-androgenic properties and are known to harm the male reproductive system in a time- (fetal, neonatal and adult), duration- and dose-dependent manner. The male reproductive system is responsible for the production of spermatozoa and enabling the male to be fertile. Testis is the site of spermatogenesis and is constituted by seminiferous tubules populated by Sertoli and germ cells. Sertoli cells are nurse cells that nourish developing germ cells to sustain spermatogenesis, which due to their non-regenerative nature are vulnerable to toxicants. In this review we discuss the effects of two commonly used plasticizer groups on Sertoli cell functions. The phthalate group of PVC additives that includes Bis- (2-ethylhexyl) phthalate (DEHP), its active metabolite Mono- (2-ethylhexyl) phthalate (MEHP) and dibutyl phthalate (DBP) has been shown to disrupt Sertoli cell cytoskeleton causing vacuolization. The inability of immature Sertoli cells to anchor germ cells resulted in an efflux of germ cells leaving behind Sertoli cell-only (SCO) tubules. DEHP has been shown to cause a decrease in testosterone synthesis resulting in delayed Sertoli cell maturation and to induce apoptosis of germ cells. The phenolic group of plasticizers that includes 4-(3', 6' dimethyl 3-heptylphenol) (Nonylphenol) and 4, 4'-dihydroxy-2, 2-diphenylpropane (Bisphenol A or BPA) has been shown to cause disassembly of Sertoli cell junctions by disrupting actin-binding proteins. Both Bisphenol A and Nonylphenol have been shown to hamper the activities of anti-oxidant enzymes and increase the levels of reactive oxygen species (ROS) leading to conditions of oxidative stress and induction of Fas/ FasL-mediated Sertoli cell apoptosis. Bisphenol A has been shown to cause sperm acrosomal abnormalities and inhibit spermatogenesis. Recent studies show that the use of plasticizers must be vigilantly monitored to avoid any adverse effects to male reproductive health.

In: Testis: Anatomy, Physiology and Pathology
Editors: Yoichi Nemoto and Norio Inaba
ISBN: 978-1-61942-739-6

Chapter 1

SPERMATOGENESIS AT THE EXTREME: OXIDATIVE STRESS AS A CONVERGING MECHANISM OF TESTICULAR DAMAGE DUE TO PATHOLOGICAL AND ENVIRONMENTAL EXPOSURE

Ricardo D. Moreno*[1]*, Juan G Reyes*[2]*, Jorge G. Farías*[3]*,
Alexis Parada-Bustamante*[4]*, Verónica Aguirre*[1]*, Andrea B. Zepeda*[3]*,
***Carolina A. Figueroa*[3] *and José A. Pino*[2]**

[1]Departamento de Fisiología, Facultad de Ciencias Biológicas,
Pontifica Universidad Católica de Chile
[2]Instituto de Química, Facultad de Ciencias, Pontificia Universidad Católica de Valparaíso, Chile
[3]Departamento de Ingeniería Química. Facultad de Ingeniería,
Ciencias y Administración. Universidad de La Frontera. Temuco, Chile
[4]Instituto de Investigaciones Materno Infantil,
Facultad de Medicina, Universidad de Chile, Chile

ABSTRACT

Mammalian spermatogenesis is a complex physiological process that takes place inside seminiferous tubules in the testis. This process involves a fine balance between cell proliferation, differentiation and apoptosis, ending up with a motile spermatozoon. In most mammals the testes are kept 4-5 °C below body core temperature in the scrotum and the spermatogenic process proceeds with a blood and oxygen supply that appears to be fairly independent of changes in other vascular beds in the body. Despite this well-controlled environment, special circumstances (i.e. genetics), lifestyle, occupational work, pathologies (e.g. diabetes, cryptorchidism and varicocele) and environmental exposure to low oxygen (hypoxia) can result in a decrease of blood flow, nutrients and oxygen supply along with increased temperature. All of these conditions, besides those that cause some pathological conditions, may lead to subfertility or infertility. However, they also represent unique conditions that help us to address some crucial questions about the cell biology and physiology of spermatogenesis: what advantage is there for the spermatogenic cell processes mentioned above taking place under mild hypothermia? What are the molecular and physiological processes that make spermatocytes especially vulnerable to high temperatures? What mechanisms of adaptation take place in the seminiferous tubules cells under hypoxia? What mechanisms lead to a decreased sperm output from spermatogenesis under hypoxia? Do these conditions have similar physiological and molecular pathways? In this chapter, we will review the available literature on human and animal models concerning "extreme" conditions for spermatogenesis, such as: heat stress, hypoxia and pathological conditions like varicocele, cryptorchidism and diabetes. Our analyses suggest that germ cell apoptosis, oxidative stress and DNA damage are common features in all of these "extreme" conditions. Furthermore, oxidative damage seems to be present in all of these conditions during the initiation step of cellular damage. This oxidative stress in the testicle is critical when it poses an imminent risk to the viability and quality of the reproductive cells of animals and humans subjected to extreme conditions. Thus, about 25% of infertile patients are diagnosed with elevated levels of reactive oxygen species (ROS) in semen samples. It is well documented that oxidative damage and elevated ROS levels in germ cells lead to apoptosis, a likely cause of hypospermatogenesis and low sperm production in these patients.

Keywords: Testis, apoptosis, oxidative damage, hypoxia, infertility, germ cell

Introduction

Oxidative and reductive chemical processes are inherent to life on earth and to the processes that use oxygen as a final electron acceptor in one-electron transference, inevitably producing reactive oxygen species (ROS) that can also lead to the formation of reactive nitrogen species (RNS), which can modify biomolecules and affect lipids, proteins and oligonucleotides. Undoubtedly, these same chemical modifications by ROS/RNS have been evolutionarily selected for as physiologically meaningful modifications and are used as signalling processes in cells. Furthermore, counteractive antioxidant mechanisms are widespread throughout biological systems and provide the necessary balance for oxidative processes to be tamed and regulated at useful levels in cells. However, many conditions that increase ROS/RNS or decrease the antioxidant capacity of cells and tissues are at the basis of many pathological situations characterized by programmed (apoptosis) or necrotic cell death and, in some cases, by carcinogenic cell transformation.

In this chapter we review some of the "extreme conditions" that the testis can be subjected to, which appear to have oxidative stress as a common denominator, leading to cell apoptosis, necrosis or carcinogenic cell transformation of testicular cells.

Human Pathologies Associated with Testicular Oxidative Stress

The causes of male infertility are extremely varied. Some infertile men have a complete absence of spermatozoa in the ejaculate that could be due to an obstruction of the deferent ducts (obstructive azoospermia) or to a failure in the spermatogenic process inside the testis (non-obstructive azoospermia), including hypospermatogenesis, maturation arrest or Sertoli cell-only syndrome. Other infertile men are able to produce spermatozoa but they have severe morphological alterations (teratozoospermia), they are completely immotile (asthenozoospermia) and/or they are produced in very low quantities (oligozoospermia).

The aetiology of male infertility due to non-obstructive conditions is as varied as the the possible diagnoses from semen analysis. Some of the factors recognized so far as being associated with non-obstructive infertility are microdeletions in the Y-chromosome (Sadeghi-Nejad and Farrokhi, 2007), failures in the hypothalamus-hypophysis-gonad axis (Sokol, 2009), exposure to certain pesticides used in agriculture (Jurewicz et al., 2009) and pathological conditions such as cryptorchidism (Chung and Brock, 2011) and varicocele (Baazeem et al., 2011). The implications of certain lifestyle factors such as laptop, Wi-Fi and cell phone usage on male infertility are still under debate (Sheynkin et al., 2005; Agarwal et al., 2008; De Luliis et al., 2009; Falzone et al., 2010, Avendaño et al, 2011).

The mechanisms by which different factors generate male infertility status are diverse. However, it has been postulated that an intratesticular and/or seminal increase in ROS levels is a common characteristic in most cases. In this first part, we will explore the hypothesis that a decrease in the testicular oxygen supply and/or an increase in gonadal temperature are causes of male infertility.

Numerous daily activities are associated with an increase in scrotal temperature, such as laptop use (Sheynkin et al., 2005) and heated car seats (Jung et al., 2008), which could negatively affect seminal parameters due to the extremely high sensitivity of germ cells to heat stress (Figure 1); however, the correct regulation of scrotal temperature and the cyclic process of spermatogenesis in healthy men prevents permanent germ cell damage caused by testicular hyperthermia (Momen et al., 2010).

On the other hand, it has been postulated that failure to maintain normal scrotal temperature and prolonged gonadal exposure to high temperatures could be part of the aetiology of male infertility, which is supported by the observation that subfertile men have a significantly higher intrascrotal temperature compared to normozoospermic men (Mieusset et al., 1987; Zorgniotti and Sealfon, 1988).

Regarding the effects of a decrease in the testicular oxygen supply on male infertility, chronic hypoxia induces a state of reversible oligozoospermia in healthy men (Verratti et al., 2008); however, if the hypoxia is permanent, it generates ischaemic damage (Gat et al., 2006). Moreover, some investigators have suggested that long-standing intratesticular hypoxia could be part of the aetiology of certain severe primary spermatogenic failures, such as maturation arrest and Sertoli cell-only syndrome (Gat et al., 2010a; Gat et al., 2010b).

The mechanism by which a permanent decrease in oxygen supply and/or increase in gonadal temperature generate germ cell impairment is most likely mediated by an increase in intratesticular or seminal ROS (Figure 1). Although these molecules have a physiological role in the spermatogenic process, a pathological increase in their concentrations would negatively affect the survival and differentiation of germ cells (Amaral et al., 2008). Indirect evidence indicates that intratesticular ROS levels in men with severe male infertility conditions, such as Sertoli cell-only syndrome and maturation arrest, are significantly increased compared to the levels detected in men with conserved spermatogenesis (Koksal et al., 2003) and that ex-cryptorchidic men with a diagnosis of oligozoospermia have greater levels of sperm DNA damage and ROS levels in their semen compared to normozoospermic healthy controls (Smith et al., 2007).

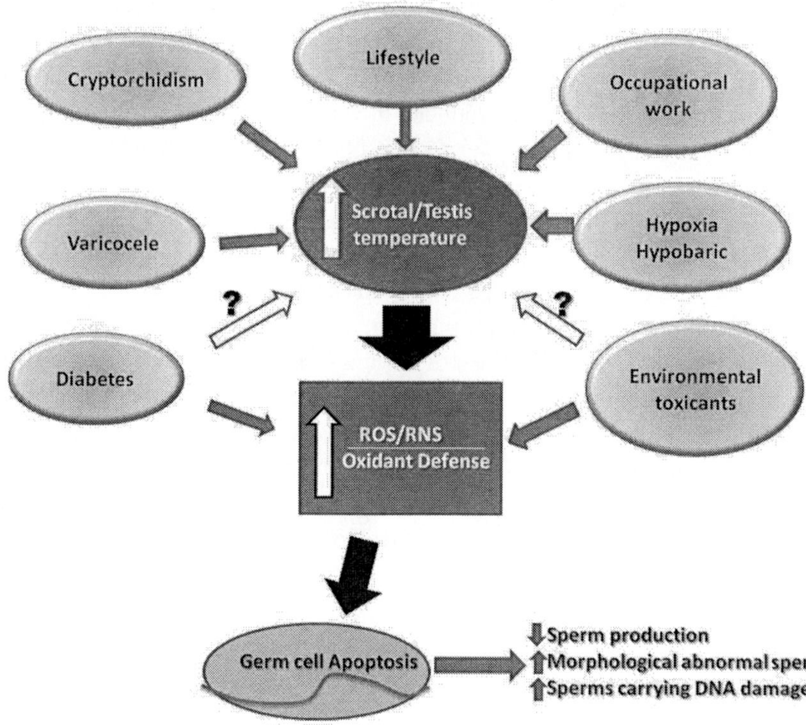

Figure 1. Pathological and environmental factors affecting spermatogenesis. Many male tract pathologies such as cryptorchidism and varicocele are strongly associated with an increase in temperature (1-2 °C) in the testes. Other pathologies, such as diabetes, can also induce an increase in testes temperature. Interestingly, other conditions such as lifestyle, occupational work and hypobaric hypoxia lead to an increase in temperature in the testes and oxidative stress, similar to varicocele and cryptorchidism. The white arrows for the diabetes and environmental toxicants indicate that no experimental data showed a role of these conditions in testes heat stress. Heat stress leads to an imbalance between the production of reactive oxygen species (ROS/RNS) and the antioxidant system (enzymatic and non-enzymatic). This oxidative stress could lead to many defects in testicular physiology; among them, an increase in germ cell apoptosis seems to be the main factor for the reduction in the number of sperm produced. In addition, oxidative stress could account for the increased levels of DNA damage and abnormal spermatozoa.

An important pathology associated with male subfertility and an increase in intratesticular and seminal ROS levels is varicocele. This pathology consists of the thickening and dilation of the pampiniform plexus above the testis, but its aetiology is still unknown. A diagnosis of varicocele is made in 35% of men with primary infertility and in approximately 80% of men with secondary infertility (Belloli et al., 1993). It is postulated that varicocele causes germ cell apoptosis by increasing the hydrostatic pressure in the testicular venous system through a malfunctioning of the testicular valves, leading to an intratesticular hypoxic environment (Gat et al., 2006). However, an alternative hypothesis is that high temperature rather than intratesticular hypoxia is the main source of oxidative stress in patients with varicocele, which is supported by three lines of evidence: 1) patients with varicocele have a higher scrotal temperature and shorter recovery period after cold stress (Merla et al., 2002); 2) varicocelectomy improves semen parameters, probably by reducing testicular temperature and ROS levels and increasing antioxidant activity in the seminal plasma (Wright et al., 1997; Mostafa et al., 2001); 3) increased scrotal temperature, but not varicocele grade, reflects testicular oxidative stress-mediated apoptosis (Shiraishi et al., 2010).

It is generally accepted that testicular and seminal ROS levels are important in the deleterious effects of varicocele on male fertility. Thus, ROS levels in semen samples from men with varicocele are significantly higher compared to those of fertile control men (Smith et al., 2006), and they are directly related to the degree of varicocele (Mostafa et al., 2011). In this regard, the damage caused by varicocele becomes worse as the time between its first appearance and varicocelectomy surgery increases (Zorba et al., 2009), indicating that the testes have intrinsic mechanisms for avoiding permanent damage under certain conditions, but that damage is inevitable when the hypoxia (or elevated temperature) is sustained over time.

Finally, in the last few years it has been proposed that some daily activities and somatic pathologies (not strictly related to fertility) such as the use of cell phone and diabetes negatively affect male infertility through an increase in intratesticular and/or seminal ROS levels via mechanisms that do not necessarily involve heat stress or hypoxia. Regarding the use of cell phones, this is one of the most conflict-ridden points. Recent studies showed that the excessive use of this device may impair some seminal parameters such as sperm count, motility, viability and normal morphology, a phenomenon that is dependent on the duration of daily exposure to cell phones and independent of initial semen quality (Agarwal et al., 2008; Gutschi et al., 2011). The mechanisms involved in this effect consist of an increase in ROS production with subsequent DNA damage in spermatozoa (De Iuliis et al., 2009), which is caused more by the radiofrequency of electromagnetic radiation than by the heat emitted from these devices (Mailankot et al., 2009). These results suggest that excessive cell phone use could be regarded as an "extreme condition" and a deleterious factor for spermatogenesis.

Obesity and diabetes have become two of the greatest threats to human health during the last century. Diabetes mellitus is a metabolic disorder characterized by insulin resistance and subsequent hyperglycaemia (Amaral et al., 2008; Cabler et al., 2010; Du Plessis et al., 2010). Diabetes I is an autoimmune disease caused by the inadequate secretion of insulin that appears in early childhood or puberty and involves the selective loss of beta-cells in the pancreas (Boitard, 2002). Diabetes II is produced by deficiencies in insulin signalling levels and is the most prevalent type of diabetes (Shulman, 2000). Obesity is considered a factor in the development of diabetes II through a mechanism associated with insulin resistance (Shulman, 2000). Diabetes and obesity are part of the cluster of metabolic diseases that, among other dysfunctions, seem to impair reproductive life (Cabler et al., 2010; Du Plessis et al., 2010). Growing evidence shows a strong link between obesity/diabetes and decreased libido, impotence and impairments in testicular functioning, which are associated with sustained hyperglycaemia (Cameron et al., 1990; Cabler et al., 2010). In this way, sperm parameters in semen such as concentration, motility and morphology are altered in obese men (Jensen et al., 2004; Hammoud et al., 2006; Hakonsen et al., 2011). Research performed on 835 diabetic men native to Qatar indicated that 35% were infertile, exhibiting primary or secondary infertility (Bener et al., 2009). Sperm parameters of diabetic men, like motility and density, are poorer than in healthy men (Sexton and Jarow, 1997; La Vignera et al., 2011). In addition, spermatozoa of diabetic men have greater levels of DNA damage and lipid peroxidation than that of normal healthy men (Kasturi et al., 2008). However, classic semen parameters do not always show subtle, functional damage in nuclear and mitochondrial sperm DNA (Agbaje et al., 2007; Agbaje et al., 2008). Furthermore, a decrease in seminiferous tubule diameter, along with germ cell exfoliation, alterations in the connection of Sertoli cells with spermatids and vacuolization of Leydig cells and Sertoli cells were observed in a study that involved ten diabetic patients (six of whom had diabetes I) (Cameron et al., 1985).

The establishment and progression of spermatogenesis depends on intratesticular concentrations of testosterone, a hormone produced by Leydig cells inside testes that works through receptors located in Sertoli cells. Lower levels of serum testosterone have been found in patients with diabetes type I compared to healthy individuals, and hyperglycaemia reduces the response of the pituitary gland when it is stimulated by gonadotropins (Distiller et al., 1975; Garcia-Diez et al., 1991). It has been reported that the conversion of testosterone to oestrogen is increased in obese individuals compared to non-obese subjects, which could be a cause of hypogonadism, presumably by the deleterious role of oestrogen in germ cell survival (Cabler et al., 2010; Du Plessis et al., 2010).

Another important element in obese men is the accumulation of adipose tissue in the suprapubic and scrotal region (Figure 2). Adipose tissue in this area can increase the temperature of the testes, which induces oxidative damage in germ cells (Kasturi et al., 2008). At this point, it is important to note that male reproductive dysfunctions in diabetes do not strictly require the simultaneous occurrence of obesity.

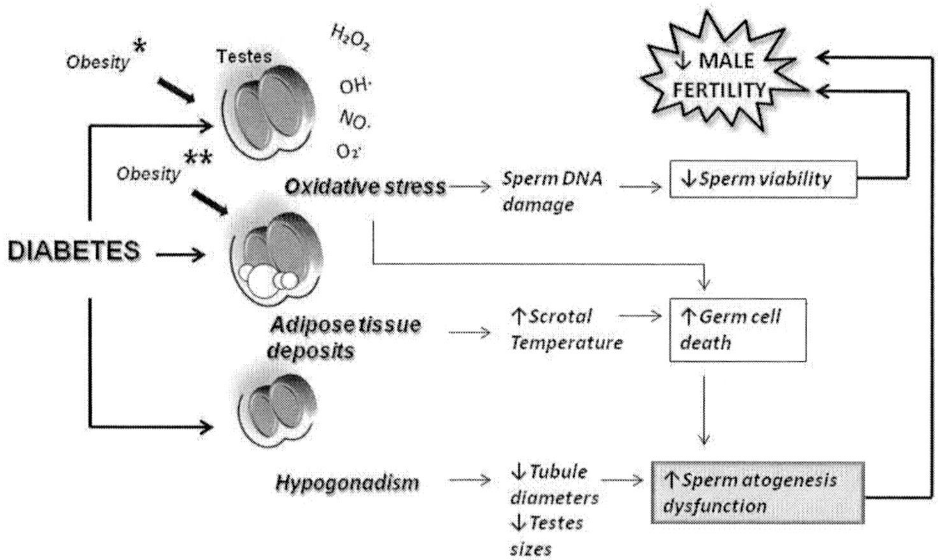

Figure 2. Mechanisms that trigger spermatogenesis dysfunctioning and the reduction of male fertility in diabetes. There is experimental evidence to show that oxidative stress is a factor that increases germ cell death, causing a dysfunction in spermatogenesis. In addition, oxidative stress damages sperm DNA, decreasing sperm viability. Hypogonadism is also an impairment that is found in diabetic subjects, which also causes sperm alterations. (*) Obesity is a factor that could contribute to spermatogenesis dysfunctioning in diabetes by increasing oxidative stress. (**) When diabetic men are obese, adipose tissue deposits build up around the testes and seminal cord, increasing the temperature.

The currently available evidence described in this section indicates that intratesticular hypoxia, increased temperature (heat stress), hyperglycaemia and possibly electromagnetic radiation exposure through the use of cell phones could lead to oxidative stress and impair spermatogenesis with a consequential increase in germ cell apoptosis and DNA damage in spermatozoa. In the next sections we will review experimental evidence using animal models in order to clarify the real contributions of hypoxia, heat stress and hyperglycaemia to the impairment of spermatogenesis through oxidative stress.

Animal Models Associated with Hypoxia

Hypoxia is a stress factor that generates a series of physiological changes in order to compensate for low oxygen tension. In studies of the effects of hypoxia in the testes, the epididymis and spermatozoa are of great relevance in the area of animal reproduction in light of current climatic changes and the increasing exposure of aquatic and terrestrial animals to extreme conditions of low oxygen tension.

Aquatic invertebrates are constantly being exposed to environmental oxygen concentration and temperature fluctuations (Gorr et al., 2010); as a consequence, reports of hypoxia have increased and are a cause of concern. In recent years, investigations that mainly focused on adult fish have shown that aquatic chronic hypoxia acts as an endocrine disruptor, leading to a decrease in gonadal growth, gametogenesis and a reduction in fertility of the Atlantic sea bass. In addition, a delay in spawning has been observed in Gulf killifish (*Fundulus grandis*), whereas in fish embryos hypoxia leads to defects in the migration of primordial germ cells to the genital ridge (Lo et al., 2011). Endocrine and reproductive dysfunctions have also been observed in fresh water species such as carp (Thomas et al., 2007). Another type of adaptation has been observed in the planktonic crustacean *Daphnia magna*, as well as in *Drosophila melanogaster*, through the regulation of different globin genes driven by the hypoxia-inducible factor (HIF), mainly influencing angiogenesis in the tracheal system (Ratcliffe et al., 1998; Gorr et al., 2010). Tracheas in insects, as well as lungs and blood vessels in mammals, are the best examples of successful adaptations that animals have shown over the course of evolution for taking up and delivering O_2 (Centanin et al., 2010).

Exposure to low levels of environmental oxygen is of great concern in domestic animals, which are not genetically adapted to altitude (GAA), unlike llamas or alpacas. The absence of chronic mountain sickness (CMS) in GAA is linked to various adaptations such as the absence or small erythrocytosis because haemoglobin has a great affinity for oxygen (Leon-Velarde and Mejia, 2008). GAA animals do not exhibit a vasoconstrictor response to hypoxia, which avoids the sustained elevation of pulmonary arterial pressure and the subsequent right ventricular hypertrophy found in humans and domestic animals at high altitudes (Leon-Velarde and Mejia, 2008). Previous studies on male rat models indicated that hypoxia reduces fertility when animals do not adapt to this condition, reducing sperm motility in semen and sperm count (Cikutovic et al., 2009; Farias et al., 2010). A reduced sperm count could be associated with an increase in apoptosis promoted by this hypoxic condition (Liao et al., 2010). The same results were observed in male rhesus monkeys (Saxena, 1995). Morphological studies have revealed that hypoxia causes degeneration of the germinal epithelium, folding of the basement membrane, degeneration and detachment of germ cells, lipid droplet sedimentation in Sertoli cells, and an increase in lipoperoxidation (Farias et al., 2005a; Liao et al., 2010). Local changes in testicles have also been observed including neovascularization, an increase in scrotal temperature, a decrease in testicular mass and an increase in interstitial space (Farias et al., 2005b). Interestingly, some of these changes have been observed in humans with varicocele (see above), suggesting that they may have a similar aetiology.

Studies on animal models indicate that varicocele induces testicular hypoxia (Wang et al., 2010). Varicocele is a dilation of the veins of the spermatic cord, determined by dilation of the spermatic vein and stasis (Fazlioglu et al., 2008). An increase in the hypoxia-inducible factor 1 alpha (HIF-1α) levels was previously observed in a rat model, which is an extrinsic marker of hypoxia, generating an increase in vascular endothelial growth factor (VEGF) and followed by angiogenesis, in addition to promoting germ cell apoptosis (Wang et al., 2010). For these reasons it is said that testicular hypoxia can affect fertility, when bilateral varicoceles are produced (Gat et al., 2006; Tekcan et al., 2011). Changes in testicular tissue have been described in both humans and animal models of varicocele, particularly in rats, including immature, amorphous and small cells (Fazlioglu et al., 2008), producing smaller testicles with a decrease in Leydig cell functioning and a low total sperm count, but with no abnormalities in the motility or morphology of the spermatozoa. The reduced sperm count is significant and directly proportional to the grade of varicocele.

As described above, environmental hypoxia affects mainly two testicular functions: first, spermatogenesis is impaired with spermatogenic cell apoptosis and, second, testosterone production is also affected by long-term hypoxia (Farias et al., 2008). Only a few studies have addressed the effects of hypoxia in isolated testicular cells. In a Leydig cell-like cell line (TM3), Lysiak et al. (2009) reported that hypoxia was able to increase the concentrations of HIF-1α and the 3β-OH steroid dehydrogenase, an enzyme in the androgen biosynthetic pathway, strongly suggesting that a direct effect of hypoxia on Leydig cell function could explain the changes in testosterone observed in animal models of hypoxia. Mitochondrial measurements in isolated spermatids from hypoxia-treated rats strongly suggested that these cells undergo lipid peroxidation. Furthermore, our group recently performed experiments to show HIF-1α responses of isolated seminiferous tubules or spermatogenic cells under chemical inhibition of prolyl hydroxylases (PDH), the enzymes that sense oxygen and control HIF-1α levels in cells. Our results strongly suggest that the prepubertal seminiferous tubules and spermatogenic cells respond with a high sensitivity to chemical hypoxia (Alliende et al., unpublished results). Regarding these aforementioned experiments, it is worth noting that inducing chemical anoxia by inhibiting mitochondrial oxidative phosphorylation is not the same as simulating hypoxia by inhibiting PDHs. The former approach is closer to a model of cellular anoxia and the latter method is closer to a model of cell hypoxia.

Animal Models Associated with High Temperature in the Testes

The most frequently used experimental protocol for inducing hyperthermia in the testes is to immerse the lower third of the animal (usually a mouse or rat) in a warm bath (normally at 43 °C) for a period of time, ranging from 15 to 30 min (to cause heat stress). It is understood that this experimental protocol is akin to the environmental conditions experienced in normal human life, such as a shower in warm water, the wearing of tight underwear, the sitting position in the workplace, and pathological conditions such as increased testicular fat or increased blood flow.

Heat stress induces a general change in the transcriptome of mice and human testes, and a total of 67 transcripts were found to be heat regulated in C57BL/6 mice (Li et al., 2009). In another study using ICR mice with a heat stress protocol of 35 °C for 24 h, it was shown that 225 genes were differentially expressed (Cammack et al., 2009). On the other hand, in humans, it was shown that 31 and 36 known proteins are differentially expressed at 2 and 9 weeks after heat treatment, respectively (Zhu et al., 2010).

Under normal conditions the highest rate of germ cell apoptosis is observed in early zygotene and ending pachytene spermatocytes (stages I and XII for rats and mice). The evaluation of germ cell apoptosis 1-2 days after heat stress showed a significant increase in apoptosis, mainly in the early (I–IV) and late (XII–XIV) stages, where pachytenes, dividing spermatocytes and early spermatids were the most frequent cell types observed undergoing apoptosis (Lue et al., 1999). In addition, a reduction in Cdc2 levels was observed in mice testes after heat stress, and in rabbit testes after experimental unilateral cryptorchidism (Kong et al., 2000; Zhang et al., 2008). Eventually, spermatogenesis recovers to levels similar to non-treated animals because spermatogonia are relatively heat resistant, with the exception of B-type spermatogonia of rams (Waites and Setchell, 1990; Lue et al., 1999) and bulls. Interestingly, isolated haploid germ cells but not somatic cells undergo apoptosis at 37°C under the same culture conditions, indicating that heat stress only activates the apoptotic pathway in germ cells (Yin et al., 1998).

The mechanism by which heat stress induces apoptosis in germ cells has yet to be defined. In rats and monkeys heat stress induces translocation of the pro-apoptotic protein BAX from the cytoplasm to the mitochondria, where it helps to release cytochrome c (Lue et al., 2002; Hikim et al., 2003; Matsuki et al., 2003; Vera et al., 2004; Jia et al., 2009). Caspase activation is a hallmark of apoptosis; during heat stress caspase-9 and 3 become active, and their pharmacological inhibition prevents germ cell death (67%), suggesting that caspases are directly linked to germ cell death after heat stress (Hikim et al., 2003; Matsuki et al., 2003; Vera et al., 2005).

The generation of ROS in the initiation of apoptosis is of paramount importance in germ cell apoptosis and DNA damage (Makker et al., 2009). Reactive oxygen species are molecules that have at least one unpaired electron and they are highly unstable and reactive in the presence of lipids, amino acids and nucleic acids (Franco et al., 2008; Hirano, 2008; Tuteja et al., 2009). At physiological levels, ROS are essential for normal reproductive functioning, acting as metabolic intermediates and regulating vascular tone, gene expression and sperm capacitation (Sikka, 2001; Franco et al., 2008; Hirano, 2008; Makker et al., 2009; Tuteja et al., 2009). Heat stress induces oxidative stress, triggering cell survival and apoptosis depending upon the cell type and the extent of the insult. Many studies on heat stress focused on ROS-generating enzymes that produce ROS as by-products of their enzymatic activity. Xanthine oxidase (XO) catalyses the conversion of hypoxanthine and xanthine to uric acid, producing hydrogen peroxide as a by-product, and XO inhibitors suppress testicular germ cell apoptosis induced by experimental cryptorchidism (Kumagai et al., 2002). However, there is a lack of information about whether or not other ROS-generating enzymes such as cyclooxygenase (COX), lipoxygenase (LOX) and NADPH oxidase (NOX) are activated after testicular heat stress. In addition, it has also been shown that the major source of non-enzymatic ROS generation in aerobic cells comes from mitochondrial sources, specifically complex I and complex III. Under normal conditions, 1-2% of all oxygen consumed during respiration undergoes a single electron reduction by leakage of electrons from quinone pools to form the superoxide radical (Raha and Robinson, 2000; Raha et al., 2002; Ott et al., 2007). Then, mitochondrial superoxide dismutase (SOD) converts superoxide into hydrogen peroxide, which is then converted to water and oxygen by catalase and glutathione peroxidase (GPx). Under stress conditions the amount of electrons that leak out is enhanced, leading to an increase in, and the accumulation of, superoxide in mitochondria. It has been shown in both fungi and skin cells that mitochondrial dysfunction and XO are the major sources of ROS production (Davidson and Schiestl, 2001; Shin et al., 2008). The enzyme GPx produces water from H_2O_2 using glutathione (GSH) as the electron donor (Meister and Anderson, 1983). The levels of GSH are maintained by glutathione reductase (GR), which recycles oxidized glutathione (GSSG) to GSH using NADPH as the electron donor. Glutathione reductase activity is modulated by ROS levels although ascorbic acid helps to prevent this effect (El-Missiry, 1999). Nitric oxide (NO) is synthesized intracellularly through the action of a family of nitric oxide synthetase (NOS) enzymes. These NOS enzymes catalyse the NADPH- and O_2-dependent oxidation of L-arginine to L-citrulline, producing NO (Hill et al., 2010). This molecule is a free radical and is chemically more stable and less reactive than other ROS such as the superoxide anion or hydrogen peroxide (Pacher et al., 2007). In monkey testes, endothelial nitric oxide synthetase (eNOS) and inducible NOS (iNOS) were found to be expressed in Sertoli and germ cells. No obvious alterations in eNOS levels were detected after heat stress, but the levels of iNOS increased 3 days after treatment compared to the controls. Immunocytochemistry showed a robust increase in iNOS expression in germ cells (Guo et al., 2009). Thus, heat stress induces NO production and it might contribute to oxidative damage in germ cells. However, the molecular targets that are modified by NO production and the consequences of this in testis physiology are unknown.

Under different conditions the production of ROS exceeds the antioxidant capacity, resulting in oxidative stress, which elicits degenerative responses such as DNA damage, necrosis, and apoptosis. Heat stress was found to increase apoptosis and ROS levels in isolated germ cells (Ikeda et al., 1999). Interestingly, oxidative damage, along with increased apoptosis, is also a hallmark of other pathologies involved in male infertility, such as varicocele and testicular torsion (Turner et al., 2004; Turner et al., 2005; Shiraishi and Naito, 2007; Shiraishi et al., 2010). Heat stress causes the upregulation of haeme oxygenase 1 (Hmox1) and the antioxidant enzymes glutathione peroxidase 1, glutathione S-transferase alpha and SOD1, consistent with a robust oxidative stress response. In agreement with the hypothesis that these enzymes participate in the antioxidant response, germ cells isolated from SOD1-knockout mice were found to be more vulnerable to apoptosis induced by heat stress than wild-type mice, suggesting a protective role of this enzyme in the oxidative stress insult induced by heat stress (Ishii et al., 2005). However, other studies reported a downregulation of mRNAs encoding for glutathione reductase 1, glutathione S-transferase alpha 2, manganese superoxide dismutase 2 (SOD2) and extracellular superoxide dismutase Cu-Zn (SOD3) (Rockett et al., 2001). Thus, it is seems that heat stress induces the upregulation of specific isoforms of stress response enzymes (SOD1 but not SOD2 or SOD3), indicating the activation of a specific genetic response programme. Peroxiredoxin-4 (Prx4) belongs to a new family of antioxidant proteins and it plays a role in regulating NF-κB (nuclear factor κB). Male Prx4-knockout mice are fertile, except for testicular atrophy and an increase in germ cell apoptosis (Iuchi et al., 2009). Interestingly, Prx-4-knockout germ cells show increased oxidation of lipids and protein thiols, and male mice show an increase in apoptosis (TUNEL-positive cells) after heat stress, suggesting that Prx4 is important in the oxidative stress response in germ cells.

Different intracellular pathways are activated downstream ROS production, among which the ASK1/p38MAPK pathway has been shown to be important in germ cell apoptosis after heat stress (Ueda et al., 2002; Matsuzawa and Ichijo, 2008). Reactive oxygen species are able to oxidize thioredoxine (Trx)-reactive thiol groups and to mediate the activation of apoptosis signal-regulating kinase 1 (ASK1)/MKKK5, a ubiquitously expressed enzyme that activates JNK and p38 MAP kinase pathways (Hsieh and Papaconstantinou, 2006; Matsuzawa and Ichijo, 2008; Hsieh et al., 2010). In rats and monkeys heat stress induces the sustained activation of both mitogen-activated protein kinase (MAPK) 1/3 and MAPK14 (p38MAPK) (Johnson et al., 2008; Jia et al., 2009; Lizama et al., 2009). Interestingly, the protection offered by caspase-2 or calpain inhibitors prevents MAPK14 (p38MAPK) activation, suggesting that caspase and calpain activation are upstream of MAPK activation (Johnson et al., 2008; Lizama et al., 2009).

Heat stress induces a gradual loss in sperm concentration and viability (Jannes et al., 1998; Setchell et al., 1998; Rockett et al., 2001; Paul et al., 2008b; Perez-Crespo et al., 2008). In monkeys, scrotal heat stress induces azoospermia or oligozoospermia 6 or 8 weeks after the first heat treatment (Lue et al., 2002), and heat stress in stallions induces increased susceptibility of spermatozoa DNA to denaturation in the absence of protamine changes (Love and Kenney, 1999). In rats, spermatocyte damage at the time of heat stress was found to result in lower sperm production 23-28 days after treatment; these sperm had reduced DNA integrity compared to the sperm of untreated rats, but spermatids at the time of heat stress showed the highest degree of DNA damage (Perez-Crespo et al., 2008). Moreover, after mating normal females to heat-exposed males, there was a reduction in the pregnancy rate and an increase in embryo reabsorption, and the surviving embryos experienced a reduction in weight during intrauterine development. *In vitro* fertilization with sperm recovered 16 h or 23 d after scrotal stress at 42°C produced embryos that experienced a block at the four-cell and blastocyst stage, suggesting a pre-implantational effect of heat stress in development and/or deficient egg activation (Paul et al., 2008a; Paul et al., 2008b). The reduction in the number and weight of embryos sired by heat-stressed males could be explained by the high levels of DNA damage, which promote abnormal embryos, yolk sacs, trophoblasts and placental development (Setchell, 1993; Setchell et al., 1998). Interestingly, a sex ratio distortion was found when spermatozoa present in the epididymis at the time of thermal stress produced embryos after mating (Perez-Crespo et al., 2008). Therefore, the available evidence clearly indicates that heat stress has a profound impact on spermatogenesis, with an increase in germ cell apoptosis and DNA damage in the spermatozoa produced by germ cells present at the time of injury. Sperm DNA damage could be induced by a strong REDOX state imbalance. Despite the upregulation of many enzymes involved in the antioxidant response, some germ cells cannot cope with elevated ROS levels and they die by apoptosis (Figure 1). However, other groups of germ cells can overcome this oxidative stress and differentiate, but sperm produced this way bears high levels of DNA fragmentation and probably other, as yet unknown, harmful modifications, which could explain the developmental abnormalities observed in embryos after heat stress.

As described above, many studies have been performed on experimental hyperthermia, showing the triggering of apoptosis in pachytene spermatocytes (Nakai et al., 2000; Somwaru et al., 2004). In contrast, few studies of hyperthermia and its associated physiological and biochemical changes have been performed in isolated cells. The only study found in the literature using prepubertal monkey Sertoli cells (Chen et al., 2008) reported that adherent junction-associated proteins are downregulated by high temperatures (43 °C). On the contrary, vimentin expression is upregulated by high temperatures. These changes in cytoskeletal and junction proteins were thought to be associated with a marked decrease in androgen receptor (AR) expression after heat treatment, as was clearly demonstrated using selective Sertoli cell AR KO mice. Testosterone is essential for spermatogenesis through its actions on Sertoli cells. Thus, Sertoli cell AR downregulation by hyperthermia explains, at least in part, spermatogenic arrest in testis subjected to high temperatures. However, evidence showing the mechanisms of AR downregulation and spermatogenic cell apoptosis under conditions of high temperature is lacking. The interspecies extrapolation that we present herein is controversial, although it could certainly provide the grounds for new research experiments. Related to testosterone, and specifically being the source of testosterone in the testis, studies of the effects of high temperature on Leydig cell functioning and testosterone production are apparently absent in the literature. Regarding isolated germ cells, Herrera et al. (2000) showed that increasing the incubating temperature of rat pachytene spermatocytes and round spermatids to 37-40°C increased intracellular [Ca^{2+}] ([Ca^{2+}]i) to levels that modify signalling in these cells (e.g., Reyes et al., 2010). The intracellular pH in these cells was found to decrease with increasing temperature. These changes occurred within 1 minute of the increase in temperature and can be classified as early events in the response of these cells to heat stress. Interestingly, the same combination of changes in these cellular parameters (increase in [Ca^{2+}]i and decrease in intracellular pH) was associated with apoptotic cells in the testis (Lizama et al., 2007), strongly suggesting that high temperatures *per se* can set physiological conditions in spermatogenic cells that make them prone to other noxious or pro-apoptotic stimuli from Sertoli cells. Furthermore, we recently found that a high temperature (40°C) induced a rapid increase in reactive oxygen and/or nitrogen species in pachytene spermatocytes but not in round spermatids (Pino et al., unpublished results), providing the noxious stimuli that could differentially trigger cell death in spermatocytes.

Overall, experimental evidence strongly suggests that experimental or pathogenic heat stress (e.g. varicocele) induces oxidative stress, which in turn could induce apoptosis or create damage in germ cells in such a way they develop into spermatozoa carrying fragmented DNA.

Animal Models in Diabetes: A Tool for Studying Spermatogenic Damage

The animal models used to study spermatogenic damage and fertility disturbances in diabetes have several advantages:

- They allow studies on main organs and tissues that would be more difficult to study in humans, such as testes, the epididymis and the vesicula seminalis.
- Rats and mice easily develop diabetes after injections of streptozotocin.
- Rodents have a short life cycle: the time taken to reach puberty, undergo spermatogenesis onset and develop the collateral effects of streptozotocin-induced diabetes is short.
- They offer the possibility of repeating experimental assays under specific conditions in order to distinguish random from non-random events.

The typical models for studying spermatogenesis in diabetes, as well as other disorders linked to diabetes, are rats and mice; the former are used more frequently than the latter because they are less resistant to streptozotocin, the drug that induces diabetes via the selective destruction of beta-pancreatic islets (Ozturk et al., 1996). These diabetic animals (induced with a single dose of 40-80 mg/kg streptozotocin) exhibit a decrease in testis and epididymal weight (Shrilatha and Muralidhara, 2007). The histological alterations include a reduction in the diameter of or a smaller diameter of seminiferous tubules, atrophy, the absence of sperm, Sertoli cell vacuolization, fewer Leydig cells and germ cell desquamation (Ballester et al., 2004; Scarano et al., 2006). Poor sperm motility and density have also been observed in rats, diabetic mice and men (Amaral et al., 2006; Scarano et al., 2006).

Excessive levels of apoptosis are related to neurodegenerative processes and a decrease in the number of beta-pancreatic islet cells, which is thought to be an underlying factor in defective insulin secretion (Butler et al., 2003). Similarly, male mice with insulitis (an illness that shows the same symptoms as diabetes I) have greater amounts of spermatocytes, spermatogonia and spermatids undergoing apoptosis, along with higher levels of phosphorylated JNK (c-Jun NH_2-terminal kinase), activated BAX and caspase-3 (Sainio-Pollanen et al., 1997; Koh, 2007). Taken together, these findings suggest the occurrence of apoptosis in the testes of diabetic rats.

Diabetes, Reactive Oxygen Species and Spermatogenesis

High levels of ROS have been found in the pancreas, liver and kidney of diabetic rats, and as well as the testes (El-Missiry, 1999; Shrilatha, 2007; Shrilatha and Muralidhara, 2007). Hyperglycaemia induces superoxide production by disrupting mitochondrial electron chain transport, which inhibits glyceraldehyde-3-phosphate dehydrogenase activity, creating a metabolic imbalance of ROS levels in the cells (Wentzel et al., 2003; Blatnik et al., 2008). On the other hand, high ROS levels could also be achieved by decreasing the antioxidant capability of the cell. Wistar rats treated with streptozotocin showed a reduction in catalase (CAT), GR, GPx and SOD after 1, 2, 4 and 6 weeks post-streptozotocin injection, while the activity of glutathione-S-transferase (GST) was significantly increased (Shrilatha, 2007). In rabbits treated with alloxane the activities of CAT, GPX, GSH and GR were increased after 10 weeks of treatment (Gumieniczek and Wilk, 2009). A reduction in GPx but not in GR was also reported in Goto-Kakizaki rats, which are currently being used as an animal model for type 2 diabetes. Cytosolic and mitochondrial fractions of diabetic adult Wistar rat testes were found to have higher levels of lipid peroxidation, as determined by the Thiobarbituric Acid Reactive Substances (TBARS) assay, and considerable amounts of ROS compared to healthy rat testes (Amaral et al., 2006; Shrilatha and Muralidhara, 2007). In addition, levels of advanced glycation end (AGE) product adducts and their receptors (RAGE) are higher in the reproductive tract of diabetic patients, and the presence of RAGE implies that they may play a role in sperm DNA damage (Mallidis et al., 2007).

In contrast, antioxidant therapy is recognized as counteracting the adverse effects of streptozotocin treatment. Antioxidants are chemicals that rapidly react with the unpaired electrons of ROS and RNS, preventing the harmful actions of these free radicals. The reproductive functioning of diabetic rats was found to be restored by the administration of C_{60} fullerene in drinking water (concentration ~30 nM) for 5 weeks (Bal et al., 2011). The authors found that this antioxidant improved sperm motility, epididymal sperm concentration, and the weights of the testis, epididymis, vesicula seminalis and prostate in diabetic rats. Furthermore, haematoxylin-eosin-stained sections of diabetic rat testes treated with C_{60} fullerene showed that the histological appearance was very similar to that of healthy rats. In other study, the activity of antioxidant enzymes in mice testes increased with the administration of daily injections of ascorbic acid compared to diabetic rats with no antioxidant treatment (Shrilatha, 2007).

Glucose and Spermatogenic Cells

Spermatogenic cells develop in a protected environment. On one hand, the lower temperature of the testis provides as yet poorly defined biochemical and physiological conditions for testicular functioning and spermatogenic cell development and, on the other, Sertoli cells provide a compartmentalized microenvironment (adluminal) for the development of meiotic and post-meiotic spermatogenic cells (Mruk and Cheng, 2004; Yan et al., 2008). The ionic, substrate and growth and death factor compositions of the adluminal compartment are still a mystery. Only a few hints have been obtained from the analysis of seminiferous tubule fluid obtained by micropuncturing (Tuck et al., 1970; Levine and Marsh, 1975; Mruk and Cheng, 2004), from the *in vitro* release of compounds by Sertoli cells in culture (Jegou, 1993) and from transport measurements (see below) and the localization of transporters on Sertoli and spermatogenic cells (see below). Regarding glucose, no reliable data are available on the concentration of this substrate in the adluminal compartment, although data from Turner et al. (1980) and Angulo et al. (1998) strongly suggest that glucose can cross the haemato-testicular barrier toward meiotic and post-meiotic spermatogenic cells. Glucose can be transported into spermatogenic cells (Rauch et al., 2006) and be metabolized by these cells. In fact, the metabolism of glucose by these cells was reported to induce a fall in intracellular ATP and an increase in intracellular AMP in round spermatids (Grootegoed et al., 1986; Nakamura et al., 1986; Reyes et al., 1990). Along with these adenine nucleotide changes, an increase in $[Ca^{2+}]i$ and a decrease in pH were reported (Herrera et al., 2000;

Reyes et al., 2002). These changes in [Ca^{2+}]i were enough to sensitize plasma membrane Ca^{2+} channels to opening by extracellular stimuli (Reyes et al., 2010). These effects of glucose were even produced at low glucose concentrations (0.5-1 mM), strongly suggesting that these glucose-driven short-term physiological changes could occur under normal glucose concentrations in the plasma. Although neither normal nor diabetic concentrations of glucose have been reported in seminiferous tubules, the glucose-driven changes in spermatogenic cells described above are clearly similar to the pro-apoptotic conditions (especially if chronically maintained) often found in cells and specifically described in apoptotic spermatogenic cells (Lizama et al., 2007). Furthermore, our unpublished data indicate that, in the absence of lactate, glucose induces apoptosis in cultured rat spermatocytes through an increase in ROS and intracellular calcium (Bustamante-Marín X and Moreno R, unpublished data). Therefore, glucose by itself seems to be an inducer of apoptosis in germ cells.

Taken together, these results suggest that an imbalance in ROS production (oxidative stress) has a role in the impairment of testicular function observed in animal models of diabetes, and it probably has a role in humans who have this pathology. However, other factors such as endocrine disorders or nutritional status must be taken into account to fully understand the complexity of these testicular pathologies.

Acknowledgments

Part of this work was supported by FONDECYT 1110267 to JGR, 11110457 to APB and 1110778 to RDM.

References

Agarwal, A., F. Deepinder, R. K. Sharma, G. Ranga and J. Li. Effect of cell phone usage on semen analysis in men attending infertility clinic: an observational study. *Fertil. Steril.*, 2008, 89, 124-128.

Agbaje, I. M., C. M. McVicar, B. C. Schock, N. McClure, A. B. Atkinson, D. Rogers and S. E. Lewis. Increased concentrations of the oxidative DNA adduct 7,8-dihydro-8-oxo-2-deoxyguanosine in the germ-line of men with type 1 diabetes. *Reprod. Biomed. Online*, 2008, 16, 401-409.

Agbaje, I. M., D. A. Rogers, C. M. McVicar, N. McClure, A. B. Atkinson, C. Mallidis and S. E. Lewis. Insulin dependant diabetes mellitus: implications for male reproductive function. *Hum. Reprod.*, 2007, 22, 1871-1877.

Amaral, S., A. J. Moreno, M. S. Santos, R. Seica and J. Ramalho-Santos. Effects of hyperglycemia on sperm and testicular cells of Goto-Kakizaki and streptozotocin-treated rat models for diabetes. *Theriogenology*, 2006, 66, 2056-2067.

Amaral, S., P. J. Oliveira and J. Ramalho-Santos. Diabetes and the impairment of reproductive function: possible role of mitochondria and reactive oxygen species. *Curr. Diabetes Rev.*, 2008, 4, 46-54.

Avendaño, C., Mata, A., Sanchez-Sarmiento, C.A., Doncel, G.F. Use of laptop computers connected to internet through Wi-Fi decreases human sperm motility and increases sperm DNA fragmentation *Fertil Steril.*, 2011, Nov 22. [Epub ahead of print] PMID: 22112647.

Baazeem, A., E. Belzile, A. Ciampi, G. Dohle, K. Jarvi, A. Salonia, W. Weidner and A. Zini. Varicocele and male factor infertility treatment: a new meta-analysis and review of the role of varicocele repair. *Eur. Urol.*, 2011, 60, 796-808.

Bal, R., G. Turk, M. Tuzcu, O. Yilmaz, I. Ozercan, T. Kuloglu, S. Gur, V. S. Nedzvetsky, A. A. Tykhomyrov, G. V. Andrievsky, G. Baydas and M. Naziroglu. Protective effects of nanostructures of hydrated C(60) fullerene on reproductive function in streptozotocin-diabetic male rats. *Toxicology*, 2011, 282, 69-81.

Ballester, J., M. C. Munoz, J. Dominguez, T. Rigau, J. J. Guinovart and J. E. Rodriguez-Gil. Insulin-dependent diabetes affects testicular function by FSH- and LH-linked mechanisms. *J. Androl.*, 2004, 25, 706-719.

Belloli, G., S. D'Agostino, C. Pesce and E. Fantuz. [Varicocele in childhood and adolescence and other testicular anomalies: an epidemiological study]. *Pediatr. Med. Chir.*, 1993, 15, 159-162.

Bener, A., A. A. Al-Ansari, M. Zirie and A. O. Al-Hamaq. Is male fertility associated with type 2 diabetes mellitus? *Int. Urol. Nephrol.*, 2009, 41, 777-784.

Blatnik, M., N. Frizzell, S. R. Thorpe and J. W. Baynes. Inactivation of glyceraldehyde-3-phosphate dehydrogenase by fumarate in diabetes: formation of S-(2-succinyl)cysteine, a novel chemical modification of protein and possible biomarker of mitochondrial stress. *Diabetes*, 2008, 57, 41-49.

Boitard, C. The origin of type 1 diabetes: an autoimmune disease? *Diabetes Metab*, 2002, 28, 263-265.

Butler, A. E., J. Janson, W. C. Soeller and P. C. Butler. Increased beta-cell apoptosis prevents adaptive increase in beta-cell mass in mouse model of type 2 diabetes: evidence for role of islet amyloid formation rather than direct action of amyloid. *Diabetes*, 2003, 52, 2304-2314.

Cabler, S., A. Agarwal, M. Flint and S. S. du Plessis. Obesity: modern man's fertility nemesis. *Asian. J. Androl.*, 2010, 12, 480-489.

Cameron, D. F., F. T. Murray and D. D. Drylie. Interstitial compartment pathology and spermatogenic disruption in testes from impotent diabetic men. *Anat. Rec.*, 1985, 213, 53-62.

Cameron, D. F., J. Rountree, R. E. Schultz, D. Repetta and F. T. Murray. Sustained hyperglycemia results in testicular dysfunction and reduced fertility potential in BBWOR diabetic rats. *Am. J. Physiol.*, 1990, 259, E881-889.

Cammack, K. M., E. Antoniou, L. Hearne and W. R. Lamberson. Testicular gene expression in male mice divergent for fertility after heat stress. *Theriogenology*, 2009, 71, 651-661.

Centanin, L., T. A. Gorr and P. Wappner. Tracheal remodelling in response to hypoxia. *J. Insect Physiol.*, 2010, 56, 447-454.

Chen, M., J. X. Yuan, Y. Q. Shi, X. S. Zhang, Z. Y. Hu, F. Gao and Y. X. Liu. Effect of 43 degrees treatment on expression of heat shock proteins 105, 70 and 60 in cultured monkey Sertoli cells. *Asian. J. Androl.*, 2008, 10, 474-485.

Chung, E. and G. B. Brock. Cryptorchidism and its impact on male fertility: a state of art review of current literature. *Can. Urol. Assoc. J.*, 2011, 5, 210-214.

Cikutovic, M., N. Fuentes and E. Bustos-Obregon. Effect of intermittent hypoxia on the reproduction of rats exposed to high altitude in the Chilean Altiplano. *High. Alt. Med. Biol.*, 2009, 10, 357-363.

Davidson, J. F. and R. H. Schiestl. Mitochondrial respiratory electron carriers are involved in oxidative stress during heat stress in Saccharomyces cerevisiae. *Mol. Cell. Biol.*, 2001, 21, 8483-8489.

De Iuliis, G. N., R. J. Newey, B. V. King and R. J. Aitken. Mobile phone radiation induces reactive oxygen species production and DNA damage in human spermatozoa in vitro. *PLoS. One*, 2009, 4, e6446.

Distiller, L. A., J. Sagel, J. E. Morley and H. C. Seftel. Pituitary responsiveness to luteinizing hormone-releasing hormone in insulin-dependent diabetes mellitus. *Diabetes*, 1975, 24, 378-380.

Du Plessis, S. S., S. Cabler, D. A. McAlister, E. Sabanegh and A. Agarwal. The effect of obesity on sperm disorders and male infertility. *Nat. Rev. Urol.*, 2010, 7, 153-161.

El-Missiry, M. A. Enhanced testicular antioxidant system by ascorbic acid in alloxan diabetic rats. *Comp Biochem Physiol C Pharmacol Toxicol Endocrinol.*, 1999, 124, 233-237.

Falzone, N., C. Huyser, D. R. Franken and D. Leszczynski. Mobile phone radiation does not induce pro-apoptosis effects in human spermatozoa. *Radiat. Res.*, 2010, 174, 169-176.

Farias JG, Bustos-Obregón E, Reyes JG. Increase in testicular temperature and vascularization induced by hypobaric hypoxia in rats. *Journal of Andrology.* 2005a;26 693-697.

Farias JG, Bustos-Obregón E, Orellana R, Bucarey JL, Quiroz E, Reyes JG. Effects of chronic hypobaric hypoxia on testis histology and round spermatid oxidative metabolism. *Andrologia.* 2005b;37: 47-52.

Farias, J. G., E. Bustos-Obregon, P. J. Tapia, E. Gutierrez, A. Zepeda, C. Juantok, G. Cruz, G. Soto, J. Benites and J. G. Reyes. Time course of endocrine changes in the hypophysis-gonad axis induced by hypobaric hypoxia in male rats. *J. Reprod. Dev.*, 2008, 54, 18-21.

Farias, J. G., M. Puebla, A. Acevedo, P. J. Tapia, E. Gutierrez, A. Zepeda, G. Calaf, C. Juantok and J. G. Reyes. Oxidative stress in rat testis and epididymis under intermittent hypobaric hypoxia: protective role of ascorbate supplementation. *J. Androl.*, 2010, 31, 314-321.

Fazlioglu, A., I. Yilmaz, O. Mete, F. Kurtulus, O. Parlakkilic, O. Guctas and M. Cek. The effect of varicocele repair on experimental varicocele-induced testicular germ cell apoptosis. *J. Androl.*, 2008, 29, 29-34.

Franco, R., O. Schoneveld, A. G. Georgakilas and M. I. Panayiotidis. Oxidative stress, DNA methylation and carcinogenesis. *Cancer. Lett.*, 2008, 266, 6-11.

Garcia-Diez, L. C., J. J. Corrales Hernandez, J. Hernandez-Diaz, M. J. Pedraz and J. M. Miralles. Semen characteristics and diabetes mellitus: significance of insulin in male infertility. *Arch. Androl.*, 1991, 26, 119-128.

Gat, Y., M. Gornish, A. Perlow, J. Chakraborty, U. Levinger, I. Ben-Shlomo and F. Pasqualotto. Azoospermia and Sertoli-cell-only syndrome: hypoxia in the sperm production site due to impairment in venous drainage of male reproductive system. *Andrologia*, 2010b, 42, 314-321.

Gat, Y., M. Gornish, J. Chakraborty, A. Perlow, U. Levinger and F. Pasqualotto. Azoospermia and maturation arrest: malfunction of valves in erect poster of humans leads to hypoxia in sperm production site. *Andrologia*, 2010a, 42, 389-394.

Gat, Y., M. Gornish, U. Navon, J. Chakraborty, G. N. Bachar and I. Ben-Shlomo. Right varicocele and hypoxia, crucial factors in male infertility: fluid mechanics analysis of the impaired testicular drainage system. *Reprod. Biomed. Online*, 2006, 13, 510-515.

Gorr, T. A., D. Wichmann, J. Hu, M. Hermes-Lima, A. F. Welker, N. Terwilliger, J. F. Wren, M. Viney, S. Morris, G. E. Nilsson, A. Deten, J. Soliz and M. Gassmann. Hypoxia tolerance in animals: biology and application. *Physiol. Biochem. Zool.*, 2010, 83, 733-752.

Grootegoed, J. A., R. Jansen and H. J. van der Molen. Effect of glucose on ATP dephosphorylation in rat spermatids. *J. Reprod. Fertil.*, 1986, 77, 99-107.

Gumieniczek, A. and M. Wilk. Nitrosative stress and glutathione redox system in four different tissues of alloxan-induced hyperglycemic animals. *Toxicol. Mech. Methods*, 2009, 19, 302-307.

Guo, J., Y. Jia, S. X. Tao, Y. C. Li, X. S. Zhang, Z. Y. Hu, N. Chiang, Y. H. Lue, A. P. Hikim, R. S. Swerdloff, C. Wang and Y. X. Liu. Expression of nitric oxide synthase during germ cell apoptosis in testis of cynomolgus monkey after testosterone and heat treatment. *J. Androl.*, 2009, 30, 190-199.

Gutschi, T., B. Mohamad Al-Ali, R. Shamloul, K. Pummer and H. Trummer. Impact of cell phone use on men's semen parameters. *Andrologia*, 2011, 43, 312-316.

Hakonsen, L. B., A. M. Thulstrup, A. S. Aggerholm, J. Olsen, J. P. Bonde, C. Y. Andersen, M. Bungum, E. H. Ernst, M. L. Hansen and C. H. Ramlau-Hansen. Does weight loss improve semen quality and reproductive hormones? Results from a cohort of severely obese men. *Reprod. Health*, 2011, 8, 24.

Hammoud, A. O., M. Gibson, C. M. Peterson, B. D. Hamilton and D. T. Carrell. Obesity and male reproductive potential. *J. Androl.*, 2006, 27, 619-626.

Herrera, E., K. Salas, N. Lagos, D. J. Benos and J. G. Reyes. Energy metabolism and its linkage to intracellular Ca2+ and pH regulation in rat spermatogenic cells. *Biol. Cell.*, 2000, 92, 429-440.

Hikim, A. P., Y. Lue, C. M. Yamamoto, Y. Vera, S. Rodriguez, P. H. Yen, K. Soeng, C. Wang and R. S. Swerdloff. Key apoptotic pathways for heat-induced programmed germ cell death in the testis. *Endocrinology*, 2003, 144, 3167-3175.

Hill, B. G., B. P. Dranka, S. M. Bailey, J. R. Lancaster, Jr. and V. M. Darley-Usmar. What part of NO don't you understand? Some answers to the cardinal questions in nitric oxide biology. *J. Biol. Chem.*, 2010, 285, 19699-19704.

Hirano, T. Repair system of 7, 8-dihydro-8-oxoguanine as a defense line against carcinogenesis. *J Radiat Res (Tokyo)*, 2008, 49, 329-340.

Hsieh, C. C. and J. Papaconstantinou. Thioredoxin-ASK1 complex levels regulate ROS-mediated p38 MAPK pathway activity in livers of aged and long-lived Snell dwarf mice. *Faseb. J.*, 2006, 20, 259-268.

Hsieh, C. C., M. Kuro-o, K. P. Rosenblatt, R. Brobey and J. Papaconstantinou. The ASK1-Signalosome regulates p38 MAPK activity in response to levels of endogenous oxidative stress in the Klotho mouse models of aging. *Aging (Albany NY)*, 2010, 2, 597-611.

Ikeda, M., H. Kodama, J. Fukuda, Y. Shimizu, M. Murata, J. Kumagai and T. Tanaka. Role of radical oxygen species in rat testicular germ cell apoptosis induced by heat stress. *Biol Reprod*, 1999, 61, 393-399.

Ishii, T., S. Matsuki, Y. Iuchi, F. Okada, S. Toyosaki, Y. Tomita, Y. Ikeda and J. Fujii. Accelerated impairment of spermatogenic cells in SOD1-knockout mice under heat stress. *Free. Radic. Res.*, 2005, 39, 697-705.

Iuchi, Y., F. Okada, S. Tsunoda, N. Kibe, N. Shirasawa, M. Ikawa, M. Okabe, Y. Ikeda and J. Fujii. Peroxiredoxin 4 knockout results in elevated spermatogenic cell death via oxidative stress. *Biochem. J.*, 2009, 419, 149-158.

Jannes, P., C. Spiessens, I. Van der Auwera, T. D'Hooghe, G. Verhoeven and D. Vanderschueren. Male subfertility induced by acute scrotal heating affects embryo quality in normal female mice. *Hum. Reprod.*, 1998, 13, 372-375.

Jegou, B. The Sertoli-germ cell communication network in mammals. *Int. Rev. Cytol.*, 1993, 147, 25-96.

Jensen, T. K., A. M. Andersson, N. Jorgensen, A. G. Andersen, E. Carlsen, J. H. Petersen and N. E. Skakkebaek. Body mass index in relation to semen quality and reproductive hormones among 1,558 Danish men. *Fertil. Steril.*, 2004, 82, 863-870.

Jia, Y., J. Castellanos, C. Wang, I. Sinha-Hikim, Y. Lue, R. S. Swerdloff and A. P. Sinha-Hikim. Mitogen-activated protein kinase signaling in male germ cell apoptosis in the rat. *Biol. Reprod.*, 2009, 80, 771-780.

Johnson, C., Y. Jia, C. Wang, Y. H. Lue, R. S. Swerdloff, X. S. Zhang, Z. Y. Hu, Y. C. Li, Y. X. Liu and A. P. Hikim. Role of caspase 2 in apoptotic signaling in primate and murine germ cells. *Biol. Reprod.*, 2008, 79, 806-814.

Jung, A., P. Strauss, H. J. Lindner and H. C. Schuppe. Influence of heating car seats on scrotal temperature. *Fertil. Steril.*, 2008, 90, 335-339.

Jurewicz, J., W. Hanke, M. Radwan and J. P. Bonde. Environmental factors and semen quality. *Int. J. Occup. Med. Environ. Health*, 2009, 22, 305-329.

Kasturi, S. S., J. Tannir and R. E. Brannigan. The metabolic syndrome and male infertility. *J Androl*, 2008, 29, 251-259.

Koh, P. O. Streptozotocin-induced diabetes increases apoptosis through JNK phosphorylation and Bax activation in rat testes. *J. Vet. Med. Sci.*, 2007, 69, 969-971.

Koksal, I. T., M. Usta, I. Orhan, S. Abbasoglu and A. Kadioglu. Potential role of reactive oxygen species on testicular pathology associated with infertility. *Asian. J. Androl.*, 2003, 5, 95-99.

Kong, W. H., G. Zheng, J. N. Lu and J. K. Tso. Temperature dependent expression of cdc2 and cyclin B1 in spermatogenic cells during spermatogenesis. *Cell. Res.*, 2000, 10, 289-302.

Kumagai, A., H. Kodama, J. Kumagai, J. Fukuda, K. Kawamura, H. Tanikawa, N. Sato and T. Tanaka. Xanthine oxidase inhibitors suppress testicular germ cell apoptosis induced by experimental cryptorchidism. *Mol. Hum. Reprod.*, 2002, 8, 118-123.

La Vignera, S., R. Condorelli, E. Vicari, R. D'Agata and A. E. Calogero. Diabetes Mellitus and Sperm Parameters: A Brief Review. *J. Androl.*, 2011, In press, jandrol.111.013193 [pii].

Leon-Velarde, F. and O. Mejia. Gene expression in chronic high altitude diseases. *High. Alt. Med. Biol.*, 2008, 9, 130-139.

Levine, N. and D. J. Marsh. Micropuncture study of the fluid composition of 'Sertoli cell-only' seminiferous tubules in rats. *J. Reprod. Fertil.*, 1975, 43, 547-549.

Li, Y., Q. Zhou, R. Hively, L. Yang, C. Small and M. D. Griswold. Differential gene expression in the testes of different murine strains under normal and hyperthermic conditions. *J. Androl.*, 2009, 30, 325-337.

Liao, W., M. Cai, J. Chen, J. Huang, F. Liu, C. Jiang and Y. Gao. Hypobaric hypoxia causes deleterious effects on spermatogenesis in rats. *Reproduction*, 2010, 139, 1031-1038.

Lizama, C., C. F. Lagos, R. Lagos-Cabre, L. Cantuarias, F. Rivera, P. Huenchunir, T. Perez-Acle, F. Carrion and R. D. Moreno. Calpain inhibitors prevent p38 MAPK activation and germ cell apoptosis after heat stress in pubertal rat testes. *J. Cell. Physiol.*, 2009, 221, 296-305.

Lizama, C., I. Alfaro, J. G. Reyes and R. D. Moreno. Up-regulation of CD95 (Apo-1/Fas) is associated with spermatocyte apoptosis during the first round of spermatogenesis in the rat. *Apoptosis*, 2007, 12, 499-512.

Lo, K. H., M. N. Hui, R. M. Yu, R. S. Wu and S. H. Cheng. Hypoxia Impairs Primordial Germ Cell Migration in Zebrafish (Danio rerio) Embryos. *PLoS One*, 2011, 6, e24540.

Love, C. C. and R. M. Kenney. Scrotal heat stress induces altered sperm chromatin structure associated with a decrease in protamine disulfide bonding in the stallion. *Biol. Reprod.*, 1999, 60, 615-620.

Lue, Y. H., A. P. Hikim, R. S. Swerdloff, P. Im, K. S. Taing, T. Bui, A. Leung and C. Wang. Single exposure to heat induces stage-specific germ cell apoptosis in rats: role of intratesticular testosterone on stage specificity. *Endocrinology*, 1999, 140, 1709-1717.

Lue, Y. H., B. L. Lasley, L. S. Laughlin, R. S. Swerdloff, A. P. Hikim, A. Leung, J. W. Overstreet and C. Wang. Mild testicular hyperthermia induces profound transitional spermatogenic suppression through increased germ cell apoptosis in adult cynomolgus monkeys (Macaca fascicularis). *J. Androl.*, 2002, 23, 799-805.

Mailankot, M., A. P. Kunnath, H. Jayalekshmi, B. Koduru and R. Valsalan. Radio frequency electromagnetic radiation (RF-EMR) from GSM (0.9/1.8GHz) mobile phones induces oxidative stress and reduces sperm motility in rats. *Clinics (Sao Paulo)*, 2009, 64, 561-565.

Makker, K., A. Agarwal and R. Sharma. Oxidative stress and male infertility. *Indian J. Med. Res.*, 2009, 129, 357-367.

Mallidis, C., I. Agbaje, D. Rogers, J. Glenn, S. McCullough, A. B. Atkinson, K. Steger, A. Stitt and N. McClure. Distribution of the receptor for advanced glycation end products in the human male reproductive tract: prevalence in men with diabetes mellitus. *Hum. Reprod.*, 2007, 22, 2169-2177.

Matsuki, S., Y. Iuchi, Y. Ikeda, I. Sasagawa, Y. Tomita and J. Fujii. Suppression of cytochrome c release and apoptosis in testes with heat stress by minocycline. *Biochem. Biophys. Res. Commun.*, 2003, 312, 843-849.

Matsuzawa, A. and H. Ichijo. Redox control of cell fate by MAP kinase: physiological roles of ASK1-MAP kinase pathway in stress signaling. *Biochim. Biophys. Acta.*, 2008, 1780, 1325-1336.

Meister, A. and M. E. Anderson. Glutathione. *Annu. Rev. Biochem.*, 1983, 52, 711-760.

Merla, A., A. Ledda, L. Di Donato, S. Di Luzio and G. L. Romani. Use of infrared functional imaging to detect impaired thermoregulatory control in men with asymptomatic varicocele. *Fertil. Steril.*, 2002, 78, 199-200.

Mieusset, R., L. Bujan, C. Mondinat, A. Mansat, F. Pontonnier and H. Grandjean. Association of scrotal hyperthermia with impaired spermatogenesis in infertile men. *Fertil. Steril.*, 1987, 48, 1006-1011.

Momen, M. N., F. B. Ananian, I. M. Fahmy and T. Mostafa. Effect of high environmental temperature on semen parameters among fertile men. *Fertil. Steril.*, 2010, 93, 1884-1886.

Mostafa, T., T. Anis, A. El Nashar, H. Imam and I. Osman. Seminal plasma reactive oxygen species-antioxidants relationship with varicocele grade. *Andrologia*, 2011.

Mostafa, T., T. H. Anis, A. El-Nashar, H. Imam and I. A. Othman. Varicocelectomy reduces reactive oxygen species levels and increases antioxidant activity of seminal plasma from infertile men with varicocele. *Int. J. Androl.*, 2001, 24, 261-265.

Mruk, D. D. and C. Y. Cheng. Sertoli-Sertoli and Sertoli-germ cell interactions and their significance in germ cell movement in the seminiferous epithelium during spermatogenesis. *Endocr. Rev.*, 2004, 25, 747-806.

Nakai, A., M. Suzuki and M. Tanabe. Arrest of spermatogenesis in mice expressing an active heat shock transcription factor 1. *Embo. J.*, 2000, 19, 1545-1554.

Nakamura, M., S. Okinaga and K. Arai. Studies of metabolism of round spermatids: glucose as unfavorable substrate. *Biol. Reprod.*, 1986, 35, 927-935.

Ott, M., V. Gogvadze, S. Orrenius and B. Zhivotovsky. Mitochondria, oxidative stress and cell death. *Apoptosis*, 2007, 12, 913-922.

Ozturk, Y., V. M. Altan and N. Yildizoglu-Ari. Effects of experimental diabetes and insulin on smooth muscle functions. *Pharmacol. Rev.*, 1996, 48, 69-112.

Pacher, P., J. S. Beckman and L. Liaudet. Nitric oxide and peroxynitrite in health and disease. *Physiol. Rev.*, 2007, 87, 315-424.

Paul, C., A. A. Murray, N. Spears and P. T. Saunders. A single, mild, transient scrotal heat stress causes DNA damage, subfertility and impairs formation of blastocysts in mice. *Reproduction*, 2008b, 136, 73-84.

Paul, C., D. W. Melton and P. T. Saunders. Do heat stress and deficits in DNA repair pathways have a negative impact on male fertility? *Mol. Hum. Reprod.*, 2008a, 14, 1-8.

Perez-Crespo, M., B. Pintado and A. Gutierrez-Adan. Scrotal heat stress effects on sperm viability, sperm DNA integrity, and the offspring sex ratio in mice. *Mol. Reprod. Dev.*, 2008, 75, 40-47.

Raha, S. and B. H. Robinson. Mitochondria, oxygen free radicals, disease and ageing. *Trends. Biochem. Sci.*, 2000, 25, 502-508.

Raha, S., A. T. Myint, L. Johnstone and B. H. Robinson. Control of oxygen free radical formation from mitochondrial complex I: roles for protein kinase A and pyruvate dehydrogenase kinase. *Free. Radic. Biol. Med.*, 2002, 32, 421-430.

Ratcliffe, P. J., J. F. O'Rourke, P. H. Maxwell and C. W. Pugh. Oxygen sensing, hypoxia-inducible factor-1 and the regulation of mammalian gene expression. *J. Exp. Biol.*, 1998, 201, 1153-1162.

Rauch, M. C., M. E. Ocampo, J. Bohle, R. Amthauer, A. J. Yanez, J. E. Rodriguez-Gil, J. C. Slebe, J. G. Reyes and Concha, II. Hexose transporters GLUT1 and GLUT3 are colocalized with hexokinase I in caveolae microdomains of rat spermatogenic cells. *J. Cell. Physiol.*, 2006, 207, 397-406.

Reyes, J. G., E. Herrera, L. Lobos, K. Salas, N. Lagos, R. A. Jorquera, P. Labarca and D. J. Benos. Dynamics of intracellular calcium induced by lactate and glucose in rat pachytene spermatocytes and round spermatids. *Reproduction*, 2002, 123, 701-710.

Reyes, J. G., M. V. Velarde, R. Ugarte and D. J. Benos. Glycolytic component of rat spermatid energy and acid-base metabolism. *Am. J. Physiol.*, 1990, 259, C660-667.

Reyes, J. G., N. Osses, M. Knox, A. Darszon and C. L. Trevino. Glucose and lactate regulate maitotoxin-activated Ca2+ entry in spermatogenic cells: the role of intracellular [Ca2+]. *FEBS Lett*, 2010, 584, 3111-3115.

Rockett, J. C., F. L. Mapp, J. B. Garges, J. C. Luft, C. Mori and D. J. Dix. Effects of hyperthermia on spermatogenesis, apoptosis, gene expression, and fertility in adult male mice. *Biol. Reprod.*, 2001, 65, 229-239.

Sadeghi-Nejad, H. and F. Farrokhi. Genetics of azoospermia: current knowledge, clinical implications, and future directions. Part II: Y chromosome microdeletions. *Urol. J.*, 2007, 4, 192-206.

Sainio-Pollanen, S., K. Henriksen, M. Parvinen, O. Simell and P. Pollanen. Stage-specific degeneration of germ cells in the seminiferous tubules of non-obese diabetic mice. *Int. J. Androl.*, 1997, 20, 243-253.

Saxena, D. K. Effect of hypoxia by intermittent altitude exposure on semen characteristics and testicular morphology of male rhesus monkeys. *Int. J. Biometeorol.*, 1995, 38, 137-140.

Scarano, W. R., A. G. Messias, S. U. Oliva, G. R. Klinefelter and W. G. Kempinas. Sexual behaviour, sperm quantity and quality after short-term streptozotocin-induced hyperglycaemia in rats. *Int. J. Androl.*, 2006, 29, 482-488.

Setchell, B. P. (1993). Spermatogenesis and spermatozoa. *Germ cells and Fertilization.* C. R. Austin and R. V. Short. Cambridge, Cambridge University Press: 63-102.

Setchell, B. P., G. Ekpe, J. L. Zupp and M. A. Surani. Transient retardation in embryo growth in normal female mice made pregnant by males whose testes had been heated. *Hum. Reprod.*, 1998, 13, 342-347.

Sexton, W. J. and J. P. Jarow. Effect of diabetes mellitus upon male reproductive function. *Urology*, 1997, 49, 508-513.

Sheynkin, Y., M. Jung, P. Yoo, D. Schulsinger and E. Komaroff. Increase in scrotal temperature in laptop computer users. *Hum. Reprod.*, 2005, 20, 452-455.

Shin, M. H., Y. J. Moon, J. E. Seo, Y. Lee, K. H. Kim and J. H. Chung. Reactive oxygen species produced by NADPH oxidase, xanthine oxidase, and mitochondrial electron transport system mediate heat shock-induced MMP-1 and MMP-9 expression. *Free. Radic. Biol. Med.*, 2008, 44, 635-645.

Shiraishi, K. and K. Naito. Nitric oxide produced in the testis is involved in dilatation of the internal spermatic vein that compromises spermatogenesis in infertile men with varicocele. *BJU Int.*, 2007, 99, 1086-1090.

Shiraishi, K., H. Takihara and H. Matsuyama. Elevated scrotal temperature, but not varicocele grade, reflects testicular oxidative stress-mediated apoptosis. *World J. Urol.*, 2010, 28, 359-364.

Shrilatha, B. and Muralidhara. Early oxidative stress in testis and epididymal sperm in streptozotocin-induced diabetic mice: its progression and genotoxic consequences. *Reprod. Toxicol.*, 2007, 23, 578-587.

Shrilatha, B. Occurrence of oxidative impairments, response of antioxidant defences and associated biochemical perturbations in male reproductive milieu in the Streptozotocin-diabetic rat. *Int. J. Androl.*, 2007, 30, 508-518.

Shulman, G. I. Cellular mechanisms of insulin resistance. *J. Clin. Invest.*, 2000, 106, 171-176.

Sikka, S. C. Relative impact of oxidative stress on male reproductive function. *Curr. Med. Chem.*, 2001, 8, 851-862.

Smith, R., H. Kaune, D. Parodi, M. Madariaga, I. Morales, R. Rios and A. Castro. [Extent of sperm DNA damage in spermatozoa from men examined for infertility. Relationship with oxidative stress]. *Rev. Med. Chil.*, 2007, 135, 279-286.

Smith, R., H. Kaune, D. Parodi, M. Madariaga, R. Rios, I. Morales and A. Castro. Increased sperm DNA damage in patients with varicocele: relationship with seminal oxidative stress. *Hum. Reprod.*, 2006, 21, 986-993.

Sokol, R. Z. Endocrinology of male infertility: evaluation and treatment. *Semin. Reprod. Med.*, 2009, 27, 149-158.

Somwaru, L., S. Li, L. Doglio, E. Goldberg and B. R. Zirkin. Heat-induced apoptosis of mouse meiotic cells is suppressed by ectopic expression of testis-specific calpastatin. *J. Androl.*, 2004, 25, 506-513.

Tekcan, M., I. T. Koksal, A. Tasatargil, O. Kutlu, E. Gungor and C. Celik-Ozenci. Potential Role of Poly(ADP-Ribose) Polymerase Activation in the Pathogenesis of Experimental Left Varicocele. *J. Androl.*, 2011.

Thomas, P., M. S. Rahman, I. A. Khan and J. A. Kummer. Widespread endocrine disruption and reproductive impairment in an estuarine fish population exposed to seasonal hypoxia. *Proc. Biol. Sci.*, 2007, 274, 2693-2701.

Tuck, R. R., B. P. Setchell, G. M. Waites and J. A. Young. The composition of fluid collected by micropuncture and catheterization from the seminiferous tubules and rete testis of rats. *Pflugers. Arch.*, 1970, 318, 225-243.

Turncr, T. T., H. J. Bang and J. J. Lysiak. Experimental testicular torsion: reperfusion blood flow and subsequent testicular venous plasma testosterone concentrations. *Urology*, 2005, 65, 390-394.

Turner, T. T., H. J. Bang and J. L. Lysiak. The molecular pathology of experimental testicular torsion suggests adjunct therapy to surgical repair. *J. Urol.*, 2004, 172, 2574-2578.

Tuteja, N., P. Ahmad, B. B. Panda and R. Tuteja. Genotoxic stress in plants: shedding light on DNA damage, repair and DNA repair helicases. *Mutat. Res.*, 2009, 681, 134-149.

Ueda, S., H. Masutani, H. Nakamura, T. Tanaka, M. Ueno and J. Yodoi. Redox control of cell death. *Antioxid Redox. Signal*, 2002, 4, 405-414.

Vera, Y., M. Diaz-Romero, S. Rodriguez, Y. Lue, C. Wang, R. S. Swerdloff and A. P. Sinha Hikim. Mitochondria-dependent pathway is involved in heat-induced male germ cell death: lessons from mutant mice. *Biol. Reprod.*, 2004, 70, 1534-1540.

Vera, Y., S. Rodriguez, M. Castanares, Y. Lue, V. Atienza, C. Wang, R. S. Swerdloff and A. P. Sinha Hikim. Functional role of caspases in heat-induced testicular germ cell apoptosis. *Biol. Reprod.*, 2005, 72, 516-522.

Verratti, V., F. Berardinelli, C. Di Giulio, G. Bosco, M. Cacchio, M. Pellicciotta, M. Nicolai, S. Martinotti and R. Tenaglia. Evidence that chronic hypoxia causes reversible impairment on male fertility. *Asian. J. Androl*, 2008, 10, 602-606.

Waites, G. M. H. and B. P. Setchell (1990). Physiology of mammalian testis. Marshall's Physiology of Reproduction. G. E. Lamming. New York, Churchill Livingstone. Vol 2 pp 1-106.

Wang, H., Y. Sun, L. Wang, C. Xu, Q. Yang, B. Liu and Z. Liu. Hypoxia-induced apoptosis in the bilateral testes of rats with left-sided varicocele: a new way to think about the varicocele. *J. Androl.*, 2010, 31, 299-305.

Wentzel, P., A. Ejdesjo and U. J. Eriksson. Maternal diabetes in vivo and high glucose in vitro diminish GAPDH activity in rat embryos. *Diabetes*, 2003, 52, 1222-1228.

Wright, E. J., G. P. Young and M. Goldstein. Reduction in testicular temperature after varicocelectomy in infertile men. *Urology*, 1997, 50, 257-259.

Yan, H. H., D. D. Mruk and C. Y. Cheng. Junction restructuring and spermatogenesis: the biology, regulation, and implication in male contraceptive development. *Curr Top Dev Biol*, 2008, 80, 57-92.

Yin, Y., B. C. Stahl, W. C. DeWolf and A. Morgentaler. Heat-induced testicular apoptosis occurs independently of hormonal depletion. *Apoptosis*, 1998, 3, 281-287.

Zhang, Y., X. Yang, H. Cao, Z. Chen, Y. Du and W. Kong. Heat stress induces Cdc2 protein decrease prior to mouse spermatogenic cell apoptosis. *Acta Histochem*, 2008, 110, 276-284.

Zhu, H., Y. Cui, J. Xie, L. Chen, X. Chen, X. Guo, Y. Zhu, X. Wang, J. Tong, Z. Zhou, Y. Jia, Y. H. Lue, A. S. Hikim, C. Wang, R. S. Swerdloff and J. Sha. Proteomic analysis of testis biopsies in men treated with transient scrotal hyperthermia reveals the potential targets for contraceptive development. *Proteomics*, 2010, 10, 3480-3493.

Zorba, U. O., O. M. Sanli, M. Tezer, F. Erdemir, S. Shavakhabov and A. Kadioglu. Effect of infertility duration on postvaricocelectomy sperm counts and pregnancy rates. *Urology*, 2009, 73, 767-771.

Zorgniotti, A. W. and A. I. Sealfon. Measurement of intrascrotal temperature in normal and subfertile men. *J. Reprod. Fertil.*, 1988, 82, 563-566.

In: Testis: Anatomy, Physiology and Pathology
Editors: Yoichi Nemoto and Norio Inaba

ISBN: 978-1-61942-739-6

Chapter 2

NEW INSIGHTS INTO THE PATHOPHYSIOLOGY OF THE TESTIS AFTER ISCHEMIA REPERFUSION INJURY

Fotios Dimitriadis and Motoaki Saito
Division of Molecular Pharmacology, Tottori University School of Medicine,
86 Nishi-machi, Yonago, Japan

ABSTRACT

Recent developments in immunology and cell biology highlighted the importance of inflammation in the pathogenesis of post-ischemic organ dysfunction due to ischemia-reperfusion injury (IRI). IRI is often observed in the testis after testicular torsion – detorsion of the spermatic cord. The inflammatory aspect of IRI includes both the cellular and humoral components. A growing body of evidence, primarily from animal models of IRI and preliminary human studies are unveiling the potential role of leukocytes and leukocyte adhesion molecules in IRI. Multiple mechanisms have been postulated for the leukocyte-mediated testicular injury following ischemia-reperfusion. Reperfusion of ischemic testis is often associated with microvascular dysfunction that is evidenced as diminished endothelium-dependent dilation in arterioles, enhanced fluid filtration and leukocyte plugging in capillaries, and the trafficking of leukocytes and plasma protein extravasation in postcapillary venules. Activated endothelial cells in all segments of the microcirculation produce more oxygen free radicals, but less nitric oxide, in the early phase of reperfusion. This imbalance leads to production and release of inflammatory mediators such as platelet-activating factor and tumor necrosis factor, which activate endothelial cells in remote organs that are not exposed to the initial ischemic insult such as the contralateral testis. The cellular and molecular mechanisms resulting to IRI are still eluding, and adjuncts to surgical intervention have received little attention. Adaptational responses to IRI including ischemic preconditioning, have been demonstrated that allow for protection of briefly ischemic tissues against the harmful effects of subsequent prolonged ischemia. Likewise, rapid intermittent interruptions of blood flow at the early phase of reperfusion, a phenomenon called postconditioning, mechanically alter reperfusion hydrodynamics in a more beneficial fashion. Moreover, pharmaceutical agents emerging from preclinical research of the basic cellular and molecular events responsible for the post-torsion testicular changes and pathology may also be usefulness as potential treatment on testes injury after ischemia and reperfusion. Understanding the cellular and molecular effects is important in order to offer better prognosis to the adult infertility that may experience males with a history of torsion.

The following chapter emphasizes current knowledge of basic science outcomes of testicular torsion and addresses the pathophysiology of testicular ischemia-reperfusion, the role of leukocytes in the post-ischemic inflammatory cascade, and the potential therapeutic alternatives and preventive manoeuvres that may diminish the post-torsion testicular damage.

Keywords: Testicular torsion, ischemia-reperfusion, ischemic preconditioning, ischemic postconditioning, free oxygen radicals, edaravone, sivelestat

INTRODUCTION

A child or adolescent with symptoms including acute scrotal pain, tenderness, or swelling should be looked upon as an emergency situation requiring prompt evaluation, differential diagnosis, and potentially immediate surgical exploration. One of the main causes of an acute scrotum in children and adolescent is testicular torsion. The occurrence of testicular torsion has been estimated to be as high as 1 in 4000 males by the age of 25, and has been implicated in testicular injury and infertility [1]. Testicular torsion and subsequent ischemia requires an emergency operation to avoid loss of germ cells and ischemic testis [2]. The surgical procedure can lead to orchiectomy of the ipsilateral torted testis, and infertility of the contralateral (not torted) testis [3]. Usually, the first signs of testicular necrosis appear within 6–12hrs of the testicular torsion crisis, and thus a delay in diagnosis and treatment can result in lower ability of spermatogenesis, or infertility. Despite improvement in early diagnosis of testicular torsion and changes in clinical management (i.e. earlier surgical intervention), infertility remains one of the main consequences [4-5]. The degree of fertility loss in an individual with testicular torsion depends on the extent of ischemia and the subsequent damage to the contralateral testis [6-8]. The primary pathophysiological event in testicular torsion is ischemia reperfusion injury (IRI) caused by the twisted spermatic cord and its release. As well, the testicular damage following the torsion of the spermatic cord is most likely mediated by reactive oxygen species (ROS) [9]. The DNA of germ cells is particularly sensitive to oxidative damage (10). In addition, torsion-detorsion has been associated with decreased spermatogenesis, alteration of the production of various hormones, and induction of infertility [11-13].

TESTICULAR ISCHEMIA REPERFUSION INJURY AND REACTIVE OXYGEN SPECIES

Reperfusion injury is an integrated response to blood flow restoration after ischemia. Moreover, reperfusion injury is initiated at the early moments of reperfusion, which can potentially last for several days [14]. IRI in the testis is related to abnormal signal transduction due to testicular torsion-detorsion and is associated with ROS over generation [15]. In fact, excessive ROS generation during reperfusion has a major role in IRI as increased ROS production inflicts significant injury on ischemic tissue by the oxidization of cell membrane lipids, protein, and DNA, leading to testicular dysfunction (3). Following that, ischemia-reperfusion contributes to cellular dysfunction and initiates the apoptosis/necrosis cascade with subsequent inflammatory infiltration [14] and cell death [3]. It has been suggested that high concentrations of ROS induce cell death by necrosis, whereas low concentrations induce cell death by apoptosis [16].

Although the basic pathogenetic mechanism underlying testicular IRI has not been completely understood, it seems that part of the basis of this pathogenetic mechanism is relied upon the action of activated neutrophils. After ischemia-reperfusion, in several organs, occurs an increase in adhesion of neutrophils to postcapillary venules [17-19] and is believed to be involved in tissue damage subsequent to reperfusion [20-21]. Neutrophils recruited to the subtunical venules may secrete inflammatory cytokines such as TNF-α, IL-1β, and IL-8 [22]. These increase the recruitment of other leukocytes and enhance expression of several endothelial cell adhesion molecules such as E-selectin and ICAM-1 [23]. The expression is maximal 3–8 hrs after stimulation and gradually decreases within 12–24 hrs [24] corresponding well with the timing of E-selectin expression seen in other models of IRI [25] or after the administration of inflammatory cytokines [24, 26].

Following testicular ischemia-reperfusion, the activated neutrophils, within the interstitium of the testis, release factors such as ROS or FasL that may directly cause apoptosis in the germ cell. Alternatively, the invading neutrophils may secrete factors that influence Sertoli cells to secrete FasL, thus indirectly effecting germ cell death. Indeed, increases in ROS [15] and FasL [27] have been previously reported after the repair of testicular torsion in the rat. In IRI of the rat testis Turner et al., [15] demonstrated that germ cell-specific apoptosis coincided with an increase in neutrophil cells margination and diapedesis [15]. An increase in ROS as assessed by thiobarbituric acid reactive substances assay and by the ability of certain reactive oxygen scavengers to partially abrogate the testicular torsion-induced apoptosis has also been observed [15]. Besides the confirmation that the pathology seen after testicular torsion is a classical IRI, these findings support also the hypothesis that neutrophils play a key role in the initiation of the molecular events leading to germ cell apoptosis [15]. In fact, the failure of testicular torsion to stimulate apoptosis in mice rendered neutropenic further supports the suggestion that neutrophils are essential for the observed pathology [28]. However, macrophages have also been documented able to release ROS [29]. Furthermore, the elimination of ROS has been shown to be beneficial in treating IRI in several organs as for example in the heart (30), in the liver [31], and in the brain [32]. In addition, enzymatic antioxidant defense systems, such as superoxide dismutase, catalase and glutathione peroxidase, protect tissues from ROS [3]. Furthermore, antioxidant pretreatment of experimental animals with superoxide dismutase, catalase, simvastatin [33], and melatonin (34) were effective to prevent testicular reperfusion injury [35].

Unilateral Testicular Ischemia Reperfusion Injury and Contralateral Testicular Function

Prolonged unilateral testicular torsion with more than 4hrs of 720 degree unilateral testicular torsion is enough to create tissue injury in both ipsilateral and contralateral testes in experimental animal models [36-37]. Also, prolonged unilateral testicular torsion is not followed by a full recovery of blood flow in the ipsilateral testis 24hrs after detorsion [38-40]. Although many studies suggest that the contralateral non-torted testis is damaged after unilateral testicular torsion [40-43], some studies have shown that this phenomenon is not always observed [38]. The physiological and biochemical mechanisms of contralateral testicular injury (including the role of ROS on such damage) are unclear [44]. Some authors have reported that decreased testicular blood flow and subsequent tissue hypoxia contribute to contralateral testicular injury after testicular torsion-detorsion [45]. Kizillican and colleagues (1992) showed that a short period of unilateral torsion (10min) produced a decrease in contralateral blood flow [46]. Furthermore, Tanyel and coworkers (1989) reported that the contralateral testis could be damaged by a reflexive decrease in blood flow from the activated sympathetic system [40]. However, our previous report strongly denied this hypothesis because in the contralateral testis the testicular blood flow did not show any variation during the ischemia period or the initial two hours of reperfusion of ipsilateral testis utilizing laser Doppler flowmeter [47]. Due to the aforementioned reports, the influence of the contralateral testis following unilateral testicular ischemia-reperfusion remains controversial. Other groups have reported the important role of immunological responses in pathogenesis [41-42]. Wallace and coworkers (1982) have suggested alternative explanations including the release of acrosomal enzymes or a neurohumoral mechanism and have also proposed the term "sympathetic orchiopathia" [43]. Moreover, Jeong and colleagues (2010) reported that puberty (ages 5 to 6 weeks) rats had more severe contralateral testicular damage than adult rats after testicular torsion because immunological, humoral and neural differentiation and maturation vary by age. Immunological protection of puberty rats for contralateral testicular damage after testicular torsion decreases at puberty due to immature Sertoli cells [48]. It might be possible that the severity of contralateral damage caused by immunological activity is different from that of adult rats [34].

Definition and Mechanism of Ischemic Preconditioning

Over two decades ago, Murry's group reported that short cycles of ischemia and reperfusion before an occlusion of a coronary artery reduced infarct size, and this was called ischemic preconditioning (IPreC) [49]. Similarly, the concurrent protection was actually found in human as IPreC causes adaptation to ischemia in all mammals [50]. IPreC limits the severity of the IRI. Thus, after IPreC, the extent of the area of a subsequent infarction, ischemia-reperfusion arrhythmias, and contractile dysfunction is reduced [51]. IPreC mechanisms of action have been extensively reviewed. Several features and pathways of this process are now clear but some elements still remain unknown. Many studies and evidence on distinct organ and species indicate the empirical knowledge about common or different mechanisms. In the literature there are inconsistencies related to differences among the animal species, tissue, and animal model. Initial IPreC protocols in the heart were unwieldy as authors usually designed four, five or six short and alternative cycles of ischemia-reperfusion. Although this procedure is very appealing, none of these studies have support for it or cannot be used to extrapolate from it to other organs. In recent years, one ischemia and one reperfusion window in IPreC protocol has been shown to have a protective effect in other organs, including the liver and the kidney [52-55]. The ischemia adaptation is biphasic, and consists of protection less than 2hrs prior to the sustained ischemia (classic preconditioning or first window of protection), and a delayed time frame 24–72hrs later [delayed preconditioning or second window of protection (SWOP)] [50]. IPreC can also be obtained by inducing ischemia on distant organs (remote preconditioning) or by pharmacological treatment prior to initial ischemia (pharmacological preconditioning) [56-61]. The benefit of IPreC relies on both infarct size reduction and functional improvement. In addition, IPreC improves endothelial function in both classic and delayed time, as a general effect as well as locally in the preconditioned organ [62-64]. Moreover, a lot of systemic stimuli by IPreC evoke a similar protection such as substances acting on G-protein coupled receptors (adenosine and bradykinin), proinflammatory substances (lipopolysaccharide, tumor necrosis factor alpha and monophosphoryl lipid A), and changes in oxygen tension (anoxia, hypoxia and hyperoxia) [50]. In fact, autacoids, such as adenosine, bradykinin, opioids and platelet activating factor produced as a response to the cycles of brief ischemia-reperfusion, play a pivotal role in IPreC protection (Figure 1). Their receptors induce signal transduction pathways that ultimately block the opening of mitochondrial permeability transition pores (mPTP) during the reperfusion phase after the infracting ischemia (Figure 1) [65-66]. Opening of mPTP can be coupled with a large amount of cell death since it completely disrupts mitochondrial function and releases ROS [67-71]. Cell death in preconditioned heart is less than that in non-preconditioned heart, which went identical ischemic insult. Thus, IPreC protection requires a complex signaling cascade, which includes the opening of sarcolemmal or mitochondrial ATP-sensitive potassium channels (sarcK_{ATP} or mitoK_{ATP}) (Figure 1) [72-77].

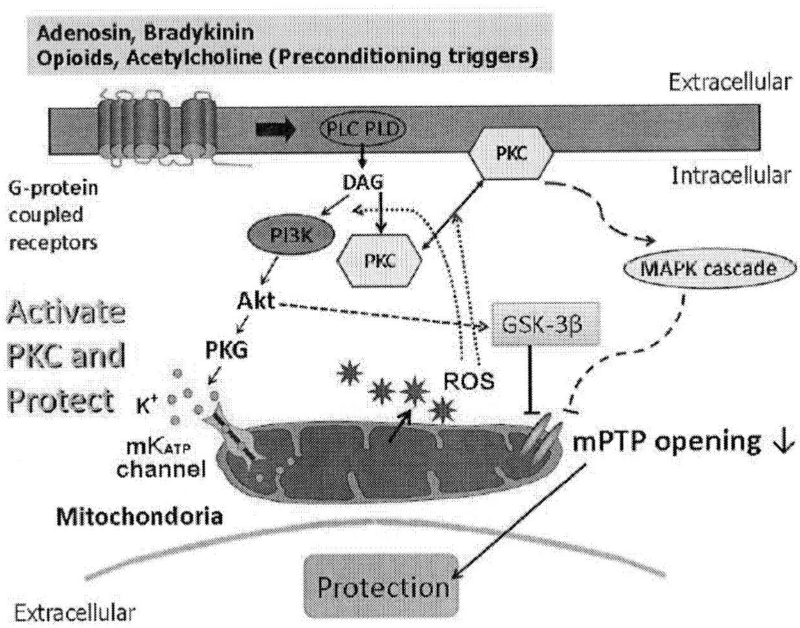

Figure 1. Possible signal transduction pathways of IPreC in the cell. PLC, phospholipase C; PLD, phospholipase D; DAG, diacyl glycerol; PKC, protein kinase C; MAPK, mitogen-activated protein kinases; mPTP, mitochondrial permeability transition pores; PI3K, phosphatidylinositol 3-kinase; Akt, protein kinase B; GSK-3β, glycogen synthase kinase 3; mKATP, mitochondrial potassium adenosine triphosphate-sensitive channels; ROS, reactive oxygen species [83].

Both of these K_{ATP} channels are regulated by PKC, which is activated by nitric oxide and also by oxygen free radicals generated after mitoK_{ATP} channel opening [78]. Diazoxide, a mitoK_{ATP} opener, pharmacologically preconditions the heart [72, 74]. Also, nicorandil is a K_{ATP} channel opener that activates the sarcK_{ATP} and mitoK_{ATP} channels. These drugs can be given before or during ischemia to prevent IRI. Hence, redox signaling is involved in other organs by preconditioning [79-80]. IPreC utilizes endogenous as well as distant mechanisms in skeletal muscle, liver, lung, kidney, intestine and brain in animal models to protect from IRI [81]. In addition, some groups have confirmed the efficacy of IPreC in cardiac surgery and percutaneous coronary interventions in humans [82]. Figure 1 shows the possible mechanisms of IPreC in the cell [83].

Definition and Mechanism of Postconditioning

Although it has been shown that IPreC can make ischemic myocardium resistant to IRI, the need for a pretreatment could limit due to its clinical application because IPreC is of little practical use as the onset of an infarction is usually unpredictable. During late 1980s and 1990s researchers intensively investigated whether or not pharmacologically modified reperfusion could reduce reperfusion injury. Meanwhile, Zhao and coworkers demonstrated that several brief cycles of ischemia and reperfusion at the start of reperfusion after sustained ischemia reduced infarct size in dogs with an efficacy comparable to that of IPreC [84-85]. This procedure has been called postconditioning. Based on the knowledge of gradual reperfusion and IPreC, Vinten-Johansen group [86] introduced the ischemic postconditioning (IPostC) treatment against IRI. In that study, the IPostC protocol was 30s of reperfusion followed by 30s of coronary occlusion, which were repeated for three cycles at the very onset of reperfusion. The IPostC concept consists of at least three factors that are the delay after which the first re-occlusion is established, the duration and number of re-occlusions, and the duration of the interspersed reperfusion [87]. IPostC still reduced infarct size when the delay to the first re-occlusion ranged from 1 to 3min. Many groups have reported that the IPostC were initiated within 1min of reperfusion, and within this 1min time frame no impact of a delay on infarct size reduction was noted [88-92]. Also, IPostC with too many cycles and/or too long duration of ischemia-reperfusion within each cycle may impair the outcome of IPostC. Additional ischemia relative to the duration of the index ischemia may limit the reduction of the infarct size. IPostC using several cycles of 5min reperfusion and 5min ischemia did not improve the damaging effect of IRI [86-87]. The efficacy of these ischemic or pharmacological interventions initiated later than 5–10min after the beginning of reperfusion resulted in markedly limited addition of cardioprotection to reperfusion per second. These mechanical interventions such as gradual reperfusion and IPostC, and several pharmacological interventions have been studied against reperfusion injury. Based on the knowledge acquired with the studies in IPreC, IPostC represents a promising tool to inhibit IRI. Recent studies demonstrate for the first time that IPostC can protect against endothelial IRI in humans [93-94]. Experimental studies suggest that IPostC is able to inhibit the detrimental effects of many of the established proponents of lethal IRI such as calcium overload, oxidative stress, rapid pH correction, endothelial dysfunction and inflammation. The main effect of IPostC-induced protection around the preservation of mitochondrial integrity via regulation of the mPTP, reduced sensitivity to the increased intracellular calcium (Ca^{2+}) levels triggered by IRI, restoration of redox balance and nitric oxide-mediated vaso-relaxation [95]. Data from many research groups have provided evidence that IPostC is able to activate cell-surface receptors such as adenosine, bradykinin and opioids that lead to protective effects via signal transduction pathways and through signaling molecules, which thereafter recruit signal transduction pathways such as the PI3K-Akt, MEK1/2-Erk (extracellular-signal regulated kinase)1/2, and cGMP-PKG kinase cascades (Figure 2).

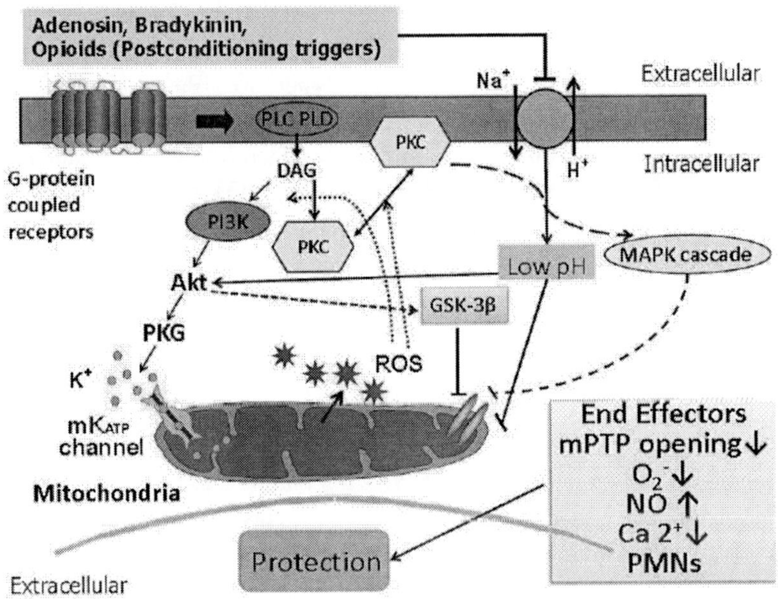

Figure 2. Possible signal transduction pathways IPostC in the cell. PLC, phospholipase C; PLD, phospholipase D; DAG, diacylglycerol; PKC, protein kinase C; MAPK, mitogen-activated protein kinases; mPTP, mitochondrial permeability transition pores; PI3K, phosphatidylinositol 3-kinase; Akt, protein kinase B; GSK-3β, glycogen synthase kinase 3; mK_{ATP}, mitochondrial potassium adenosine triphosphate-sensitive channels; ROS, reactive oxygen species; NO, nitric oxide; PMNs, polymorphonuclears [83].

The above signal transduction pathways are known to terminate on the mitochondria. Early acidosis and kinases such as GSK-3beta prevents mPTP opening (Figure 2) [96-100].

In other words, the first few minutes of reperfusion represents a window of opportunity for triggering the many mediators, which in concert will lead to protection against reperfusion injury. Figure 2 shows the possible mechanisms of IPostC in the cell.

Similarities and Differences in Cellular Signal Transduction Between Ischemic Preconditioning and Postconditioning

Although understanding the precise cellular signaling events is still in evolution, similarities exist between IPreC and IPostC despite the fundamental differences in the timing of protection. In particular, the first few minutes of reperfusion following the ischemia appear crucial to both IPreC and IPostC induced protection. Much evidence indicates that components of the so-called RISK (reperfusion injury salvage kinase) pathway play a role both in IPreC and in IPostC. IPreC and IPostC also reduce the oxidant-induced injury. Moreover, they attenuate the local inflammatory response to reperfusion (84, 88, 92). IPreC and IPostC activate a signal transduction pathway involving the PI3K-Akt and Erk1/2, which has been termed the RISK pathway. The RISK pathway terminates with the inhibition of the MET (a membrane receptor that is essential for embryonic development and wound healing) opening at reperfusion to afford protection in both IPreC and IPostC [96-100]. However, some differences between the pathways activated by IPreC and IPostC also exist [84]. It is likely that the ROS signaling involved in pre- and post-ischemic phases are not the same. Since exogenous ROS are able to induce IPreC but not IPostC, it is also likely that compartmentalization plays a pivotal role in the latter case. In particular, the concomitance of acidosis, NO formation, mPTP inhibition, and ROS generation seems mandatory in IPostC [51]. In addition, Yang and colleagues (2004) showed that Erk is involved in IPostC, but not in IPreC [90]. Some groups showed that a redox signaling may be involved in IPostC, but the ROS involved may not be the same of those involved in IPreC [101-102]. (see Figures 1 and 2).

Pharmacological Postconditioning

As the mechanisms regulating IPostC have been completely unraveled, the possibility to induce IPostC pharmacologically has arisen. In fact, several studies are focused on the effects of protective drugs administered either before, or during the index ischemia or at the onset of reperfusion. Kin and coworkers (2005) provided strong evidence to support the involvement of some adenosine receptor subtypes in IPostC [103].

Hausenloy and Yellon (2007) reported that an increasing number of agents including insulin, erythropoietin, adipocytokines, adenosine, volatile anesthetics natriuretic peptides and 'statins' when administered specifically at the time of myocardial reperfusion, reduce myocardial infarct size through the activation of the RISK pathway [100]. Successful pharmacological IPostC in humans in the surgical setting has been reported by Jin and coworkers (2007) using adenosine given within 1min of aortic cross-clamp removal [104]. Understanding the IPostC mechanisms may improve the protective results effect of drug administration that is otherwise limited by the systemic hemodynamic side effects or other harmful or undesirous side effects of these agents.

Ischemic Preconditioning and Postconditioning as Protective Measures against Testicular Ischemia Reperfusion Injury

Similarly, some researchers reported the effects of IPreC on testicular ischemia-reperfusion induced damage. Ceylan and colleagues (2005) noted no protective effects of IPreC in rat testes during 90min of 720-degree torsion [105], while Sahinkanat and coworkers (2007) reported that IPreC protects testicular tissue [106]. Although some studies show that

IPreC is effective, especially in the reperfusion phase in other tissue, these reports did not include observations in the reperfusion phase. Akcora et al. (2008) reported that gradual detorsion has a tendency to decrease testicular IRI in the rat torsion-detorsion model [107]. Their results showed that the gradual detorsion (controlled reperfusion) of ischemic testis may be a method for preventing reperfusion injury. Accordingly a study generated from our laboratory investigated the hypothesis that IPostC, which is a variation of controlled reperfusion requiring a similar surgical manipulation presents protective effect against IRI in the testis. Recently, our study showed that IPreC and IPostC demonstrated protective effects against ischemia-reperfusion induced biochemical and histological changes in rat testes including observations in the reperfusion [108]. However, IPreC is clinically feasible only when testicular torsion is predictable [81]. The concept of IPostC is attractive from a testicular surgical point of view. Interventions at the time of reperfusion are easy to perform when surgical repair of patients with testicular torsion. Many groups suggest that the early moments of reperfusion are important in the pathogenesis of post-ischemic injury and that early manipulation of reperfusion phase can reduce ischemia-reperfusion related injury [85, 109]. Recently, we have demonstrated that IPostC after unilateral testicular IRI has protective effect on ipsilateral and contralateral testes [110]. IPreC as well as IPostC inhibit production of ROS and neutrophil infiltration in the testis [19]. In a previous study of our laboratory, an IPostC protocol was applied, which consisted of five cycles of 10s of reperfusion followed by 10s of ischemia [108]. However, the optimal number and duration of the intermitted interruptions of blood flow during testicular IPostC remains unknown. It has been shown that among the different experimental protocols, IPostC 3-30 protocol (three cycles of 30s reperfusion-30s ischemia) presented the maximal protective effect against ischemia-reperfusion-induced biochemical and histological alterations in both ipsilateral and contralateral testes. IPostC 3-30 protocol significantly inhibited these parameters. We reported that the IPostC 3-30 protocol significantly decreased the tissue levels of lipid peroxidation, neutrophil infiltration and apoptosis in both ipsilateral and contralateral testes caused by unilateral IRI. Figures 3 and 4 show data of MDA and MPO concentrations, respectively, in the experimental testis.

However, it has not been reported whether the deleterious effects of IRI were attenuated or whether some beneficial mechanisms were triggered following testicular IPostC compensating the IRI-related damage.

Further studies are needed to clarify the potential mechanisms responsible for the beneficial effect of IPostC in both ipsilateral and contralateral testes after unilateral testicular IRI. Although among the different IPostC protocols the IPostC 3-30 protocol showed the maximal protective effect to bilateral testes, it is still unclear if this protocol is the ideal one to offer the maximal protective effect against testicular IRI (Figures 5-7). Extensive tubular vacuolation, necrosis and loss of maturation of germ cells were observed in the ischemia-reperfusion group (Figure 6). IPostC 3-30 treatment dramatically reduced bilaterally the alterations observed in the ischemia-reperfusion group (Figure 7). Apoptosis in bilateral testicular samples was characterized by TUNEL technique. A large number of TUNEL-positive germinal cells mostly at the spermatogonium and spematocyte stage were observed in testicular samples bilaterally in ischemia-reperfusion group (Figure 6). TUNEL-positive germ cells in bilateral testicular samples in the group IPostC 3-30 were significantly lower compared with ischemia-reperfusion group (Figures 6 and 7).

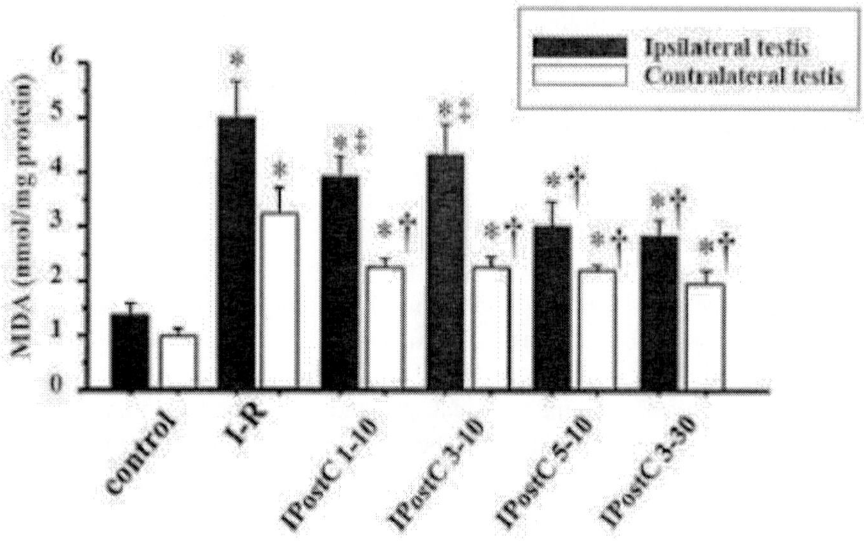

Figure 3. Mean values of tissue MDA concentration in both ipsilateral and contralateral testes of all groups. MDA concentration was normalized with protein content. Data are shown as mean ± SEM of six separate determinations in each group. * significantly different from control group. ($p<0.05$) † significantly different from ischemia-reperfusion group. ($p<0.05$) ‡ significantly different from contralateral testis in the same group. ($p<0.05$) [110].

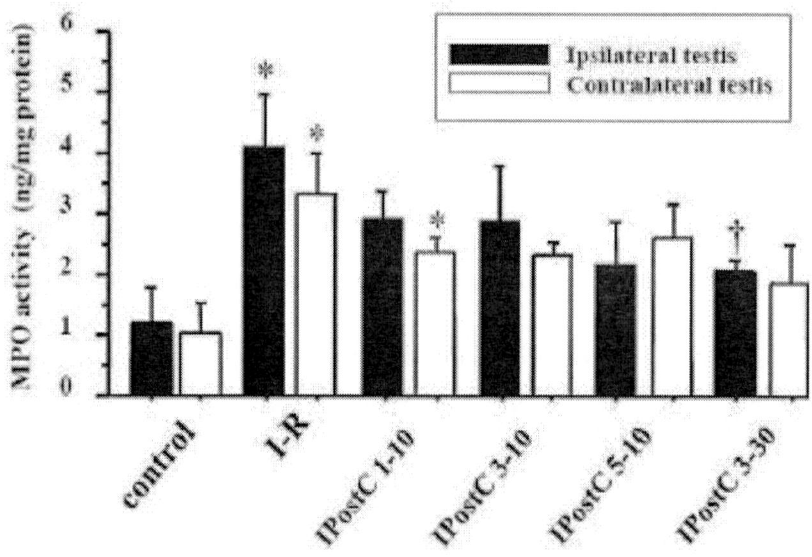

Figure 4. Mean values of tissue MPO activity in both ipsilateral and contralateral testis of all groups. MPO activity was normalized with protein content. Data are shown as mean ± SEM of six separate determinations in each group. * significantly different from control group. ($p<0.05$) † significantly different from ischemia-reperfusion group. ($p<0.05$) ‡ significantly different from contralateral testis in the same group. ($p<0.05$) [110].

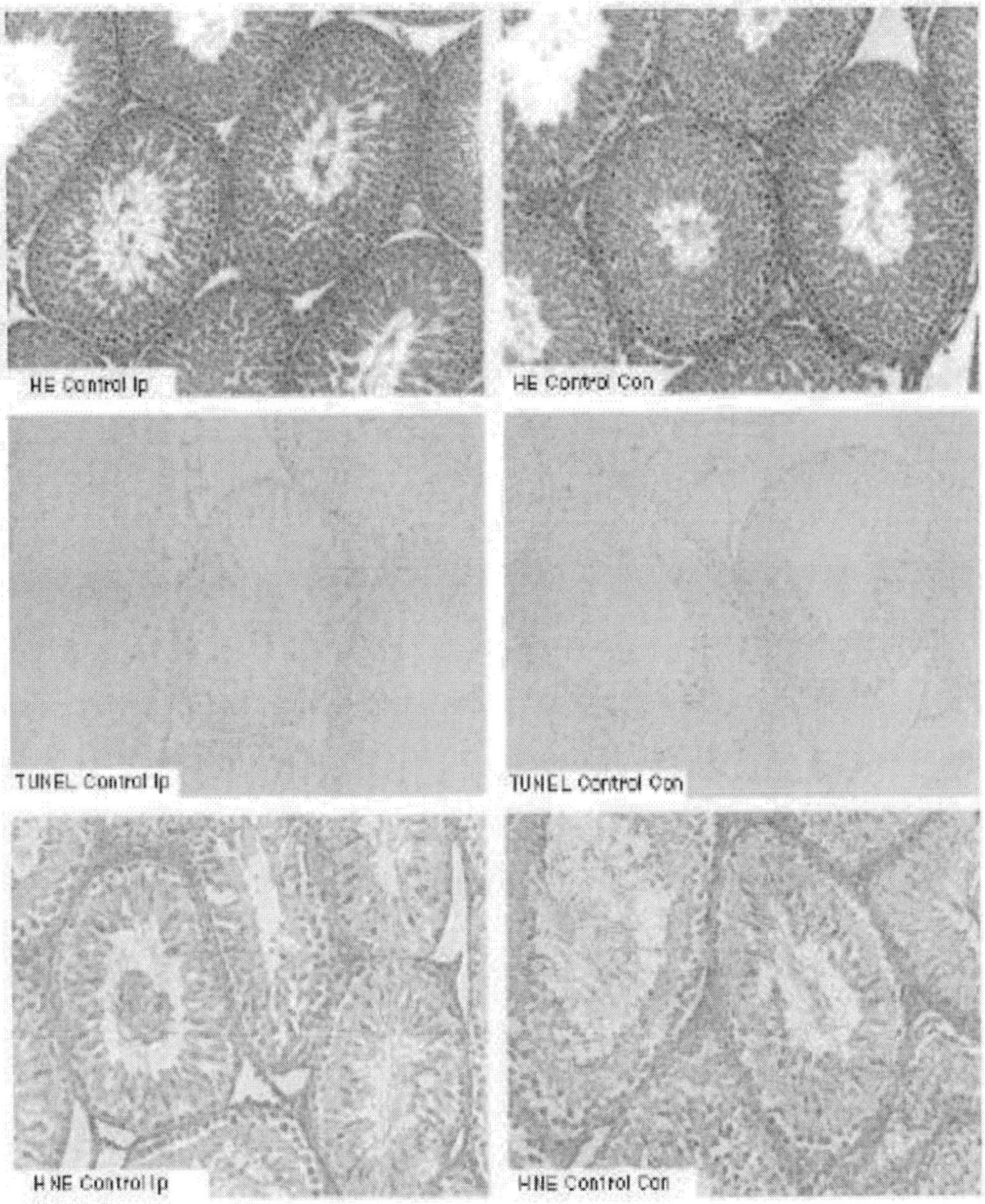

Figure 5. Hematoxylin-eosin (HE), Terminal deoxynucleotidyl transferase mediated dUTP Nick End Labeling (TUNEL) and immunohistochemical staining of 4-Hydroxy-2-Nonenal (4-HNE) in both ipsilateral and contralateral testis of the control group. Original magnification: x200. Ip: ipsilateral testis, Con: contralateral testis, IPostC: ischemic postconditioning, HNE: 4-HNE [110].

In bilateral testicular samples of ischemia-reperfusion group, 4-HNE immunoreactive cells in the basement membrane of the seminiferous tubules, germ cells, and Leydig cells were greatly increased compared with the control group (Figures 5 and 6). 4-HNE immunoreactivity in IPostC 3-30 group was decreased compared with ischemia-reperfusion group (Figure 7).

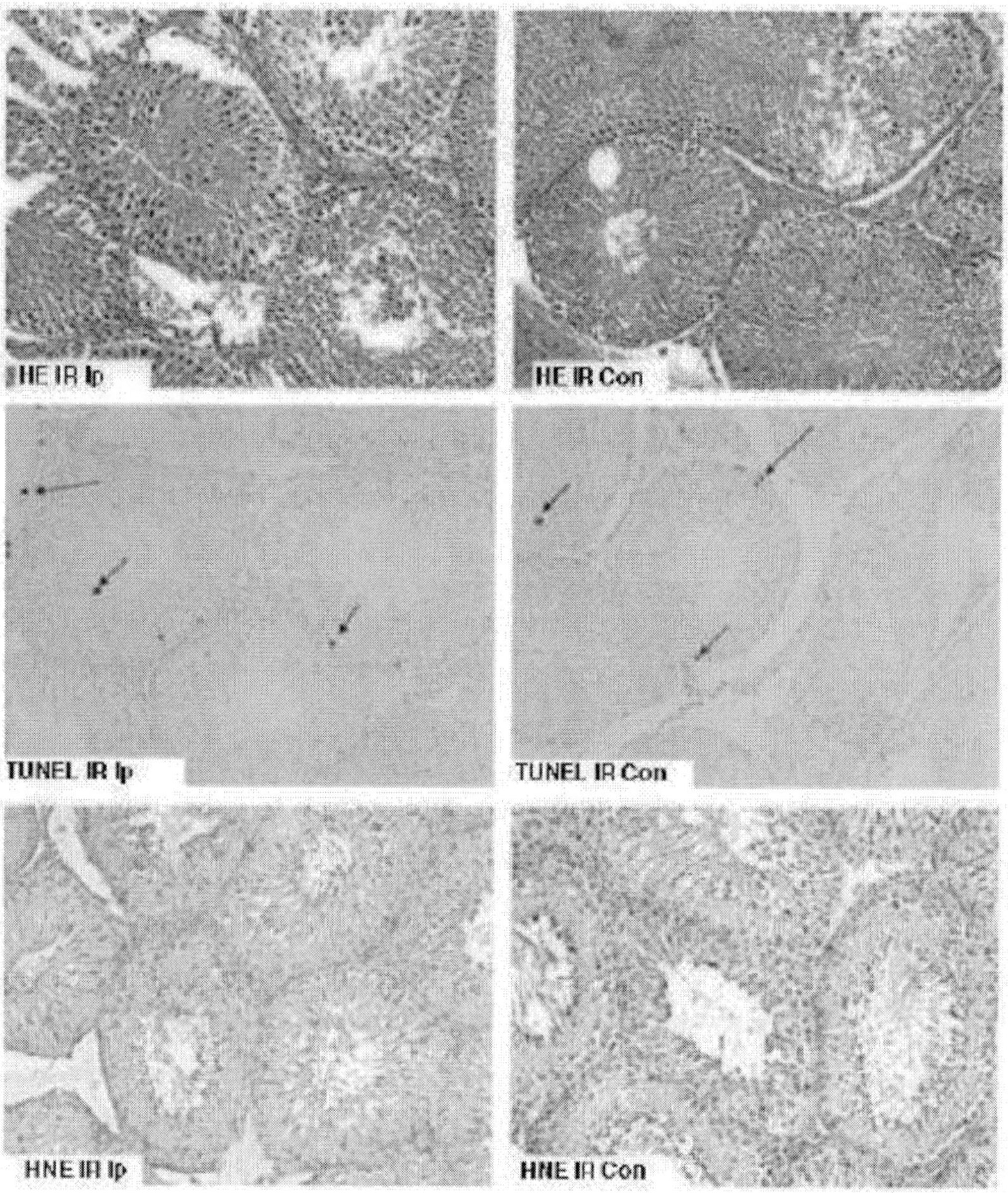

Figure 6. Hematoxylin-eosin (HE), Terminal deoxynucleotidyl transferase mediated dUTP Nick End Labeling (TUNEL) and immunohistochemical staining of 4-Hydroxy-2-Nonenal (4-HNE) in both ipsilateral and contralateral testes of the ischemia-reperfusion group. TUNEL-positive germinal cells in the seminiferous tubules (black arrows). Original magnification: x200. Ip: ipsilateral testis, Con: contralateral testis, IPostC: ischemic postconditioning, HNE: 4-HNE [110].

Additional investigations are required to identify the most appropriate time intervals and duration as well as the number of cycles during IPostC management [110].

To date, extensive investigatory efforts have aimed to find effective strategies and drugs to ameliorate or even prevent testicular IRI. However, apart from cooling the scrotum, no other method has thus far been successfully applied in clinical practice [111].

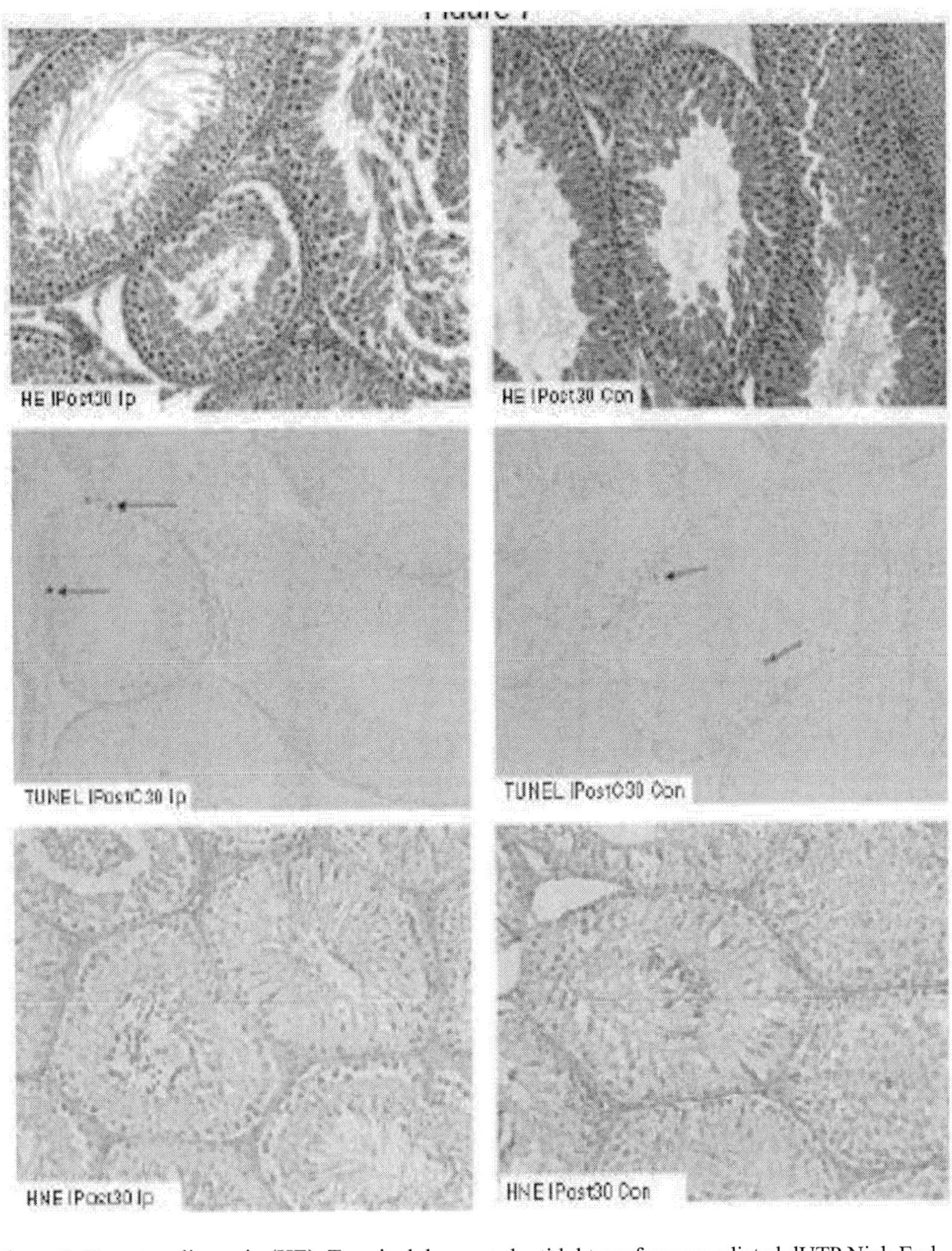

Figure 7. Hematoxylin-eosin (HE), Terminal deoxynucleotidyl transferase mediated dUTP Nick End Labeling (TUNEL) and immunohistochemical staining of 4-Hydroxy-2-Nonenal (4-HNE) in both ipsilateral and contralateral testes of the IPostC 3-30 group. TUNEL-positive germinal cells in the seminiferous tubules (black arrows). Original magnification: x200. Ip: ipsilateral testis, Con: contralateral testis, IPostC: ischemic postconditioning, HNE: 4-HNE (110).

The application of IPostC appears to be a simple and promising strategy to reduce testicular IRI.

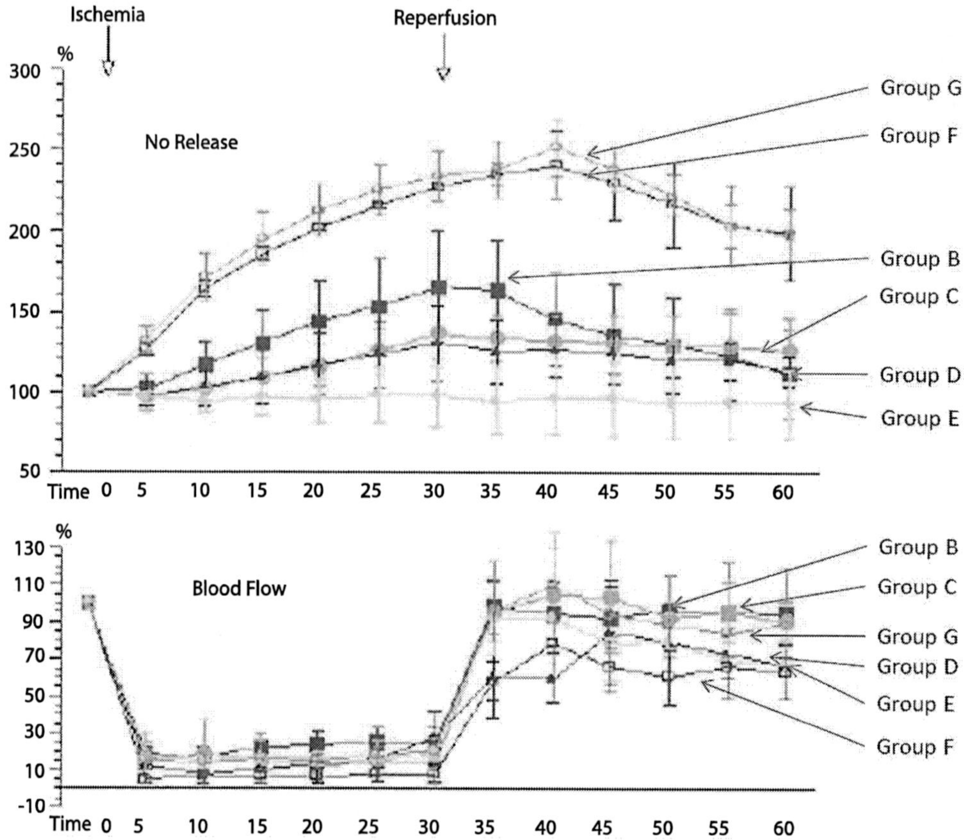

Figure 8. Blood flow and NO release during ischemia-reperfusion (IR) in the testis. B: 30min ischemia-30min reperfusion (IR) rats C: ischemia-reperfusion rats treated with L-NAME (10 mg/kg i.p.) D: ischemia-reperfusion rats treated with L-NAME (30 mg/kg i.p.) E: ischemia-reperfusion rats treated with L-NAME (100 mg/kg i.p.) F: ischemia-reperfusion rats treated with L-Arg (10 mg/kg i.p.) G: ischemia-reperfusion rats treated with L-Arg (30 mg/kg i.p.). Blood flow and NO release were expressed as % of the basal level. Data are shown as mean ± SEM of six to eight separated determinations in each group [116].

Pharmacological Agents for the Protection against Testicular Ischemia Reperfusion Injury

Several reports describe the protective effects of pharmacological agents against testicular IRI. Sarica and coworkers (2001) reported that a calcium-channel blocker, verapamil, may act beneficially against unilateral testicular torsion injury [112]. Moreover, Sarioglu-Buke and colleagues (2001) reported that capsaicin effectively prevented apoptosis in the both ipsilateral and contralateral testis after unilateral testicular torsion [113]. Subsequently, effects of dexamethasone (glucocorticoid class of steroid), molsidomine (vasodilator and NO donor), selenium and sildenafil (phosphodiesterase type 5 inhibitor) against testicular torsion-detorsion injury have been reported [7, 114-115]. In previous published works from our laboratory, it was demonstrated that L-arginine significantly, an NO donor, ameliorated ischemia-reperfusion induced injury in the testis, suggesting that NO has a cytoprotective effect against IRI in the testis [116]. Figure 8 shows a real time monitoring of NO and blood flow in the ipsilateral testis during ischemia-reperfusion. Clamping of the left testicular artery in the rat resulted in a decreased blood flow of 5-20% compared to the basal level measured before clamping (Figure 8). After removal of the clip, the blood flow recovered from 50 to 100% of the basal level within one minute in all groups. Immediately following clamping of the testicular artery, NO release rapidly increased, reaching a plateau within approximately 30min (Figure 8). When a NO electrode was inserted into the rat testis treated with 10, 30 and 100mg/kg i.p. of L-NAME, a non-selective inhibitor of nitric oxide synthase, NO release was decreased in a dose-dependent manner. Groups C, D and E correspond to 10, 30 and 100mg/kg, respectively (Figure 8). In contrast to treatment with L-NAME, L-arginine treatment (10 or 30mg/kg i.p.) significantly increased NO release in a dose-dependent manner (groups F or G) (Figure 8).

After removing the clip, NO release treated with L-NAME returned almost to basal levels whereas NO release treated with L-arginine (10 or 30mg/kg i.p.) remained significantly higher than basal levels during these 30minutes (Figure 8).

The role of NO during ischemia-reperfusion is complicated and sometimes has been controversial. Ozokutan and associates (2000) have reported that NO plays an important role in damaging the testis in ischemia-reperfusion [117]. In contrast, some reports have indicated that increased in NO levels in the testis significantly prevent ischemia-reperfusion or torsion detorsion injury [118-120]. Possible mechanisms of testicular dysfunction in ischemia may include the impairment of oxygen and nutrient supplies and the removal of waste products through the circulatory system. Decreases in the intracellular content of ATP and glycogen and an increase in intracellular Ca^{2+} may play important roles in testicular injury. Generation of these reactive oxygen species is attributed to IRI. Peroxynitrite has also been reported to be a powerful oxidative product with deleterious effects on various cells and tissues [121-122]. In contrast, ischemia rapidly decreases the extracellular pH during the ischemic condition. The reduction of NO_2 to NO is promoted by ischemia-induced acidosis as well as enzymatic catalysis. NO donors protect against ischemia reperfusion damage in *in vitro* models of these tissues [123-125]. Moreover, reactive oxygen species inactivate the relaxing NO and promote a reduction in blood flow. Attenuation of NO mediated vasodilation has been reported to be dependent on the inactivation of NO by superoxide anion generated by endothelial xanthine oxidase [126]. Because NO interacts with free oxygen radicals, the decreased NO release during reperfusion may be the result of oxidant species that react with NO, possibly causing a decrease in NO concentrations in the reperfused testis [118].

Edaravone, a free-radical scavenger, is used for the clinical treatment of cerebral ischemia in Japan. Edaravone ameliorates cerebral ischemia by supplying individual free-radical molecules with one of its electrons, and thereby detoxifying them [127]. Edaravone is an especially strong scavenger of hydroxyl radicals, and thus has been approved as a neuroprotective agent for the treatment of acute cerebral infarction by the Japanese Health Organization since 2001 [128]. In rat cerebral ischemia-reperfusion, edaravone has been shown to protect neurones through the early free radical scavenging pathway and a late anti-inflammatory response [129-130]. Several other reports have shown that edaravone protects against IRI of the brain, heart, liver, and small intestine in animal models [129-133]. Tamamura and coworkers (2010) reported that edaravone significantly ameliorated ischemia-reperfusion induced testicular damage by reducing the oxidative stress (see Table 1) [13].

Table 1. Malondialdehyde (MDA), 8-hydroxydeoxyguanosine (8-OHdG) and myeloperoxidase (MPO) levels in the testis

	MDA (nmol/mg protein)	8-OHdG (pg/μg DNA)	MPO (ng/mg protein)
Cont	1.02 ± 0.09	4.84 ± 0.46	0.57 ± 0.04
I-R(0)	2.30 ± 0.35 *	6.74 ± 0.23 *	8.53 ± 2.69 *
I-R(1)	1.71 ± 0.39	4.96 ± 0.72	5.43 ± 2.76 †
I-R(10)	1.46 ± 0.20	5.15 ± 0.34	4.09 ± 1.06 †

Cont, control group; I-R(0), ischemia-reperfusion group; I-R(1), ischemia-reperfusion group plus 1mg/Kg of edaravone i.p.; I-R(10), ischemia-reperfusion group plus 10mg/Kg of edaravone i.p. *significantly different ($P<0.05$) from control group and I-R10 group; †significantly different from control group [13].

Figure 9 shows the histological data presented in the report. Extensive cell swelling, tubular vacuolation, necrosis, and loss of germ cell maturation were observed in the ischemia-reperfusion groups (IR(0) and IR(1) groups). In contrast, high-dose treatment with edaravone (IR(10) group) significantly reduced these ischemia-reperfusion-induced changes. In the breakdown of microcirculation it is clear that the change of interaction between vascular endothelial cells and leukocytes triggers I-R injury. Testicular torsion itself causes a significant increase in neutrophil adhesion to the testicular venous endothelium [28].

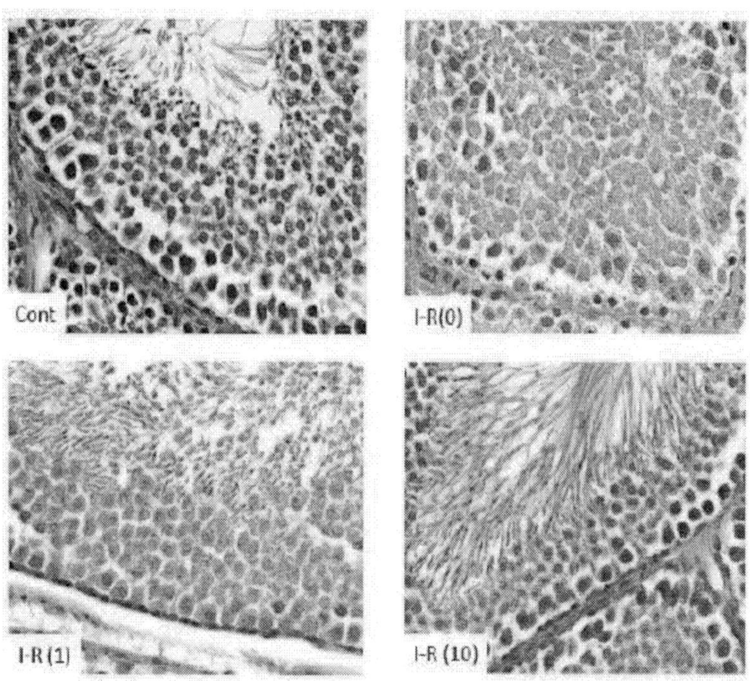

Figure 9. Histological changes evaluated by hematoxylin-eosin (HE) staining.A sham-operated control group administered edaravone at 10 mg/kg i.p. (Cont group); a group administered vehicle and then subjected to induction of 30-min ischemia and 60-min reperfusion (IR(0) group); and groups administered edaravone at 1 or 10 mg/kg i.p. and then subjected to 30-min ischemia and 60-min reperfusion (IR(1) and IR(10) groups, respectively). 60min prior to induction of ischemia, edaravone was administrated intraperitonally. Original magnification: ×400 [13].

Table 2. Measurement of testosterone (T) malondialdehyde (MDA) levels, expression of heat-shock protein-70 (HSP-70) and myeloperoxidase (MPO) activity in both ipsilateral (RT) and contralateral (LT) rat testis

		Control	I-R-A	I-R15-A	I-R60-A	I-R-B	I-R15-B	I-R60-B
T	RT	17.80±10.22	-	-	-	1.30±0.75 ^{a}	2.16±1.73 ^{a}	4.70±4.05 ^{a}
	LT	17.55±10.8	-	-	-	1.01±0.47 ^{a}	2.81±1.42 ^{a}	0.49±0.28 ^{a}
MDA	RT	2.37±0.22	4.60±0.41 ^{a}	4.61±0.37 ^{a}	3.66±0.38 ^{a}	10.43±0.82 ^{a,b}	10.31±0.43 ^{a,b}	6.72±1.22 ^{a}
	LT	2.37±0.22	4.42±0.35 ^{a}	4.25±0.29 ^{a}	3.26±0.35 ^{a}	7.60±0.35 ^{a,c}	5.19±0.85 ^{a,c}	2.85±0.22 ^{a,c}
HSP-70	RT	2.52±0.27	9.92±1.26 ^{a}	9.38±1.17 ^{a}	11.81±1.10 ^{a}	11.34±0.79 ^{a}	15.52±1.07 ^{a}	14.19±0.83 ^{a}
	LT	2.52±0.27	10.93±1.11 ^{a}	8.00±1.18 ^{a}	10.85±1.16 ^{a}	13.06±1.23 ^{a}	12.16±0.62 ^{a}	12.16±0.77 ^{a}
MPO	RT	43.80±6.71	350.74±133.39 ^{a}	37.53±13.78 ^{d}	97.10±42.73	94.00±24.72 ^{a}	52.24±11.50	69.38±12.89
	LT	43.80±6.71	119.49±60.46	29.26±5.32	29.30±13.52	141.97±62.14	35.59±6.37	61.78±8.60

I-R-A, ischemia followed by 2 hours of reperfusion.
I-R15-A, ischemia followed by 2 hours of reperfusion plus administration of 15mg/Kg of sivelestat.
I-R60-A, ischemia followed by 2 hours of reperfusion plus administration of 60mg/Kg of sivelestat.
I-R-B, ischemia followed by 48 hours of reperfusion.
I-R15-B, ischemia followed by 48 hours of reperfusion plus administration of 15mg/Kg of sivelestat.
I-R60-B, ischemia followed by 48 hours of reperfusion plus administration of 60mg/Kg of sivelestat.
^{a} Significantly different from the control group ($P<0.05$). ^{b} Significantly different from group I-R60-B ($P<0.05$). ^{c} Significantly different ($P<0.05$) from any of the other cells sharing the same superscript. ^{d} Significantly different from group I-R-A ($P<0.05$). The data are shown as mean±SD [47].

It has been reported that neutrophils recruited to the testes after detorsion are potent generators of ROS [28]. In the study by Tamamura and coworkers (2010), neutrophil infiltration was estimated by measuring MPO concentrations in the testes [13].

Treatment with edaravone significantly prevented neutrophil infiltration into the I-R-damaged testes. In microvessels, it is known that neutrophils induce ROS and tissue injury by two different mechanisms, i.e. free radicals and pro-inflammatory cytokines. In the first phase, free radicals contribute to the oxidative injury of lipids in vascular endothelial cells, proteins and nucleic acids.

It is important to prevent neutrophil adhesion to inhibit both mechanisms, i.e. free radicals and the pro-inflammatory pathway. It has been demonstrated that edaravone affects the latter phase, i.e. the pro-inflammatory pathway [134].

Sivelestat sodium aminoacetate tetrahydrate is a synthetic, specific, low-molecular weight neutrophil elastase inhibitor [135]. The drug is intravenously active, and competitively inhibits the activity of neutrophil elastase in humans, hamsters and dogs, but does not affect other proteases such as plasmin, thrombin, kallikrein, cathepsin B, or collagenase I [135]. Several studies demonstrated that sivelestat protects against IRI on the lung, liver, renal and transplanted organs [136-139]. Although the mechanisms of sivelestat on IRI are unclear, the main mechanism is considered to be that sivelestat selectively and competitively inhibits the release of neutrophil elastase [138]. Tsounapi and coworkers (2011) reported that sivelestat, a neutrophil elastase inhibitor, directly inhibits the accumulation and activation of neutrophils [47]. Additionally, sivelestat offers efficient protection against the production of oxygen radicals and cytokines not only in the ipsilateral but also in the contralateral testis (Table 2) [47]. Human neutrophil elastase degrades extracellular matrix components and is involved in tissue destruction in several inflammatory states. The extracellular space contains very high concentrations of proteinase inhibitors such as α1-proteinase inhibitor (α1-PI) and α2-macroglobulin (α2-MG), which normally prevent connective tissue damage caused by the released polymorphonuclear proteases.

Therefore, there are two ways for proteolytic tissue injury to be produced by human neutrophil elastase: (i) human neutrophil elastase must be present in quantities that exceed the proteinase inhibitor capacity of the local tissue environment – as might happen in the case that polymorphonuclears are in contact with the tissue substrate, or (ii) the effectiveness of proteinase inhibitor must be impaired [140]. In contrast to these antiproteinases, a low molecular weight human neutrophil elastase inhibitor might be delivered to achieve close contact [141], suggesting the benefit of a low molecular weight human neutrophil elastase inhibitor acting as a therapeutic agent. Neutrophil elastase has a substantial role on ischemia-reperfusion injury by releasing toxic mediators such as oxygen-free radicals. These oxygen-free radicals initiate a chain reaction that leads to damage of the cell membrane by lipid peroxidation [142]. This irreversible process takes place primarily by the peroxidation of unsaturated fatty acids that are essential parts of the cell membrane. As aforementioned, during ischemia-reperfusion or inflammation, polymorphonuclears are accumulated, reactivated, and lead to leucocyte endothelial interaction, emigration, and subsequent tissue damage. Accumulated and activated leucocytes produce a second burst of oxygen radicals, along with other neutrophil-derived products, which cause further and maybe more severe damage [142]. A reliable biomarker to measure the extent of lipid peroxidation is the expression of MDA on the tissue. In the study by Tsounapi and coworkers (2011), the testicular MDA concentrations bilaterally were significantly increased in ischemia-reperfusion groups compared with those of the control group [47]. Treatment with sivelestat significantly decreased the bilateral testicular MDA production caused by ischemia-reperfusion [47].

To date, extensive investigatory efforts aim to find effective strategies and drugs to ameliorate or even prevent testicular ischemia-reperfusion injury. However, apart from cooling the scrotum, no other method has thus far been successfully applied in clinical practice [143]. The pathophysiological events during the IRI share common mechanisms between experimental animals and humans and the cornerstone of this pathophysiology appears to be the generation of ROS during the reperfusion period [3, 144]. Thus the above studies may also have to a certain degree of relevance to the clinical practice as well.

As for this, further clinical trials are mandatory to confirm the above hypothesis. On a theoretical basis, and if a specific pharmaceutical treatment is proved appropriate for clinical application, an immediate administration of that pharmacological agent right after the diagnosis of testicular torsion and while the patient is being prepared for the surgical room, would minimize the testicular damage, offering ultimately a better prognostics for the future testicular function.

Conclusion

There is still a need to find new treatments in order to improve testicular protection during open testis surgery. However, it is obscure whether the principle of IPostC is a suitable method to achieve this goal. Although it has been reported that experimental IPostC effectively protects testicular IRI, it was not checked if this procedure would be the same protective during routine use in human testicular surgery. Further work is clearly required to assess the potential benefit of IPostC in humans. If IPostC on testicular torsion detorsion should become an important and widespread technique of testicular protection, large-scale studies are necessary to provide strong evidence of the beneficial effects of this procedure in human testes as well as in other organs. However, there is always the potential danger to damage the testicular artery by the repeated clamping and releasing.

For this reason, IPostC might never gain widespread acceptance as a routine technique in the majority of patients. The key is to find pharmacological ways to induce IPostC. Pharmacological PostC has the potential advantage of reducing the requirement for invasive therapy associated with unavoidable endothelial trauma and possible embolic events. Thus, it is important to reveal the underlying IPostC signal transduction of protection and induce this pharmacologically. More experimental studies providing mechanistic insights are required.

REFERENCES

[1] Sigman M, Jarow JP. Disorders of spermatogenesis. In: Walsh PC, Retik AB, Vaughan ED, Wein AJ, editors. Campbell's Urology. Eighth edition ed. Philadelphia: *Saunders*, 2002. p. 15046-8.

[2] Dokmeci D. Testicular torsion, oxidative stress and the role of antioxidant therapy. *Folia. Med.*, (Plovdiv) 2006;48(3-4):16-21.

[3] Filho DW, Torres MA, Bordin AL, Crezcynski-Pasa TB, Boveris A. Spermatic cord torsion, reactive oxygen and nitrogen species and ischemia-reperfusion injury. *Mol. Aspects. Med.,* 2004 Feb-Apr;25(1-2):199-210.

[4] Bartsch G, Frank S, Marberger H, Mikuz G. Testicular torsion: late results with special regard to fertility and endocrine function. *J. Urol.*, 1980 Sep;124(3):375-8.

[5] Heindel RM, Pakyz RE, Reinking LN, Cosentino MJ. The effect of various degrees of unilateral spermatic cord torsion on fertility in the rat. *J. Urol.,* 1990 Aug;144(2 Pt 1):366-9.

[6] Prillaman HM, Turner TT. Rescue of testicular function after acute experimental torsion. *J. Urol.,* 1997 Jan;157(1):340-5.

[7] Avlan D, Erdougan K, Cimen B, Dusmez Apa D, Cinel I, Aksoyek S. The protective effect of selenium on ipsilateral and contralateral testes in testicular reperfusion injury. *Pediatr. Surg. Int.*, 2005 Apr;21(4):274-8.

[8] Costabile RA, Choyke PL, Frank JA, Girton ME, Diggs R, Billups KL, et al. Variability of ischemia during spermatic cord torsion in the rat. *J. Urol.,* 1994 Apr;151(4):1070-2.

[9] Anim JT, Kehinde EO, Prasad A, Varghese R. Morphological responses of the rabbit testis to ischemic/reperfusion injury due to torsion. Urol Int 2005;75(3):258-63.

[10] Fujii J, Iuchi Y, Matsuki S, Ishii T. Cooperative function of antioxidant and redox systems against oxidative stress in male reproductive tissues. *Asian. J. Androl.,* 2003 Sep;5(3):231-42.

[11] Turner TT, Brown KJ. Spermatic cord torsion: loss of spermatogenesis despite return of blood flow. *Biol. Reprod.,* 1993 Aug;49(2):401-7.

[12] Becker EJ, Jr., Turner TT. Endocrine and exocrine effects of testicular torsion in the prepubertal and adult rat. *J. Androl.*, 1995 Jul-Aug;16(4):342-51.
[13] Tamamura M, Saito M, Kinoshita Y, Shimizu S, Satoh I, Shomori K, et al. Protective effect of edaravone, a free-radical scavenger, on ischaemia-reperfusion injury in the rat testis. *BJU Int.*, 2010 Mar;105(6):870-6.
[14] Zhao ZQ, Velez DA, Wang NP, Hewan-Lowe KO, Nakamura M, Guyton RA, et al. Progressively developed myocardial apoptotic cell death during late phase of reperfusion. *Apoptosis*, 2001 Aug;6(4):279-90.
[15] Turner TT, Tung KS, Tomomasa H, Wilson LW. Acute testicular ischemia results in germ cell-specific apoptosis in the rat. *Biol. Reprod.*, 1997 Dec;57(6):1267-74.
[16] Packham G, Ashmun RA, Cleveland JL. Cytokines suppress apoptosis independent of increases in reactive oxygen levels. *J. Immunol.*, 1996 Apr 15;156(8):2792-800.
[17] Menger MD, Vollmar B. In vivo analysis of microvascular reperfusion injury in striated muscle and skin. *Microsurgery*, 1994;15(6):383-9.
[18] Kaminski KA, Bonda TA, Korecki J, Musial WJ. Oxidative stress and neutrophil activation--the two keystones of ischemia/reperfusion injury. *Int. J. Cardiol.*, 2002 Nov;86(1):41-59.
[19] Dimitriadis F, Saito M. Neutrophils: Focus in Andrology and Male Infertility. In: DeFranco, editor. Neutrophils: Lifespan, Functions and Roles in Disease. New York, (NY): *NovaScience*, 2010. p. 1-76.
[20] Springer TA. Traffic signals on endothelium for lymphocyte recirculation and leukocyte emigration. *Annu. Rev. Physiol.*, 1995;57:827-72.
[21] Weyrich AS, Ma XY, Lefer DJ, Albertine KH, Lefer AM. In vivo neutralization of P-selectin protects feline heart and endothelium in myocardial ischemia and reperfusion injury. *J. Clin. Invest.*, 1993 Jun;91(6):2620-9.
[22] Derevianko A, D'Amico R, Simms H. Polymorphonuclear leucocyte (PMN)-derived inflammatory cytokines--regulation by oxygen tension and extracellular matrix. *Clin. Exp. Immunol.*, 1996 Dec;106(3):560-7.
[23] Fassbender K, Kaptur S, Becker P, Groschl J, Hennerici M. Adhesion molecules in tissue injury: kinetics of expression and shedding and association with cytokine release in humans. *Clin. Immunol. Immunopathol.,* 1998 Oct;89(1):54-60.
[24] Weller A, Isenmann S, Vestweber D. Cloning of the mouse endothelial selectins. Expression of both E- and P-selectin is inducible by tumor necrosis factor alpha. *J. Biol. Chem.*, 1992 Jul 25;267(21):15176-83.
[25] Takada M, Nadeau KC, Shaw GD, Marquette KA, Tilney NL. The cytokine-adhesion molecule cascade in ischemia/reperfusion injury of the rat kidney. Inhibition by a soluble P-selectin ligand. *J. Clin. Invest.*, 1997 Jun 1;99(11):2682-90.
[26] Keelan ET, Licence ST, Peters AM, Binns RM, Haskard DO. Characterization of E-selectin expression in vivo with use of a radiolabeled monoclonal antibody. *Am. J. Physiol.*, 1994 Jan;266(1 Pt 2):H278-90.
[27] Lysiak JJ, Turner SD, Turner TT. Molecular pathway of germ cell apoptosis following ischemia/reperfusion of the rat testis. *Biol. Reprod.*, 2000 Nov;63(5):1465-72.
[28] Lysiak JJ, Turner SD, Nguyen QA, Singbartl K, Ley K, Turner TT. Essential role of neutrophils in germ cell-specific apoptosis following ischemia/reperfusion injury of the mouse testis. *Biol. Reprod.*, 2001 Sep;65(3):718-25.

[29] Nathan CF, Root RK. Hydrogen peroxide release from mouse peritoneal macrophages: dependence on sequential activation and triggering. *J. Exp. Med.,* 1977 Dec 1;146(6):1648-62.

[30] Milei J, Ferreira R, Llesuy S, Forcada P, Covarrubias J, Boveris A. Reduction of reperfusion injury with preoperative rapid intravenous infusion of taurine during myocardial revascularization. *Am. Heart. J.,* 1992 Feb;123(2):339-45.

[31] Tong L, Li J, Qiao H, Jiang H, Meng F, Sun X. Taurine protects against ischemia-reperfusion injury in rabbit livers. *Transplant. Proc*., 2006 Jun;38(5):1575-9.

[32] Wang GH, Jiang ZL, Fan XJ, Zhang L, Li X, Ke KF. Neuroprotective effect of taurine against focal cerebral ischemia in rats possibly mediated by activation of both GABAA and glycine receptors. *Neuropharmacology*, 2007 Apr;52(5):1199-209.

[33] Yang S, Shih HJ, Chow YC, Wang TY, Tsai PS, Huang CJ. Simvastatin attenuates testicular injury induced by torsion-detorsion. *J. Urol*., 2010 Aug;184(2):750-6.

[34] Jeong SJ, Choi WS, Chung JS, Baek M, Hong SK, Choi H. Preventive effects of cyclosporine a combined with prednisolone and melatonin on contralateral testicular damage after ipsilateral torsion-detorsion in pubertal and adult rats. *J. Urol*., 2010 Aug;184(2):790-6.

[35] Marotto ME, Thurman RG, Lemasters JJ. Early midzonal cell death during low-flow hypoxia in the isolated, perfused rat liver: protection by allopurinol. *Hepatology*, 1988 May-Jun;8(3):585-90.

[36] Akgur FM, Kilinc K, Tanyel FC, Buyukpamukcu N, Hicsonmez A. Ipsilateral and contralateral testicular biochemical acute changes after unilateral testicular torsion and detorsion. *Urology*, 1994 Sep;44(3):413-8.

[37] Lievano G, Nguyen L, Radhakrishnan J, Fornell L, John E. New animal model to evaluate testicular blood flow during testicular torsion. *J. Pediatr. Surg*., 1999 Jun;34(6):1004-6.

[38] Turner TT. Acute experimental testicular torsion. No effect on the contralateral testis. *J. Androl*., 1985 Jan-Feb;6(1):65-72.

[39] Cosentino MJ, Nishida M, Rabinowitz R, Cockett AT. Histological changes occurring in the contralateral testes of prepubertal rats subjected to various durations of unilateral spermatic cord torsion. *J. Urol*., 1985 May;133(5):906-11.

[40] Tanyel FC, Buyukpamukcu N, Hicsonmez A. Contralateral testicular blood flow during unilateral testicular torsion. *Br. J. Urol*., 1989 May;63(5):522-4.

[41] Harrison RG, Lewis-Jones DI, Moreno de Marval MJ, Connolly RC. Mechanism of damage to the contralateral testis in rats with an ischaemic testis. *Lancet*, 1981 Oct 3;2(8249):723-5.

[42] Nagler HM, White RD. The effect of testicular torsion on the contralateral testis. *J. Urol*., 1982 Dec;128(6):1343-8.

[43] Wallace DM, Gunter PA, Landon GV, Pugh RC, Hendry WF. Sympathetic orchiopathia--an experimental and clinical study. *Br. J. Urol.,* 1982 Dec;54(6):765-8.

[44] Blank ML, O'Neill PJ, Steigman CK, Cobb LM, Wilde RA, Havenstein PJ, et al. Reperfusion injury following testicular torsion and detorsion in prepubertal rats. *Urol. Res*., 1993;21(6):389-93.

[45] Andiran F, Okur DH, Kilinc A, Gediko, gmacr, lu G, et al. Do experimentally induced ipsilateral testicular torsion, vas deferens obstruction, intra-abdominal testis or venous

obstruction damage the contralateral testis through a common mechanism? *BJU Int.*, 2000 Feb;85(3):330-5.

[46] Kizilcan F, Bernay I, Tanyel FC, Buyukpamukcu N, Bekdik C, Hicsonmez A. Ipsilateral and contralateral testicular blood flows during unilateral testicular torsion by 133Xe clearance technique. *Int. Urol. Nephrol.,* 1992;24(5):515-20.

[47] Tsounapi P, Saito M, Dimitriadis F, Shimizu S, Kinoshita Y, Shomori K, et al. Protective effect of sivelestat, a neutrophil elastase inhibitor, on ipsilateral and contralateral testes after unilateral testicular ischaemia-reperfusion injury in rats. *BJU Int.*, 2011 Jan;107(2):329-36.

[48] Jeong SJ, Choi WS, Ha SB, Jeong MS, Chung JS, Baek M, et al. The different effects of testicular torsion on the contralateral testis between pubertal and adult rats. *Korean J. Urol.*, 2009;50:704-10.

[49] Murry CE, Jennings RB, Reimer KA. Preconditioning with ischemia: a delay of lethal cell injury in ischemic myocardium. *Circulation*, 1986 Nov;74(5):1124-36.

[50] Valen G, Vaage J. Pre- and postconditioning during cardiac surgery. *Basic Res. Cardiol.*, 2005 May;100(3):179-86.

[51] Penna C, Mancardi D, Rastaldo R, Pagliaro P. Cardioprotection: a radical view Free radicals in pre and postconditioning. *Biochim. Biophys. Acta.,* 2009 Jul;1787(7):781-93.

[52] Torras J, Herrero-Fresneda I, Lloberas N, Riera M, Ma Cruzado J, Ma Grinyo J. Promising effects of ischemic preconditioning in renal transplantation. *Kidney Int.,* 2002 Jun;61(6):2218-27.

[53] Riera M, Herrero I, Torras J, Cruzado JM, Fatjo M, Lloberas N, et al. Ischemic preconditioning improves postischemic acute renal failure. *Transplant Proc.*, 1999 Sep;31(6):2346-7.

[54] Peralta C, Hotter G, Closa D, Gelpi E, Bulbena O, Rosello-Catafau J. Protective effect of preconditioning on the injury associated to hepatic ischemia-reperfusion in the rat: role of nitric oxide and adenosine. *Hepatology*, 1997 Apr;25(4):934-7.

[55] Sindram D, Rudiger HA, Upadhya AG, Strasberg SM, Clavien PA. Ischemic preconditioning protects against cold ischemic injury through an oxidative stress dependent mechanism. *J. Hepatol.*, 2002 Jan;36(1):78-84.

[56] Bolli R. Cardioprotective function of inducible nitric oxide synthase and role of nitric oxide in myocardial ischemia and preconditioning: an overview of a decade of research. *J. Mol. Cell Cardiol.*, 2001 Nov;33(11):1897-918.

[57] Hausenloy DJ, Yellon DM. Preconditioning and postconditioning: new strategies for cardioprotection. *Diabetes Obes. Metab.*, 2008 Jun;10(6):451-9.

[58] Hausenloy DJ, Yellon DM. Preconditioning and postconditioning: united at reperfusion. *Pharmacol Ther.*, 2007 Nov;116(2):173-91.

[59] Yellon DM, Hausenloy DJ. Myocardial reperfusion injury. *N. Engl. J. Med.,* 2007 Sep 13;357(11):1121-35.

[60] Penna C, Mancardi D, Raimondo S, Geuna S, Pagliaro P. The paradigm of postconditioning to protect the heart. *J. Cell Mol. Med.*, 2008 Apr;12(2):435-58.

[61] Gross ER, Gross GJ. Ligand triggers of classical preconditioning and postconditioning. *Cardiovasc. Res.*, 2006 May 1;70(2):212-21.

[62] Laude K, Beauchamp P, Thuillez C, Richard V. Endothelial protective effects of preconditioning. *Cardiovasc. Res.*, 2002 Aug 15;55(3):466-73.

[63] Tokuno S, Chen F, Pernow J, Jiang J, Valen G. Effects of spontaneous or induced brain ischemia on vessel reactivity: the role of inducible nitric oxide synthase. *Life Sci.*, 2002 Jun 28;71(6):679-92.

[64] Tahepold P, Elfstrom P, Eha I, Kals J, Taal G, Talonpoika A, et al. Exposure of rats to hyperoxia enhances relaxation of isolated aortic rings and reduces infarct size of isolated hearts. *Acta. Physiol. Scand.*, 2002 Aug;175(4):271-7.

[65] Juhaszova M, Zorov DB, Kim SH, Pepe S, Fu Q, Fishbein KW, et al. Glycogen synthase kinase-3beta mediates convergence of protection signaling to inhibit the mitochondrial permeability transition pore. *J. Clin. Invest.*, 2004 Jun;113(11):1535-49.

[66] Weiss JN, Korge P, Honda HM, Ping P. Role of the mitochondrial permeability transition in myocardial disease. *Circ. Res.*, 2003 Aug 22;93(4):292-301.

[67] Borutaite V, Jekabsone A, Morkuniene R, Brown GC. Inhibition of mitochondrial permeability transition prevents mitochondrial dysfunction, cytochrome c release and apoptosis induced by heart ischemia. *J. Mol. Cell Cardiol.*, 2003 Apr;35(4):357-66.

[68] Cohen MV, Yang XM, Downey JM. The pH hypothesis of postconditioning: staccato reperfusion reintroduces oxygen and perpetuates myocardial acidosis. *Circulation*, 2007 Apr 10;115(14):1895-903.

[69] Hausenloy DJ, Yellon DM. The mitochondrial permeability transition pore: its fundamental role in mediating cell death during ischaemia and reperfusion. *J. Mol. Cell Cardiol.*, 2003 Apr;35(4):339-41.

[70] Murphy E. Primary and secondary signaling pathways in early preconditioning that converge on the mitochondria to produce cardioprotection. *Circ. Res.*, 2004 Jan 9;94(1):7-16.

[71] Costa AD, Jakob R, Costa CL, Andrukhiv K, West IC, Garlid KD. The mechanism by which the mitochondrial ATP-sensitive K+ channel opening and H2O2 inhibit the mitochondrial permeability transition. *J. Biol. Chem.,* 2006 Jul 28;281(30):20801-8.

[72] Carroll R, Gant VA, Yellon DM. Mitochondrial K(ATP) channel opening protects a human atrial-derived cell line by a mechanism involving free radical generation. *Cardiovasc. Res.*, 2001 Sep;51(4):691-700.

[73] Cohen MV, Yang XM, Liu GS, Heusch G, Downey JM. Acetylcholine, bradykinin, opioids, and phenylephrine, but not adenosine, trigger preconditioning by generating free radicals and opening mitochondrial K(ATP) channels. *Circ. Res.*, 2001 Aug 3;89(3):273-8.

[74] Forbes RA, Steenbergen C, Murphy E. Diazoxide-induced cardioprotection requires signaling through a redox-sensitive mechanism. *Circ. Res.*, 2001 Apr 27;88(8):802-9.

[75] O'Rourke B. Myocardial K(ATP) channels in preconditioning. *Circ. Res.,* 2000 Nov 10;87(10):845-55.

[76] Oldenburg O, Cohen MV, Yellon DM, Downey JM. Mitochondrial K(ATP) channels: role in cardioprotection. *Cardiovasc. Res.*, 2002 Aug 15;55(3):429-37.

[77] Oldenburg O, Qin Q, Krieg T, Yang XM, Philipp S, Critz SD, et al. Bradykinin induces mitochondrial ROS generation via NO, cGMP, PKG, and mitoKATP channel opening and leads to cardioprotection. *Am. J. Physiol. Heart Circ. Physiol.*, 2004 Jan;286(1):H468-76.

[78] Harada N, Miura T, Dairaku Y, Kametani R, Shibuya M, Wang R, et al. NO donor-activated PKC-delta plays a pivotal role in ischemic myocardial protection through

accelerated opening of mitochondrial K-ATP channels. *J. Cardiovasc. Pharmacol.*, 2004 Jul;44(1):35-41.
[79] Ohmasa F, Saito M, Shimizu S, Taniguchi S, Dimitriadis F, Satoh I, et al. The role of ATP-sensitive potassium channel on acute urinary retention and subsequent catheterization in the rat. *Eur. J. Pharmacol.*, 2010 Jun 10;635(1-3):194-7.
[80] Sun Z, Zhang X, Ito K, Li Y, Montgomery RA, Tachibana S, et al. Amelioration of oxidative mitochondrial DNA damage and deletion after renal ischemic injury by the KATP channel opener diazoxide. *Am. J. Physiol. Renal. Physiol.*, 2008 Mar;294(3):F491-8.
[81] Ambros JT, Herrero-Fresneda I, Borau OG, Boira JM. Ischemic preconditioning in solid organ transplantation: from experimental to clinics. *Transpl. Int.*, 2007 Mar;20(3):219-29.
[82] Cohen MV, Baines CP, Downey JM. Ischemic preconditioning: from adenosine receptor to KATP channel. *Annu. Rev. Physiol.*, 2000;62:79-109.
[83] Shimizu S, Martin DT, Dimitriadis F, Satoh K, Saito M. The effect of ischemic preconditioning and postconditioning on testicular torsion-detorsion injury. *Global Journal of Biochemistry*:Advance Online Publication, In press.
[84] Zhao ZQ, Corvera JS, Halkos ME, Kerendi F, Wang NP, Guyton RA, et al. Inhibition of myocardial injury by ischemic postconditioning during reperfusion: comparison with ischemic preconditioning. *Am. J. Physiol. Heart Circ. Physiol.,* 2003 Aug;285(2):H579-88.
[85] Zhao H. The protective effect of ischemic postconditioning against ischemic injury: from the heart to the brain. *J. Neuroimmune. Pharmacol.,* 2007 Dec;2(4):313-8.
[86] Vinten-Johansen J, Yellon DM, Opie LH. Postconditioning: a simple, clinically applicable procedure to improve revascularization in acute myocardial infarction. *Circulation*, 2005 Oct 4;112(14):2085-8.
[87] Skyschally A, van Caster P, Iliodromitis EK, Schulz R, Kremastinos DT, Heusch G. Ischemic postconditioning: experimental models and protocol algorithms. *Basic. Res. Cardiol.*, 2009 Sep;104(5):469-83.
[88] Kin H, Zhao ZQ, Sun HY, Wang NP, Corvera JS, Halkos ME, et al. Postconditioning attenuates myocardial ischemia-reperfusion injury by inhibiting events in the early minutes of reperfusion. *Cardiovasc. Res.*, 2004 Apr 1;62(1):74-85.
[89] Philipp S, Yang XM, Cui L, Davis AM, Downey JM, Cohen MV. Postconditioning protects rabbit hearts through a protein kinase C-adenosine A2b receptor cascade. *Cardiovasc. Res.*, 2006 May 1;70(2):308-14.
[90] Yang XM, Proctor JB, Cui L, Krieg T, Downey JM, Cohen MV. Multiple, brief coronary occlusions during early reperfusion protect rabbit hearts by targeting cell signaling pathways. *J. Am. Coll Cardiol.*, 2004 Sep 1;44(5):1103-10.
[91] Vinten-Johansen J, Zhao ZQ, Zatta AJ, Kin H, Halkos ME, Kerendi F. Postconditioning--A new link in nature's armor against myocardial ischemia-reperfusion injury. *Basic. Res. Cardiol.*, 2005 Jul;100(4):295-310.
[92] Zhao ZQ, Vinten-Johansen J. Postconditioning: reduction of reperfusion-induced injury. *Cardiovasc. Res.*, 2006 May 1;70(2):200-11.
[93] Loukogeorgakis SP, Panagiotidou AT, Yellon DM, Deanfield JE, MacAllister RJ. Postconditioning protects against endothelial ischemia-reperfusion injury in the human forearm. *Circulation*, 2006 Feb 21;113(7):1015-9.

[94] Luo W, Li B, Chen R, Huang R, Lin G. Effect of ischemic postconditioning in adult valve replacement. *Eur. J. Cardiothorac. Surg.*, 2008 Feb;33(2):203-8.

[95] Mockford KA, Girn HR, Homer-Vanniasinkam S. Postconditioning: current controversies and clinical implications. *Eur. J. Vasc. Endovasc. Surg.*, 2009 Apr;37(4):437-42.

[96] Hausenloy DJ, Ong SB, Yellon DM. The mitochondrial permeability transition pore as a target for preconditioning and postconditioning. *Basic. Res. Cardiol.*, 2009 Mar;104(2):189-202.

[97] Lim SY, Davidson SM, Hausenloy DJ, Yellon DM. Preconditioning and postconditioning: the essential role of the mitochondrial permeability transition pore. *Cardiovasc. Res.*, 2007 Aug 1;75(3):530-5.

[98] Yellon DM, Downey JM. Preconditioning the myocardium: from cellular physiology to clinical cardiology. *Physiol. Rev.*, 2003 Oct;83(4):1113-51.

[99] Sivaraman V, Mudalagiri NR, Di Salvo C, Kolvekar S, Hayward M, Yap J, et al. Postconditioning protects human atrial muscle through the activation of the RISK pathway. *Basic. Res. Cardiol.*, 2007 Sep;102(5):453-9.

[100] Hausenloy DJ, Yellon DM. Reperfusion injury salvage kinase signalling: taking a RISK for cardioprotection. *Heart Fail Rev.*, 2007 Dec;12(3-4):217-34.

[101] Penna C, Mancardi D, Rastaldo R, Losano G, Pagliaro P. Intermittent activation of bradykinin B2 receptors and mitochondrial KATP channels trigger cardiac postconditioning through redox signaling. *Cardiovasc Res.*, 2007 Jul 1;75(1):168-77.

[102] Yang XM, Philipp S, Downey JM, Cohen MV. Postconditioning's protection is not dependent on circulating blood factors or cells but involves adenosine receptors and requires PI3-kinase and guanylyl cyclase activation. *Basic Res. Cardiol.*, 2005 Jan;100(1):57-63.

[103] Kin H, Zatta AJ, Lofye MT, Amerson BS, Halkos ME, Kerendi F, et al. Postconditioning reduces infarct size via adenosine receptor activation by endogenous adenosine. *Cardiovasc. Res.*, 2005 Jul 1;67(1):124-33.

[104] Jin ZX, Zhou JJ, Xin M, Peng DR, Wang XM, Bi SH, et al. Postconditioning the human heart with adenosine in heart valve replacement surgery. *Ann. Thorac. Surg.*, 2007 Jun;83(6):2066-72.

[105] Ceylan H, Yuncu M, Armutcu F, Gurel A, Bagci C, Demiryurek AT. Effects of early phase of preconditioning on rat testicular ischemia. *Urol. Int.*, 2005;74(2):166-72.

[106] Sahinkanat T, Ozkan KU, Tolun FI, Ciralik H, Imrek SS. The protective effect of ischemic preconditioning on rat testis. *Reprod. Biol. Endocrinol.*, 2007;5:47.

[107] Akcora B, Altug ME, Balci A, Hakverdi S, Yonden Z, Akbas A, et al. Gradual detorsion of torsioned rat testis attenuates ischemia reperfusion injury. *J. Pediatr. Surg.*, 2008 Oct;43(10):1879-84.

[108] Shimizu S, Saito M, Kinoshita Y, Shomori K, Satoh I, Satoh K. Ischemic preconditioning and post-conditioning to decrease testicular torsion-detorsion injury. *J. Urol.*, 2009 Oct;182(4):1637-43.

[109] Chen H, Xing B, Liu X, Zhan B, Zhou J, Zhu H, et al. Ischemic postconditioning inhibits apoptosis after renal ischemia/reperfusion injury in rat. *Transpl. Int.*, 2008 Apr;21(4):364-71.

[110] Shimizu S, Saito M, Dimitriadis F, Kinoshita Y, Shomori K, Satoh I, et al. Protective effect of ischaemic post-conditioning on ipsilateral and contralateral testes after

unilateral testicular ischaemia-reperfusion injury. *Int. J. Androl.*, 2011 Jun;34(3):268-75.
[111] Visser AJ, Heyns C, F. Testicular function after torsion of the spermatic cord. *BJU Int.*, 2003;92: 200-3.
[112] Sarica K, Bakir K, Erbagci A, Yagci F, Uysal O, Ucak R. Unilateral testicular torsion: evaluation of bcl-2, p-53 and PCNA expression in contralateral testes. *Urol. Int.*, 2001;66(2):94-9.
[113] Sarioglu-Buke A, Erdem S, Gedikoglu G, Bingol-Kologlu M, Tanyel FC. Capsaicin effectively prevents apoptosis in the contralateral testis after ipsilateral testicular torsion. *BJU Int.*, 2001 Nov;88(7):787-9.
[114] Mogilner JG, Elenberg Y, Lurie M, Shiloni E, Coran AG, Sukhotnik I. Effect of dexamethasone on germ cell apoptosis in the contralateral testis after testicular ischemia-reperfusion injury in the rat. *Fertil. Steril.*, 2006 Apr;85 Suppl 1:1111-7.
[115] Dokucu AI, Ozturk H, Tuncer MC, Yilmaz F. The effects of molsidomine on hypoxia inducible factor alpha and Sonic hedgehog in testicular ischemia/reperfusion injury in rats. *Int. Urol. Nephrol.*, 2009;41(1):101-8.
[116] Kono T, Saito M, Kinoshita Y, Satoh I, Shinbori C, Satoh K. Real-time monitoring of nitric oxide and blood flow during ischemia-reperfusion in the rat testis. *Mol. Cell Biochem.*, 2006 Jun;286(1-2):139-45.
[117] Ozokutan BH, Kucukaydin M, Muhtaroglu S, Tekin Y. The role of nitric oxide in testicular ischemia-reperfusion injury. *J. Pediatr. Surg.*, 2000 Jan;35(1):101-3.
[118] Koltuksuz U, Irmak MK, Karaman A, Uz E, Var A, Ozyurt H, et al. Testicular nitric oxide levels after unilateral testicular torsion/detorsion in rats pretreated with caffeic acid phenethyl ester. *Urol. Res.*, 2000 Dec;28(6):360-3.
[119] Barlas M, Hatiboglu C. The effect of nitric oxide in testicular ischemia-reperfusion injury. *Int. Urol. Nephrol.*, 2002;34(1):81-6.
[120] Sukhotnik I, Helou H, Mogilner J, Lurie M, Bernsteyn A, Coran AG, et al. Oral arginine improves intestinal recovery following ischemia-reperfusion injury in rat. *Pediatr. Surg. Int.*, 2005 Mar;21(3):191-6.
[121] Darley-Usmar V, Wiseman H, Halliwell B. Nitric oxide and oxygen radicals: a question of balance. *FEBS Lett.*, 1995 Aug 7;369(2-3):131-5.
[122] Muijsers RB, Folkerts G, Henricks PA, Sadeghi-Hashjin G, Nijkamp FP. Peroxynitrite: a two-faced metabolite of nitric oxide. *Life Sci.*, 1997;60(21):1833-45.
[123] Sola A, Palacios L, Lopez-Marti J, Ivorra A, Noguera N, Gomez R, et al. Multiparametric monitoring of ischemia-reperfusion in rat kidney: effect of ischemic preconditioning. *Transplantation*, 2003 Mar 27;75(6):744-9.
[124] Webb A, Bond R, McLean P, Uppal R, Benjamin N, Ahluwalia A. Reduction of nitrite to nitric oxide during ischemia protects against myocardial ischemia-reperfusion damage. *Proc. Natl. Acad. Sci. USA*,2004 Sep 14;101(37):13683-8.
[125] Okamoto M, Tsuchiya K, Kanematsu Y, Izawa Y, Yoshizumi M, Kagawa S, et al. Nitrite-derived nitric oxide formation following ischemia-reperfusion injury in kidney. *Am. J. Physiol. Renal. Physiol.*, 2005 Jan;288(1):F182-7.
[126] Seki S, Flavahan NA, Smedira NG, Murray PA. Superoxide anion scavengers restore NO-mediated pulmonary vasodilation after lung transplantation. *Am. J. Physiol.*, 1999 Jan;276(1 Pt 2):H42-6.

[127] Watanabe K, Morinaka Y, Iseki K, Watanabe T, Yuki S, Nishi H. Structure-activity relationship of 3-methyl-1-phenyl-2-pyrazolin-5-one (edaravone). *Redox. Rep.*, 2003;8(3):151-5.

[128] Yamamoto T, Yuki S, Watanabe T, Mitsuka M, Saito KI, Kogure K. Delayed neuronal death prevented by inhibition of increased hydroxyl radical formation in a transient cerebral ischemia. *Brain Res.*, 1997 Jul 11;762(1-2):240-2.

[129] Nakashima M, Niwa M, Iwai T, Uematsu T. Involvement of free radicals in cerebral vascular reperfusion injury evaluated in a transient focal cerebral ischemia model of rat. *Free Radic. Biol. Med.*, 1999 Mar;26(5-6):722-9.

[130] Zhang N, Komine-Kobayashi M, Tanaka R, Liu M, Mizuno Y, Urabe T. Edaravone reduces early accumulation of oxidative products and sequential inflammatory responses after transient focal ischemia in mice brain. *Stroke*, 2005 Oct;36(10):2220-5.

[131] Minhaz U, Tanaka M, Tsukamoto H, Watanabe K, Koide S, Shohtsu A, et al. Effect of MCI-186 on postischemic reperfusion injury in isolated rat heart. *Free Radic. Res.*, 1996 May;24(5):361-7.

[132] Higashi Y, Jitsuiki D, Chayama K, Yoshizumi M. Edaravone (3-methyl-1-phenyl-2-pyrazolin-5-one), a novel free radical scavenger, for treatment of cardiovascular diseases. Recent Pat Cardiovasc *Drug Discov.,* 2006 Jan;1(1):85-93.

[133] Abe T, Unno M, Takeuchi H, Kakita T, Katayose Y, Rikiyama T, et al. A new free radical scavenger, edaravone, ameliorates oxidative liver damage due to ischemia-reperfusion in vitro and in vivo. *J. Gastrointest. Surg.,*2004 Jul-Aug;8(5):604-15.

[134] Nishiyama T, Ogawa M. Intrathecal edaravone, a free radical scavenger, is effective on inflammatory-induced pain in rats. *Acta. Anaesthesiol. Scand.,* 2005 Feb;49(2):147-51.

[135] Nakao S, Matsumoto S, Yamada A. Studies on the in vitro, ex vivo and in vivo pharmacological profile of a neutrophil elastase inhibitor ONO-5046-Na. *Kiso To Rinsho,* 1997;31:3347-56.

[136] Takayama M, Ishibashi M, Ishii H, Kuraki T, Nishida T, Yoshida M. Effects of neutrophil elastase inhibitor (ONO-5046) on lung injury after intestinal ischemia-reperfusion. *J. Appl. Physiol.*,2001 Oct;91(4):1800-7.

[137] Hayama T, Matsuyama M, Funao K, Tanaka T, Tsuchida K, Takemoto Y, et al. Benefical effect of neutrophil elastase inhibitor on renal warm ischemia-reperfusion injury in the rat. *Transplant. Proc.*, 2006 Sep;38(7):2201-2.

[138] Soejima Y, Yanaga K, Nishizaki T, Yoshizumi T, Uchiyama H, Sugimachi K. Effect of specific neutrophil elastase inhibitor on ischemia/reperfusion injury in rat liver transplantation. *J. Surg. Res.*, 1999 Sep;86(1):150-4.

[139] Aoki T, Tsuchida M, Takekubo M, Saito M, Sato K, Hayashi J. Neutrophil elastase inhibitor ameliorates reperfusion injury in a canine model of lung transplantation. *Eur. Surg. Res.*, 2005 Sep-Oct;37(5):274-80.

[140] Campbell EJ, Senior RM, McDonald JA, Cox DL. Proteolysis by neutrophils. Relative importance of cell-substrate contact and oxidative inactivation of proteinase inhibitors in vitro. *J. Clin. Invest.*, 1982 Oct;70(4):845-52.

[141] Weitz JI, Huang AJ, Landman SL, Nicholson SC, Silverstein SC. Elastase-mediated fibrinogenolysis by chemoattractant-stimulated neutrophils occurs in the presence of physiologic concentrations of antiproteinases. *J. Exp. Med.*, 1987 Dec 1;166(6):1836-50.

[142] McCord JM. Oxygen-derived free radicals in postischemic tissue injury. *N. Engl. J. Med.*, 1985 Jan 17;312(3):159-63.

[143] Visser AJ, Heyns CF. Testicular function after torsion of the spermatic cord. *BJU Int.*, 2003 Aug;92(3):200-3.

[144] Kehinde EO, Mojiminiyi OA, Mahmoud AH, Al-Awadi KA, Al-Hunayan A, Omu AE. The significance of measuring the time course of serum malondialdehyde concentration in patients with torsion of the testis. *J. Urol.*, 2003 Jun;169(6):2177-80.

In: Testis: Anatomy, Physiology and Pathology
Editors: Yoichi Nemoto and Norio Inaba
ISBN: 978-1-61942-739-6

Chapter 3

Roles and Regulatory Mechanism of Proton Pumping V-ATPase in Spermatozoa and Epididymis Physiology

***Mayumi Nakanishi-Matsui*[1], *Sylvie Breton*[2, 3], *Haruko Okamoto*[1] *and Masamitsu Futai*[1]**

[1]Department of Biochemistry, Faculty of Pharmaceutical Sciences, Iwate Medical University, Iwate, Japan
[2]Program in Membrane Biology, Center for Systems Biology and Nephrology Division, Massachusetts General Hospital, Massachusetts, US
[3]Harvard Medical School, Boston, Massachusetts, US

Abstract

The regulation of pH is critical for a wide variety of biological processes, including fertilization and spermatogenesis. Acrosomes in spermatozoa are acidic inside and contain hydrolytic enzymes essential for penetrating the *zona pellucida* around the eggs. The lumen of epididymis and vas deferens is also acidic, which is required for the maturation and storage of spermatozoa in a quiescent state. The proton pumping vacuolar-type ATPase (V-ATPase) is responsible for acidification of organelles and tissues. V-ATPase is a large multi-subunit enzyme with structural variations: six out of 12 subunits of the mammalian enzyme have more than two isoforms that are specific for cell and/or organelle. We found that the E subunit has two isoforms E1 and E2, which are expressed specifically in testis and ubiquitously in all cells, respectively. V-ATPase with E1 isoform is localized in the acrosome of spermatozoa and is necessary for assembly of the entire enzyme. In the epididymis and vas deferens, V-ATPase is localized in the plasma membrane of narrow and clear cells. In these cells, proton secretion is regulated via recycling of this enzyme: alkaline luminal pH triggers the accumulation of V-ATPase molecules in the apical membrane, whereas lower pH reduces their accumulation. In this review, we summarize and discuss possible roles and regulatory mechanism(s) of V-ATPase in fertilization and spermatogenesis.

Introduction

The pH is regulated in organelles and cells to establish a suitable environment for their specific function (For reviews, see [24, 25, 98, 101]). Organelles, such as endosome, lysosome, Golgi apparatus, synaptic vesicle, and secretory vesicle, have their own pH, ranging from 4.5 to 6.5 [24, 98]. The lysosome lumen is kept acidic with a pH ~ 4.5, which is optimal for its enzymes to hydrolyze macromolecules [97]. The lumen of synaptic vesicles is also acidic, which is critical for the accumulation of neurotransmitters [24, 25, 59]. Acidification of these intracellular organelles is achieved by the proton pumping vacuolar ATPase (V-ATPase) [24, 25, 98, 101]. In addition to its intracellular location, V-ATPase is also expressed in the plasma membrane of specialized proton-secreting cells [11, 24, 25, 97, 101, 107]. The osteoclast is an example of such cells that transport protons outside. Osteoclasts attach tightly to the bone surface and secrete protons into the bone resorption lacuna, a process that is essential for bone resorption. V-ATPase rich acid-secreting cells are also present in the kidney, where they are involved in the maintenance of systemic acid/base balance [11, 107]. V-ATPase subunit mutations cause defective proton secretion by renal intercalated cells leading to distal tubular acidosis [45, 91].

Acidic environments are also essential for the fertilization and maturation of spermatozoa [85, 97, 98]. The acrosomes are spermatozoa-specific secretory vesicles, lying in front of compressed haploid nucleus in the head sector (Figure 1A, red). During spermatogenesis, numerous small proacrosomal vesicles fuse together, forming a large acrosome. They are derived from the Golgi apparatus and considered to be modified lysosomes, since they contain hydrolytic enzymes capable of digesting proteins and complex sugars. The interaction of spermatozoa and the *zona pellucida* (a gelatinous coat that covers the egg) triggers Ca^{+} influx into the cytosol, which causes exocytosis of the acrosome and release of its enzymes. This process is known as the acrosomal reaction. Secreted enzymes digest the *zona pellucida* and assist the spermatozoa in penetrating the egg. The acrosome lumen is kept acidic, which is critical for processing protease zymogens.

The lumen of the epididymis and vas deferens is also acidic compared to blood (pH 6.6-6.8) [19, 20, 53]. These organs are the sites, where functionally immature spermatozoa from seminiferous tubules acquire the ability to move to fertilize the egg (Figure 2A). The acidity of the luminal fluid and a low bicarbonate concentration in these tissues help keep spermatozoa in a quiescent state during their maturation and storage in these organs [87]. Inhibition of luminal acidification by environmental factors, such as tobacco smoke and heavy metals [13, 31], induces a reduction in male fertility in men. The importance of luminal acidification in the establishment of male fertility was further demonstrated in two mouse models. Male mice that are deficient in the c-*ros* [111] and *Foxi1* [4, 105] genes have elevated epididymal luminal pH and are infertile.

The V-ATPase transports protons across the membrane, using the energy of ATP hydrolysis. It is a large multi-subunit enzyme composed of two sectors: the V_o sector forms the membrane proton pathway, and the V_1 sector corresponds to the catalytic domain (Figure 3) [3, 61, 64, 82, 101]. Mammalian V-ATPase subunits have cell and/or organelle specific isoforms [60, 93, 94, 96, 98, 99, 102, 103]. This structural variation probably contributes to a wide range of luminal pH of organelles or compartments. Sun-Wada, Futai and coworkers found that the E subunit located in the peripheral stalks has two isoforms, E1 and E2. E1 isoform is specifically expressed in the testis, whereas the E2 is ubiquitous [93]. V-ATPase with E1 is localized in the acrosomal membrane. Further studies of E1 have revealed a role of the E subunit in reversible change of V_o and V_1 association [29].

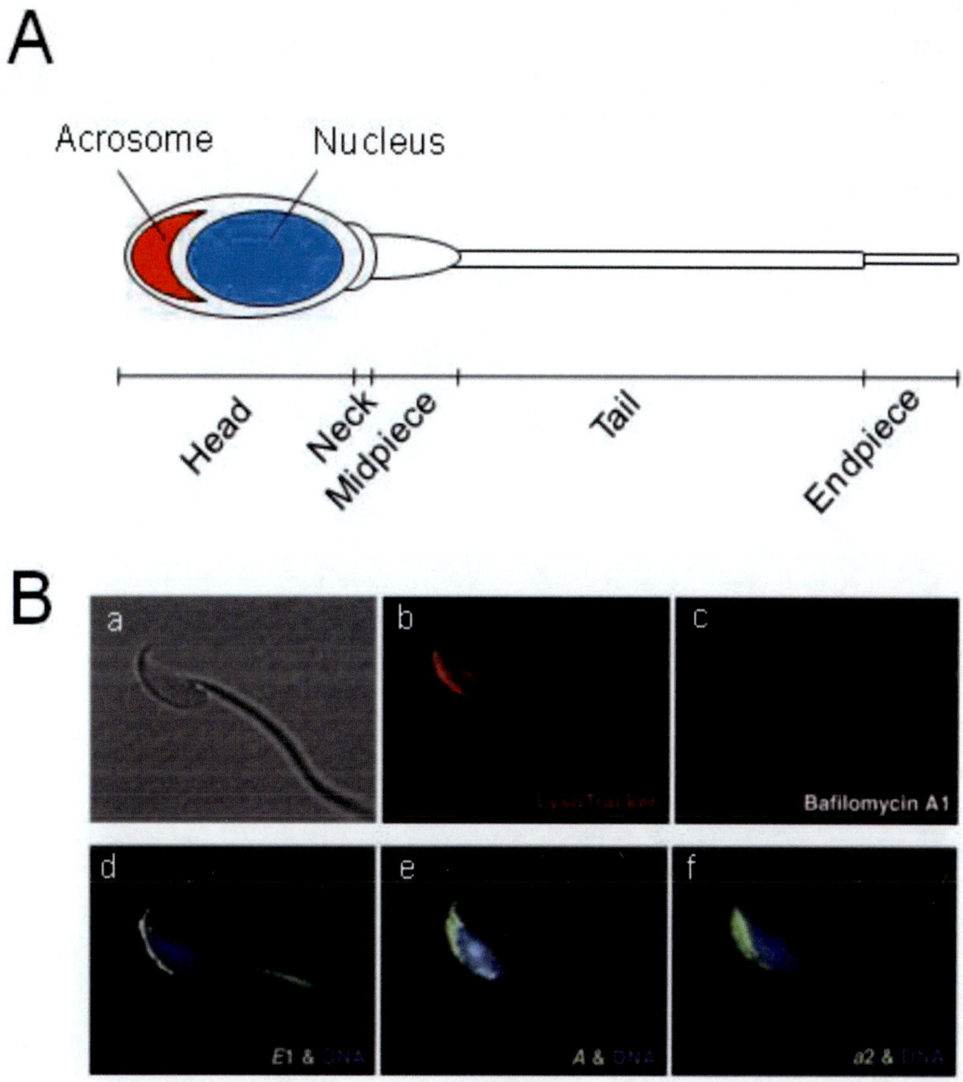

Figure 1. Localization of E1 isoform of V-ATPase in spermatozoa. A. Schematic illustration of spermatozoa. Acrosome is a large acidic organelle lying in front of compressed haploid nucleus in the head. B. Immunofluorescence labeling of spermatozoa using specific antibodies against E1, A, and *a*2 subunits. A phase-contrast image (a) is shown together with a living epididymal spermatozoa stained with LysoTracker Red (b). Spermatozoa were also stained with LysoTracker after incubation with 10 nM bafilomycin A1 for 30 min in Krebs-Ringer bicarbonate buffer (c). For immunochemical identification of the E1(d), A, (e) and *a*2 (f) subunits, spermatozoa were fixed and labeled with corresponding antibodies. Merged images (d – f) with DNA visualized using the fluorescent dye 4,6-diamidino-2-phenylindole are shown. Cited from Sun-Wada *et al.* [93].

The V-ATPase is localized in the apical plasma membrane of a subset of epithelial cells, the narrow and clear cells in the epididymis and vas deferens, and is required to establish an acidic luminal pH [1, 7, 10, 30, 70, 72, 77]. The regulation of V-ATPase dependent acidification includes recycling this enzyme to and from the apical plasma membrane. It has been shown recently that this recycling is controlled via a complex interplay between the different cell types that compose the epididymal epithelium [85, 86].

In this chapter, we summarize the physiological roles of V-ATPase in the acrosomal vesicles of spermatozoa and in the epithelium lining parts of the male reproductive tract. We also discuss selected aspects of the regulatory mechanisms of luminal acidification of these organelles and tissues.

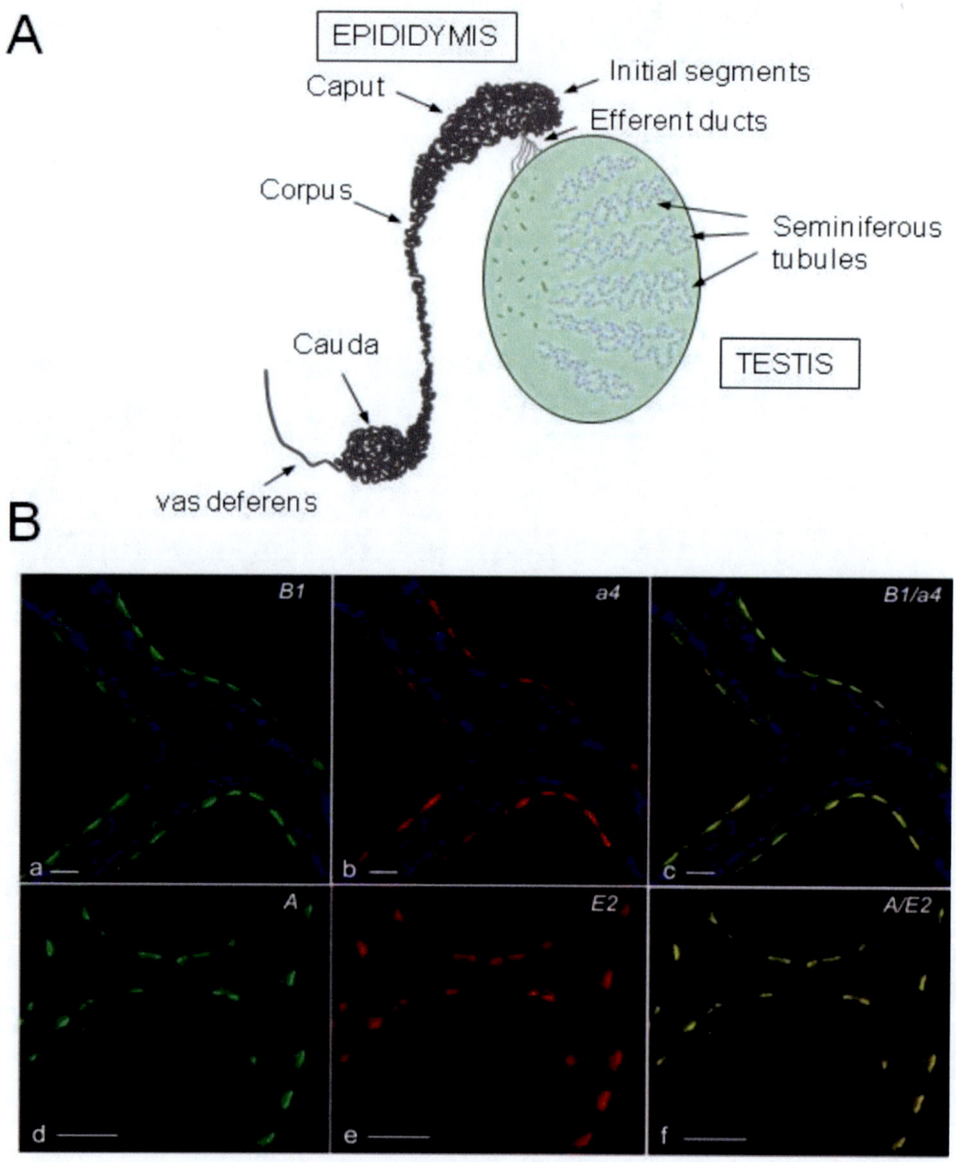

C

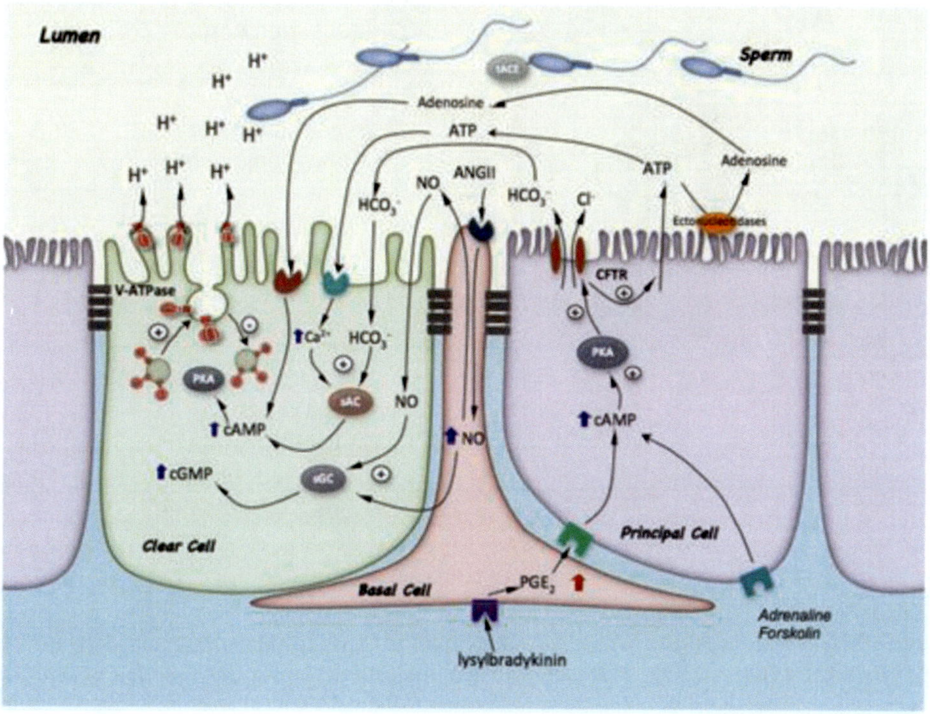

Figure 2. Localization of V-ATPase in epididymis. **A.** Schematic illustration of part of the male reproductive tract. The epididymis connects the testis to the vas deferens via the efferent ducts. Spermatogenesis occurs in the seminiferous tubules of the testis. The epididymis is divided into four major regions: initial segments, caput, corpus and cauda. Spermatozoa undergo their final maturation and are stored in the epididymis. **B.** Localization of V-ATPase in clear cells in epididymis. Rat cauda epididymis was stained using affinity-purified antibodies against V-ATPase subunit isoforms B1 (panel a; green), *a*4 (b; red), A (d; green) and E2 (e; red). Panels c and f show merged images from panels a and b, and panels d and e, respectively. All these subunit isoforms are detected in the apical pole of clear cells. A faint B1, A and E2 staining is also detected in the cytosol of clear cells, consistent with their localization in the V_0 sector of the V-ATPase. Nuclei and spermatozoa are stained in blue with DAPI in panels a-c. Scale bars = 20 μm (a-c), 50 μm (d-f). **C.** Regulation of V-ATPase-dependent proton secretion in clear cells via cell-cell crosstalk. Principal cells secrete bicarbonate and ATP upon basolateral stimulation with several factors including adrenaline. Both processes are mediated by cystic fibrosis transmembrane conductance regulator (CFTR). Bicarbonate activates soluble adenylyl cyclase (sAC) in clear cells, followed by an increase in cAMP concentration and activation of protein kinase A (PKA). This induces the accumulation of V-ATPase in apical microvilli of clear cells via either inhibition of endocytosis or activation of exocytosis. Purinergic activation by ATP and adenosine trigger the calcium- and cAMP-pathway, respectively, in clear cells, and induce V-ATPase apical membrane accumulation. Luminal angiotensin II (ANGII) is produced from testicular angiotensin converting enzyme (tACE). Basal cells extend a narrow body projection that crosses the tight junction barrier. ANGII binding to ANGII type II receptor in these cells (AT2) triggers the production of nitric oxide, which then diffuses out to reach clear cells where it activates soluble guanylate cyclase (sGC). An increase in cGMP also induces the apical accumulation of V-ATPase and stimulates proton secretion. Stimulation of basal cells by basolateral factors including lysylbradykinin activates principal cells via the production of prostaglandin E2 (PGE_2). Modified from [87].

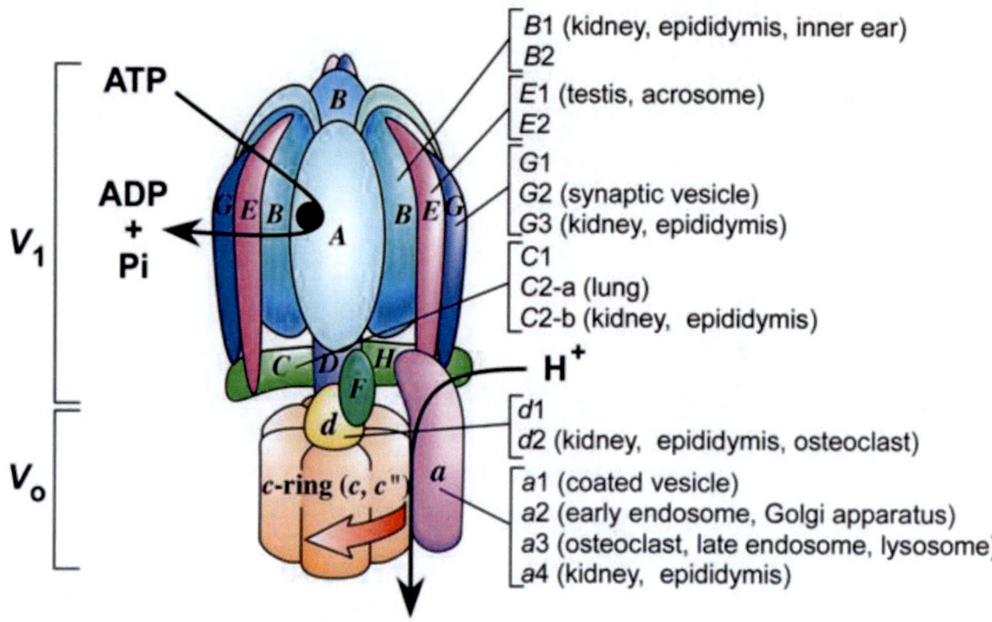

Figure 3. Schematic illustration of V-ATPase. The structure of mammalian V-ATPase based on that of yeast enzyme is shown together with catalysis and proton transport. The membrane integrated (V_o) and peripheral (V_1) sectors, catalytic hexamer, stalk regions, proton pathway, and subunit isoforms are indicated. Red arrow illustrates rotation of the central stalk and *c*-ring against the other part of the enzyme. Isoforms with cells or organelles in parentheses are expressed specifically, and the others are ubiquitous. Subunit isoforms include those expressed epididymis and acrosome discussed in the text.

Tissue and Organelle Specific Structural Variation of V-ATPase

As mentioned above, V-ATPase is composed of a membrane embedded proton pumping V_o and a catalytic V_1 sector (Figure 3). The nucleotide binding subunits (A_3B_3 in V_1) and the proton pathway subunits in the membrane (V_o) are connected by the central (DF*d*) and peripheral (CE_3G_3Ha) stalks [61, 101, 113]. Chemistry (ATP hydrolysis) and proton transport are coupled through subunit rotation [34, 62, 63]: the central stalk and proton-transporting *c*-ring rotate together against other subunits. Deletion of mammalian V_o subunit *c*, encoded by a single gene, has been shown to cause an embryonic lethal phenotype, indicating that V-ATPase is essential for normal embryogenesis [37, 95].

Six out of 12 subunits of mammalian V-ATPase have isoforms specific for tissue and intracellular organelle (Figure 3) [25, 98]. We describe here the specific functions of selected isoform briefly. The B1, C2-b, G3, *a*4, and *d*2 isoforms were initially found to be expressed in the kidney and were originally labeled as "kidney specific" [41, 67, 90, 94, 99]. They were later described in the plasma membrane of epididymal clear cells [18, 20, 73, 77]. The B2 isoform is expressed in the plasma membrane of osteoclasts [47] and proximal tubule epithelial cells [9, 65]. The V-ATPase is responsible for acid secretion by renal intercalated cells and mutations in the human B1 and *a*4 genes cause distal renal tubular acidosis, a condition characterized by impaired renal acid secretion resulting in metabolic acidosis [45, 91].

The *d2* isoform was originally described in the kidney [99], and later, found induced during differentiation of osteoclasts [48, 90]. Progenitor cells from *d2* gene knock-out mouse form only small osteoclasts [48]. The *a3* is a ubiquitous isoform localized in the lysosomal membrane. The *a3* and *d2* subunits are induced during osteoclastogenesis and became components of V-ATPase localized in the osteoclast plasma membrane (Matsumoto *et al.* unpublished observation). Progenitors from mice with defective *a3* form morphologically normal osteoclasts but without bone resorption activity, resulting in osteopetrosis [54]. Expressions of C2-a and G2 are lung and synaptic vesicle specific, respectively [60, 94]. The V-ATPase with *a1*, *a2*, and *a3* isoforms are expressed ubiquitously, and specifically localized in the intercellular organelles: those with *a1* in coated vesicles, *a2* in early endosomes and the Golgi apparatus, and *a3* in late endosomes and the lysosomes. Thus, isoforms may be involved in targeting V-ATPase to specific organelles or to the plasma membrane, together with regulating luminal acidification of each organelle.

Testis Specific E1 Isoform of V-ATPase

Similar to other subunits of V-ATPase, mouse and human E subunit, one of the components of peripheral stalks, has two isoforms, spermatozoa-specific E1 and ubiquitous E2 (Figure 3), encoded by the *Atp6e1* (*Atp6v1e2*) and *Atp6e2* (*Atp6v1e1*) genes, respectively [36, 93]. Nomenclatures shown in parentheses are by Human Genome Organisation. In the testis, E2 is expressed from early embryonic stages, whereas E1 expression is detected only in adult testis [93]. The E1 transcript appears about 3 weeks after birth, corresponding to the start of meiosis, and is expressed exclusively in round spermatids in seminiferous tubules. Immunohistochemistry and electron microscopy with isoform-specific antibodies revealed that E1 is localized specifically in developing acrosomes of spermatids and acrosomes in mature spermatozoa. On the other hand, E2 is ubiquitously present in the perinuclear compartments.

The *a* subunit is a component that forms the V-ATPase proton pathway together with the *c* and *c"* subunits in the V_o sector (Figure 3). Three *a* subunit isoforms (*a1*, *a2*, and *a3*) are ubiquitously expressed including testis. However, their respective distributions are different from each other [93]: *a1* isoform is expressed in almost all cells except the spermatozoa. The isoform found in the acrosomes of elongated spermatids is *a2*, and *a3* is expressed specifically in the Sertoli cells, which produce the nutrients required for the spermatogenesis. Immunoprecipitation experiment confirmed that both E1 and *a2* isoforms are present in the same V-ATPase complex [93]. The V-ATPase specific inhibitor, bafilomycin A1, abolishes acidic pH in acrosomes (Figure 1B), indicating that this unique V-ATPase with E1 is responsible for establishing luminal acidic pH (about 5.3), which is essential for activation of protease zymogens to digest the *zona pellucida*.

Possible Roles of the Mouse E1 Isoform in V-ATPase Assembly

V-ATPase with spermatozoa-specific E1 may be a key enzyme for understanding the role of acrosomes. However, the biochemical properties of a specific V-ATPase in mammalian tissue are difficult to establish because the same cell contains those with different isoforms. Using a genetic approach, the hybrid enzyme formed from a mammalian isoform and other yeast subunits has been useful to study the properties of the specific V-ATPase [29, 60, 66, 93, 99].

The mouse E1 and E2 exhibit more than 70% amino acid identity to each other, and 36 and 33% with the yeast counterpart VMA4, respectively. Both of them could functionally complement a null mutation (*Δvma4*) of *VMA4*. The mouse E subunit/yeast hybrid enzymes formed in the mutant cell show slightly lower Km than yeast V-ATPase [93].

A null mutant harboring cDNA for the E1 gene can grow at 30°C. However, the same cells cannot grow at 37°C, although those with E2 cDNA can [29, 93]. Consistent with the temperature-sensitive growth of *Δvma4* expressing the E1, vacuolar membrane vesicles exhibit temperature-sensitive coupling between ATP hydrolysis and proton transport [93]. These results suggest that the E1 is essential for the energy coupling involved in the acidification of acrosomes.

We found that the E1/yeast hybrid V-ATPase shows a reversible change of V_o and V_1 association depending on the temperature shift [29]. The subunit *a* epitope is exposed to the corresponding antibody at 37°C, whereas it is not at 30°C (Figure 4A) possibly covered with the peripheral stalk in V_1 sector. This result suggests that assembly of V_o and V_1 sectors in the E1/yeast hybrid V-ATPase is altered depending on temperature. However, immunoprecipitation experiment revealed that V_1 and V_o sectors of the hybrid V-ATPase are associated, even after the epitope is exposed at 37°C [29]. Consistent with the association of the two sectors, proton-pumping activity of the hybrid enzyme recovered rapidly upon shift to lower temperature (Figure 4B) [29].

Altered assembly of V_o and V_1 sectors at 37°C also depends on the pH; upon shifting the medium from pH 7.5 to pH 5.0, the subunit *a* epitope became inaccessible to the antibody [29], possibly due to the reassembly of V-ATPase. Furthermore, analysis of the E1/Vma4p chimeric subunits indicated that the amino terminal domain between Lys26 and Val83 of the E1 is responsible for the negative growth of yeast with the hybrid and defective proton transport due to the assembly change [29].

The subunit structure of V-ATPase supports the role of E1 in V_o and V_1 assembly. The E subunit is one of the components of peripheral stalks that connect the catalytic V_1 sector and proton translocation pathway V_o sector (Figure 3): as shown by yeast studies, the E subunit is an elongated protein forming a heterodimer with the G subunit [39]. The amino terminal domain interacts with the subunits C, H, and *a*, and the carboxyl terminal domain reaching the top of the subunit B [22, 40, 57, 68, 113]. Thus, the amino terminal domain of E1 plays an important role in assembly probably through interaction with other subunit(s) of V-ATPase.

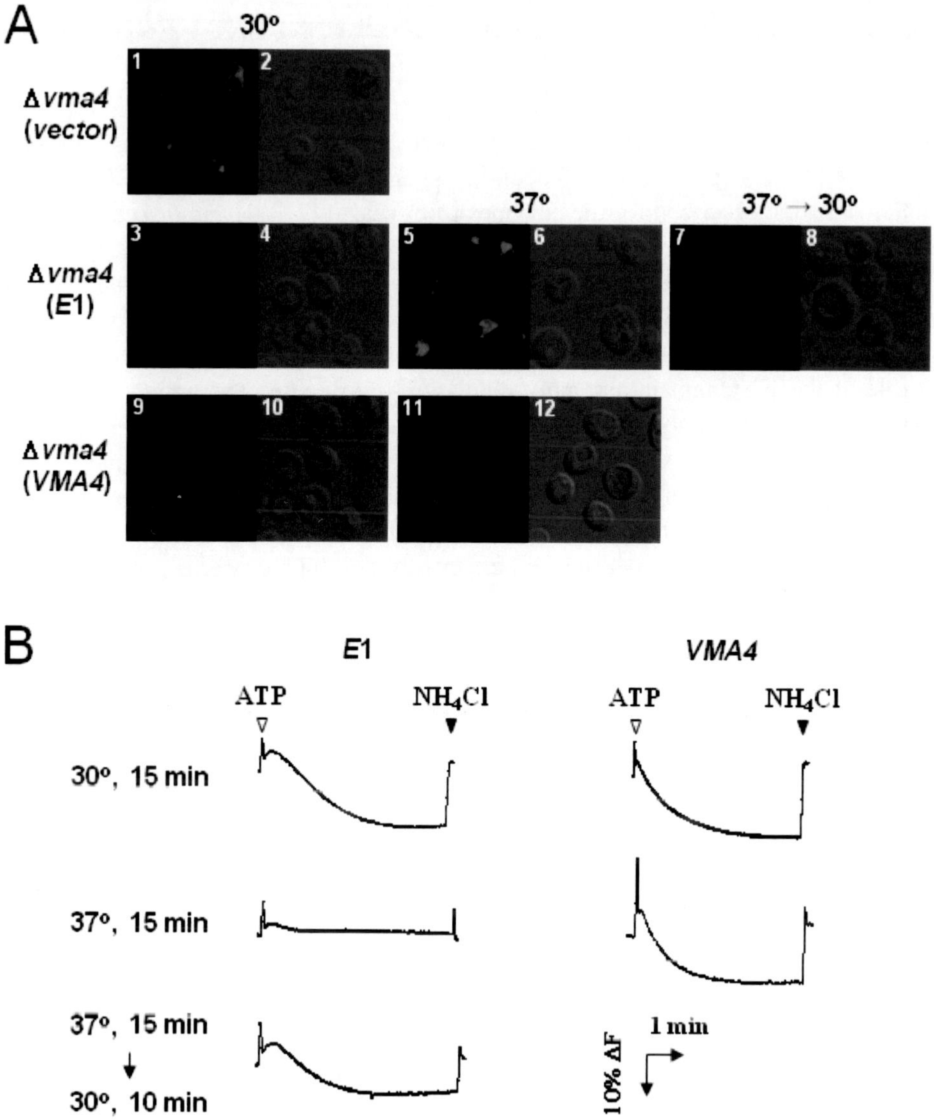

Figure 4. Temperature-dependent reversible change of assembly of E1/yeast hybrid V-ATPase V_1 and V_o sectors. A. Yeast *Δvma4* expressing mouse testis specific E1 or yeast VMA4 were suspended in YEPD medium pH7.5, and then incubated for 15 min at 30°C or 37°C. They were also incubated in the presence of 100 μg/ml cycloheximide at 37°C for 15 min in pH 7.5 medium, followed by 15 min at 30°C (37° → 30°). The control [*Δvma4*(vector)] was *Δvma4* cells harboring the vector without E1 cDNA or *VMA4* cDNA inserted. All cells were fixed overnight with 3.7% formaldehyde, and then subjected to immunohistochemistry using monoclonal antibody 10D7 against yeast subunit *a* (vph1p), and fluorescent images (odd numbered panels) are shown together with Normarski ones (even numbered panels). B. Formation of an electrochemical proton gradient in vacuolar vesicles expressing the mouse E1/yeast hybrid V-ATPase. Vacuolar vesicles (10 μg protein) derived from *Δvma4*(E1) and *Δvma4*(*VMA4*) cells carrying mouse E1 and yeast *VMA4*, respectively, were incubated at 30 or 37°C for 15 min in pH 7.5 buffer; or incubated at 37°C for 15 min followed by a further 10 min at 30°C (37°, 15 min → 30°, 10 min). The incubation temperatures are indicated together with the addition of ATP (open arrowhead) or NH_4Cl (closed arrowhead). Cited from Hayashi *et al.* [29].

ROLE OF THE E SUBUNIT IN GLUCOSE-DEPENDENT REGULATION OF V-ATPASE ASSEMBLY

Finding of E1 isoform could be extended to the role of the E subunit in assembly regulation. Glucose-depletion from medium is known to dissociate V_1 from V_o. This regulation was first described for the enzymes from yeast [42 - 44] and insect [92], and more recently also found in higher animals [21].

The E1/yeast hybrid V-ATPase may have altered assembly regulation, since the hybrid changed assembly depending on the temperature and pH of the medium. As expected, the hybrid did not show the dissociation upon glucose depletion [29]. This finding prompted us to study role of the E subunit in assembly regulation by glucose. The amino terminal region (Lys33 – Lys83, yeast numbering) of E (Vma4p) should contain domain or residues essential for glucose dependent assembly regulation, since the mouse/yeast chimera with the corresponding mouse region exhibited altered assembly. We replaced a series of amino acid residues in Vma4p different from E1, and analyzed assembly regulation. Yeast V-ATPase with replacement of Glu44 to Ala showed essentially the same properties as E1/yeast hybrid V-ATPase, suggesting that this residue or its vicinity is pertinent for the dissociation of V_1 from V_0 upon glucose depletion (Okamoto and Futai, to be published). Asn39 in E1 corresponded to yeast Glu44 when they were aligned, suggesting that the minimal change in this region affects V-ATPase assembly. Further studies will address physiological significance of assembly regulation in acrosomal V-ATPase with E1.

A regulatory role of the E subunit is also suggested by the multiple interactions with other proteins including the glycolytic enzyme aldolase [55, 56] and the RAVE (regulator of the H^+-ATPase of vacuolar and endosomal membranes) complex [44, 88, 89]. RAVE complex was shown to associate with subunit E in the V_1 sector released from V-ATPase [88]. Thus, it will be of interest to know that Glu44 and its vicinity of the E subunit have a role in these interactions.

V-ATPASE IN THE MALE REPRODUCTIVE TRACT

The spermatozoa released from the seminiferous tubules of testis are functionally immature, even after completion of normal spermatogenesis. They acquire the ability to move up the female reproductive tract and to fertilize the egg during their transit through the tubule in the epididymis [17, 33, 38, 69, 78, 112]. Acidic luminal pH and low concentration of bicarbonate in the epididymis and vas deferens is essential for the maturation of spermatozoa and their storage in a quiescent state [5, 7, 19, 72, 85]. The proto-oncogene tyrosine kinase c-*ros* knock-out mice are infertile and have abnormally elevated epididymal luminal pH [111]. Male mice deficient in the transcription factor Foxi1 also have an increased epididymal luminal pH and their spermatozoa show impaired mobility [4].

The epididymis is formed by a coiled tubule that is composed of functionally distinct segments, the initial segments, caput, corpus, and cauda (Figure 2A). There are four cell types in the epithelium lining the epididymis lumen: narrow, clear, principal, and basal cells [33, 38, 69, 78, 85]. Narrow cells are present exclusively in the initial segments, whereas clear cells are present in all other epididymal regions. Principal and basal cells are observed in all segments of the epididymis. These cell types contribute to maintain the unique luminal environment of the epididymis tubule.

As mentioned above, a particular set of V-ATPase subunit isoforms is exclusively and abundantly expressed in the apical plasma membrane of clear cells, which are responsible for net proton secretion in the distal region of the epididymis and proximal vas deferens. The inhibitors for V-ATPase, bafilomycin A1 and concanamycin A, abolish proton secretion in vas deferens [5, 7]. In addition to rat and mice, clear cells of human epididymis also express the V-ATPase [30]. In rat clear cells, the plasma membrane V-ATPase is formed by the subunit isoforms, A, B1, *a*4, and E2 (Figure 2B) [10, 20, 77]. Interestingly, the transcription factor Foxi1 is expressed specifically in clear cells where it directly regulates *a*4 expression [105]. Several V-ATPase subunits are absent from *Foxi1* knock-out mice. It is noteworthy that the clear cell plasma membrane V-ATPase has ubiquitous E2 and "kidney specific" *a*4 isoforms, whereas in the acrosomal vesicle it is composed of testis specific E1 and ubiquitous *a*2. These differences of isoform composition may be important for targeting this enzyme to appropriate localization and for regulating its proton transport activity.

Regulation of Epididymal Luminal pH via V-ATPase Recycling

Breton, Brown, and coworkers have intensively studied the mechanism(s) involved in the regulation of epididymal luminal pH. They have established *in vivo* perfusion techniques, and have shown that the luminal acidification in epididymis is controlled via recycling of V-ATPase to and from the apical plasma membrane [87]. V-ATPase is colocalized with endosomes in clear cells at the physiological acidic pH of 6.5. However, it is accumulated in the plasma membrane when luminal pH is elevated by perfusing the lumen *in vivo*. This targeting also occurs by introducing bicarbonate or a cAMP analog into the lumen [70, 71]. These reagents induced high expression of soluble adenylyl cyclase (sAC), a chemosensor mediating bicarbonate-dependent elevation of cAMP, in epididymal clear cells. Inhibition of sAC abolishes the V-ATPase targeting that is triggered by luminal alkalinization or addition of bicarbonate. These results indicate that sAC senses elevated luminal pH or bicarbonate, and triggers the redistribution of V-ATPase to the plasma membrane through the production of cAMP, followed by protein kinase A (PKA) activation.

V-ATPase recycling in clear cells is regulated via modulation of the actin and microtubule cytoskeleton. The V-ATPase is completely redistributed from the apical pole of clear cells to intracellular vesicles after disruption of the microtubule network by colchicine [6]. The V-ATPase isoforms B1, B2 and C interact either directly or indirectly with the actin cytoskeleton [8, 15, 35, 106]. The actin-severing and actin-capping protein, gelsolin, is abundantly expressed in clear cells and is a key regulator of V-ATPase recycling [1]. In addition, depolymerization of the cortical actin cytoskeleton after inhibition of RhoA or ROCKII induces the accumulation of the V-ATPase to the apical membrane in clear cells [84]. Finally, V-ATPase recycling requires intracellular calcium and active phospholipase C [1].

V-ATPase Recycling is Regulated via Cell-Cell Cross-Talk

As mentioned above, V-ATPase recycling is regulated by cross-talk between the different cell types lining the epididymal epithelium (Figure 2C). Principal cells secrete bicarbonate upon basolateral stimulation, resulting in increased luminal pH [14, 28, 49, 74, 75, 83]. A transient increase in bicarbonate concentration following principal cell stimulation was proposed to prime spermatozoa prior to ejaculation [12, 14, 74]. Thus, the bicarbonate-activated V-ATPase accumulation that occurs in clear cells would provide a feedback mechanism for the re-establishment of the epididymal lumen to its resting acidic value [87]. ATP is also released from principal cells upon basolateral stimulation [79], and induces the accumulation of V-ATPase in the apical membrane of clear cells [2]. Both ATP and bicarbonate release are mediated by CFTR (cystic fibrosis transmembrane conductance regulator) in some cells, including airway epithelial cells [114]. Mutations in CFTR cause cystic fibrosis, which often leads to male infertility [32, 104, 108, 110]. CFTR is highly expressed in the apical membrane of epididymal principal cells [76, 80, 85], where it mediates bicarbonate [51] and ATP [79] secretion. Thus, impaired ATP and bicarbonate signaling in the epididymis due to CFTR mutations might lead to defective regulation of clear cells in cystic fibrosis.

V-ATPase recycling in clear cells is also regulated in a hormonal manner: *in vivo* luminal perfusion of rat epididymis with angiotensin II (ANG II) increases V-ATPase apical accumulation and activates V-ATPase-dependent proton secretion from clear cells [86]. This process is mediated via activation of the ANGII type II receptor (AGTR2). It is known that the epididymal luminal fluid contains ANG I and ANG II [27, 46, 52, 81, 109]. ANG II is produced from ANG I by angiotensin I converting enzyme (ACE), and testicular ACE (t-ACE) knock-out male mice are infertile due to dysfunctional spermatozoa [23, 27, 46]. Interestingly, AGTR2 is not present in clear cells, whereas it is exclusively present in basal cells [86]. Epididymal basal cells have the ability to elongate their body, which can then cross the tight junction barrier to reach the luminal compartment. Shum *et al.* proposed a model of cross-talk between basal and clear cells: basal cells sense luminal ANG II via the AGTR2, which triggers the production and release of nitric oxide (NO) [86]. NO reaches clear cells and induces the accumulation of V-ATPase in the apical membrane, via activation of the guanylate cyclase and elevation of cGMP. Luminal ANGII production requires t-ACE, which is bound to the membrane of immature spermatozoa [26, 58, 100]. During their maturation in the epididymis, spermatozoa release t-ACE into the luminal fluid. Thus, the regulation of V-ATPase recycling in clear cells by the luminal hormone ANGII depends on the complex interactions between spermatozoa, principal cells and clear cells. In addition, basolateral stimulation of basal cells activates anion secretion by principal cells [16, 50] further illustrating the complexity of the intercellular networks that are put into place to control transepithelial transport in the epididymis.

CONCLUSION

Organelle- or tissue-specific V-ATPases acidify lumen of acrosome, epididymis, and vas deferens, which is essential for fertilization and spermatogenesis. Proton transport by V-ATPase is regulated by several mechanisms including: 1) Control of reversible change of V_o and V_1 assembly; 2) Expression of V-ATPase isoforms in specialized cells; 3) Modulation of the coupling ratio between ATP hydrolysis and proton transport. In spermatozoa, V-ATPase activity may be controlled by the reversible change of assembly of V_o and V_1 sectors, which is mediated by the E1 isoform in a temperature dependent manner. In epididymal clear cells, V-ATPase recycling to and from the apical membrane depends on several luminal factors including pH, bicarbonate and ANGII. Whether the V-ATPase can also be regulated via association/dissociation or via modulation of the coupling ratio between ATP hydrolysis and proton transport in these cells will require future investigations.

REFERENCES

[1] Beaulieu, V., Da Silva, N., Pastor-Soler, N., Brown, C. R., Smith, P. J., Brown, D. & Breton, S. (2005). Modulation of the actin cytoskeleton via gelsolin regulates vacuolar H^+ATPase (V-ATPase) recycling. *J Biol Chem*, 280, 8452-8463.

[2] Belleannee, C., Da Silva, N., Shum W. W., Brown, D. & Breton, S. (2010). Role of purinergic signaling pathways in V-ATPase recruitment to apical membrane of acidifying epididymal clear cells. *Am J Physiol Cell Physiol*, 298, C817-830.

[3] Beyenbach, K. W. & Wieczorek, H. (2006). The V-type H^+ ATPase: molecular structure and function, physiological roles and regulation. *J Exp Biol*, 209, 577-589.

[4] Blomqvist, S. R., Vidarsson, H., Soder, O. & Enerbäck, S. (2006). Epididymal expression of the forkhead transcription factor Foxi1 is required for male fertility. *EMBO J*, 25, 4131-4141.

[5] Breton, S., Hammar, K., Smith, P. J. & Brown, D. (1998). Proton secretion in the male reproductive tract: involvement of Cl^-- independent HCO_3^- transport. *Am J Physiol*, 275, C1134-1142.

[6] Breton, S., Nsumu, N. N., Galli, T., Sabolic, I., Smith, P. J. & Brown, D. (2000). Tetanus toxin-mediated cleavage of cellubrevin inhibits proton secretion in the male reproductive tract. *Am J Physiol Renal Physiol*, 278, F717-725.

[7] Breton, S., Smith, P. J., Lui, B. & Brown, D. (1996). Acidification of the male reproductive tract by a proton pumping H^+- ATPase. *Nat Med*, 2, 470-472.

[8] Breton, S., Wiederhold, T., Marshansky, V., Nsumu, N. N., Ramesh, V. & Brown, D. (2000). The B1 subunit of the H^+ATPase is a PDZ domain-binding protein. Colocalization with NHE-RF in renal B-intercalated cells. *J Biol Chem*, 275, 18219-18224.

[9] Brown, D., Hirsch, S. & Gluck, S. (1988). Localization of a proton-pumping ATPase in rat kidney. *J Clin Invest*, 82, 2114-2126.

[10] Brown, D., Lui, B., Gluck, S. & Sabolic, I. (1992). A plasma membrane proton ATPase in specialized cells of rat epididymis. *Am J Physiol*, 263, C913-916.

[11] Brown, D., Paunescu, T. G., Breton, S. & Marshansky, V. (2009). Regulation of the V-ATPase in kidney epithelial cells: dual role in acid-base homeostasis and vesicle trafficking. *J Exp Biol*, 212, 1762-1772.

[12] Caflisch, C. R. (1992). Acidification of testicular and epididymal fluids in the rat after surgically-induced varicocele. *Int J Androl*, 15, 238-245.

[13] Caflisch, C. R. & DuBose T. D. Jr. (1991). Cadmium-induced changes in luminal fluid pH in testis and epididymis of the rat *in vivo*. *J Toxicol Environ Health*, 32, 49-57.

[14] Carlin, R. W., Lee, J. H., Marcus, D. C. & Schultz, B. D. (2003). Adenosine stimulates anion secretion across cultured and native adult human vas deferens epithelia. *Biol Reprod*, 68, 1027-1034.

[15] Chen, S. H., Bubb, M. R., Yarmola, E. G., Zuo, J., Jiang, J., Lee, B. S., Lu, M., Gluck, S. L., Hurst, I. R. & Holliday, L. S. (2004). Vacuolar H^+-ATPase binding to microfilaments: regulation in response to phosphatidylinositol 3-kinase activity and detailed characterization of the actin-binding site in subunit B. *J Biol Chem*, 279, 7988-7998.

[16] Cheung, K. H., Leung, G. P., Leung, M. C., Shum, W. W., Zhou, W. L. & Wong, P. Y. (2005). Cell-cell interaction underlies formation of fluid in the male reproductive tract of the rat. *J Gen Physiol*, 125, 443-454.

[17] Cornwall, G. A. (2009). New insights into epididymal biology and function. *Hum Reprod Update*, 15, 213-227.

[18] Da Silva, N., Pisitkun, T., Miller, R. L., Nelson, R. D., Knepper, M. A., Brown, D. & Breton, S. (2010) Proteomic analysis of proton-transporting epididymal celar cells and renal intercalated cells. *Am J Physiol Cell Physiol*, 298, C1326-C1342.

[19] Da Silva, N., Shum, W. W. & Breton, S. (2007). Regulation of vacuolar proton pumping ATPase-dependent luminal acidification in the epididymis. *Asian J Androl*, 9, 476-482.

[20] Da Silva, N., Shum, W. W., El-Annan, J., Paunescu, T. G., McKee, M., Smith, P. J., Brown, D. & Breton, S. (2007). Relocalization of the V-ATPase B2 subunit to the apical membrane of epididymal clear cells of mice deficient in the B1 subunit. *Am J Physiol Cell Physiol*, 293, C199-210.

[21] Dechant, R., Binda, M., Lee, S. S., Pelet, S., Winderickx, J. & Peter, M. (2010). Cytosolic pH is a second messenger for glucose and regulates the PKA pathway through V-ATPase. *EMBO J*, 29, 2515-2526.

[22] Diab, H., Ohira, M., Liu, M., Cobb, E. & Kane, P. M. (2009). Subunit interactions and requirements for inhibition of the yeast V_1-ATPase. *J Biol Chem*, 284, 13316-13325.

[23] Esther, C. R., Jr., Howard, T. E., Marino, E. M., Goddard, J. M., Capecchi, M. R. & Bernstein, K. E. (1996). Mice lacking angiotensin-converting enzyme have low blood pressure, renal pathology, and reduced male fertility. *Lab Invest*, 74, 953-965.

[24] Futai, M., Oka, T., Sun-Wada, G.-H., Moriyama, Y., Kanazawa, H. & Wada, Y. (2000). Luminal acidification of diverse organelles by V-ATPase in animal cells. *J Exp Biol*, 203, 107-116.

[25] Forgac, M. (2007). Vacuolar ATPases: rotary proton pumps in physiology and pathophysiology. *Nat Rev Mol Cell Biol*, 8, 917-929.

[26] Gatti, J. L., Druart, X., Guerin, Y., Dacheux, F., & Dacheux, J. L. (1999). A 105- to 94-kilodalton protein in the epididymal fluids of domestic mammals is angiotensin I-

converting enzyme (ACE); evidence that sperm are the source of this ACE. *Biol Reprod*, 60, 937-945.

[27] Hagaman, J. R., Moyer, J. S., Bachman, E. S., Sibony, M., Magyar, P. L., Welch, J. E., Smithies, O., Krege, J. H. & O'Brien, D. A. (1998). Angiotensin-converting enzyme and male fertility. *Proc Natl Acad Sci U S A*, 95, 2552-2557.

[28] Hagedorn, T. M., Carlin, R. W. & Schultz, B. D. (2007). Oxytocin and vasopressin stimulate anion secretion by human and porcine vas deferens epithelia. *Biol Reprod*, 77, 416-424.

[29] Hayashi, K., Sun-Wada, G.-H., Wada, Y., Nakanishi-Matsui, M. & Futai, M. (2008). Defective assembly of a hybrid vacuolar H^+-ATPase containing the mouse testis-specific E1 isoform and yeast subunits. *Biochim Biophys Acta*, 1777, 1370-1377.

[30] Herak-Kramberger, C. M., Breton, S., Brown, D., Kraus, O. & Sabolic, I. (2001). Distribution of the vacuolar H^+ATPase along the rat and human male reproductive tract. *Biol Reprod*, 64, 1699-1707.

[31] Herak-Kramberger, C. M., Sabolic, I., Blanusa, M., Smith, P. J., Brown, D. & Breton, S. (2000). Cadmium inhibits vacuolar H^+ATPase-mediated acidification in the rat epididymis. *Biol Reprod*, 63, 599-606.

[32] Hernandez-Gonzalez, E. O., Trevino, C. L., Castellano, L. E., de la Vega-Beltran, J. L., Ocampo, A. Y., Wertheimer, E., Visconti, P. E. & Darszon, A. (2007). Involvement of cystic fibrosis transmembrane conductance regulator in mouse sperm capacitation. *J Biol Chem*, 282, 24397-24406.

[33] Hinton, B. T., Palladino, M. A., Rudolph, D., Lan, Z. J. & Labus, J. C. (1996). The role of the epididymis in the protection of spermatozoa. *Curr Top Dev Biol*, 33, 61-102.

[34] Hirata, T., Iwamoto-Kihara, A., Sun-Wada, G.-H., Okajima, T., Wada, Y. & Futai, M. (2003). Subunit rotation of vacuolar-type proton pumping ATPase: relative rotation of the G and *c* subunits. *J Biol Chem*, 278, 23714-23719.

[35] Holliday, L. S., Lu, M., Lee, B. S., Nelson, R. D., Solivan, S., Zhang, L. & Gluck, S. L. (2000). The amino-terminal domain of the B subunit of vacuolar H^+-ATPase contains a filamentous actin binding site. *J Biol Chem*, 275, 32331-32337.

[36] Imai-Senga, Y., Sun-Wada, G.-H., Wada, Y. & Futai, M. (2002). A human gene, *ATP6E1*, encoding a testis-specific isoform of H^+-ATPase subunit E. *Gene*, 289, 7-12.

[37] Inoue, H., Noumi, T., Nagata, M., Murakami, H. & Kanazawa, H. (1999). Targeted disruption of the gene encoding the preteolipid subunit of mouse vacuolar H^+-ATPase leads to early embryonic lethality. *Biochim Biophys Acta*, 1413, 130-138.

[38] Jones, R. C. & Murdoch, R. N. (1996). Regulation of the motility and metabolism of spermatozoa for storage in the epididymis of eutherian and marsupial mammals. *Reprod Fertil*, Dev 8, 553-568.

[39] Jones, R. P, Durose, L. J., Phillips, C., Keen, J. N., Findlay, J. B. & Harrison, M. A. (2010). A site-directed cross-linking approach to the characterization of subunit E-subunit G contacts in the vacuolar H^+-ATPase stator. *Mol Membr Biol*, 27, 147-159.

[40] Jones, R. P, Durose, L. J., Findlay, J. B. & Harrison, M. A. (2005). Defined sites of interaction between subunits E (Vma4p), C (Vma5p), and G (Vma10p) within the stator structure of the vacuolar H^+-ATPase. *Biochemistry*, 44, 3933-3941.

[41] Jouret, F., Auzanneau, C., Debaix, H., Wada, G. H., Pretto, C., Marbaix, E., Karet, F. E., Courtoy, P. J. & Devuyst, O. (2005). Ubiquitous and kidney-specific subunits of

vacuolar H^+-ATPase are differentially expressed during nephrogenesis. *J Am Soc Nephrol*, 16, 3235-3246.

[42] Kane, P. M. (1995). Disassembly and reassembly of the yeast vacuolar H^+-ATPase *in vivo*. *J Biol Chem*, 270, 17025-17032.

[43] Kane, P. M. (2006). The where, when, and how of organelle acidification by the yeast vacuolar H^+-ATPase. *Microbiol Mol Biol Rev*, 70, 177-191.

[44] Kane, P. M. & Smardon, A. M. (2003). Assembly and regulation of the yeast vacuolar H^+-ATPase. *J Bioenerg Biomembr*, 35, 313-321.

[45] Karet, F. E., Finberg, K. E., Nelson, R. D., Nayir, A., Mocan, H., Sanjad, S. A., Rodriguez-Soriano, J., Santos, F., Cremers, C. W., Di Pietro, A., Hoffbrand, B. I., Winiarski, J., Bakkaloglu, A., Ozen, S., Dusunsel, R., Goodyer, P., Hulton, S. A., Wu, D. K., Skvorak, A. B., Morton, C. C., Cunningham, M. J., Jha, V. & Lifton, R. P. (1999). Mutations in the gene encoding B1 subunit of H^+-ATPase cause renal tubular acidosis with sensorineural deafness. *Nat Genet*, 21, 84-90.

[46] Krege, J. H., John, S. W., Langenbach, L. L., Hodgin, J. B., Hagaman, J. R., Bachman, E. S., Jennette, J. C., O'Brien, D. A. & Smithies, O. (1995). Male-female differences in fertility and blood pressure in ACE-deficient mice. *Nature*, 375, 146-148.

[47] Lee, B. S., Holliday, L. S., Ojikutu, B., Krits, I. & Gluck, S. L. (1996). Osteoclasts express the B2 isoform of vacuolar H^+-ATPase intracellularly and on their plasma membranes. *Am J Physiol*, 270, C382-388.

[48] Lee S.-H., Rho, J., Jeong, D., Sul, J.-Y., Kim, T., Kim, N., Kang, J.-S., Miyamoto, T., Suda, T., Lee, S.-K., Pignolo, R. J., Koczon-Jaremko, B., Lorenzo J. & Choi, Y. (2006). v-ATPase V_o subunit *d*2-deficient mice exhibit impaired osteoclast fusion and increased bone formation. *Nat Med*, 12, 1403-1409.

[49] Leung, A. Y., Yip, W. K., & Wong, P. Y. (1992). Characterization of adrenoceptors involved in the electrogenic chloride secretion by cultured rat epididymal epithelium. *Br J Pharmacol*, 107, 146-151.

[50] Leung, G. P., Cheung, K. H., Leung, C. T., Tsang, M. W. & Wong, P. Y. (2004). Regulation of epididymal principal cell functions by basal cells: role of transient receptor potential (Trp) proteins and cyclooxygenase-1 (COX-1). *Mol Cell Endocrinol*, 216, 5-13.

[51] Leung, G. P. & Wong, P. Y. (2000). Activation of cystic fibrosis transmembrane conductance regulator in rat epididymal epithelium by genistein. *Biol Reprod*, 62, 143-149.

[52] Leung, P. S. & Sernia, C. (2003). The renin-angiotensin system and male reproduction: new functions for old hormones. *J Mol Endocrinol*, 30, 263-270.

[53] Levine, N. & Marsh, D. J. (1971). Micropuncture studies of the electrochemical aspects of fluid and electrolyte transport in individual seminiferous tubules, the epididymis and the vas deferens in rats. *J Physiol*, 213, 557-570.

[54] Li, Y.-P., Chen, W., Liang, Y., Li, E. & Stashenko, P. (1999). *Atp6i*-deficient mice exhibit severe osteopetrosis due to loss of osteoclast-mediated extracellular acidification. *Nat Genet*, 23, 447-451.

[55] Lu, M., Ammar, D., Ives, H., Albrecht, F. & Gluck, S. L. (2007). Physical interaction between aldolase and vacuolar H^+-ATPase is essential for the assembly and activity of the proton pump. *J Biol Chem*, 282, 24495-24503.

[56] Lu, M., Holliday L. S., Zhang, L., Dunn, W. A. Jr. & Gluck, S. L. (2001). Interaction between aldolase and vacuolar H^+-ATPase: evidence for direct coupling of glycolysis to the ATP-hydrolyzing proton pump. *J Biol Chem*, 276, 30407-30413.

[57] Lu, M., Vergara, S., Zhang, L., Holliday L. S., Aris, J. & Gluck, S. L. (2002). The amino-terminal domain of the E subunit of vacuolar H^+-ATPase (V-ATPase) interacts with the H subunit and is required for V-ATPase function. *J Biol Chem*, 277, 38409-38415.

[58] Metayer, S., Dacheux, F., Dacheux, J. L., & Gatti, J. L. (2002). Germinal angiotensin I-converting enzyme is totally shed from the rodent sperm membrane during epididymal maturation. *Biol Reprod*, 67, 1763-1767.

[59] Moriyama, Y., Maeda, M. & Futai, M. (1992). The role of V-ATPase in neuronal and endocrine systems. *J Exp Biol*, 172, 171-178.

[60] Murata, Y., Sun-Wada, G.-H., Yoshimizu, T., Yamamoto, A., Wada, Y. & Futai, M. (2002) Differential localization of the vacuolar H^+ pump with G subunit isoforms (G1 and G2) in mouse neurons. *J Biol Chem*, 277, 36296-36303.

[61] Muench, S. P., Trinick, J. & Harrison, M. A. (2011). Structural divergence of the rotary ATPases. *Q Rev Biophys*, 44, 311-356.

[62] Nakanishi-Matsui, M. & Futai, M. (2006). Stochastic proton pumping ATPases: from single molecules to diverse physiological roles. *IUBMB Life*, 58, 318-322.

[63] Nakanishi-Matsui, M., Sekiya, M., Nakamoto, R. K. & Futai, M. (2010). The mechanism of rotating proton pumping ATPases. *Biochim Biophys Acta*, 1797, 1343-1352.

[64] Nelson, N. & Harvey, W. R. (1999). Vacuolar and plasma membrane proton-adenosinetriphosphatases. *Physiol Rev*, 79, 361-385.

[65] Nelson, R. D., Guo, X. L., Masood, K., Brown, D., Kalkbrenner, M. & Gluck, S. (1992). Selectively amplified expression of an isoform of the vacuolar H^+-ATPase 56-kilodalton subunit in renal intercalated cells. *Proc Natl Acad Sci U S A*, 89, 3541-3545.

[66] Nishi, T., Kawasaki-Nishi, S. & Forgac, M. (2003). Expression and function of the mouse V-ATPase *d* subunit isoforms. *J Biol Chem*, 278, 46396-46402.

[67] Oka, T., Murata, Y., Namba, M., Yoshimizu, T., Toyomura, T., Yamamoto, A., Sun-Wada, G. H., Hamasaki, N., Wada, Y. & Futai, M. (2001). *a*4, a unique kidney-specific isoform of mouse vacuolar H^+-ATPase subunit *a*. *J Biol Chem*, 276, 40050-40054.

[68] Oot, R. A. & Wilkens, S. (2010). Domain characterization and intercation of the yeast vacuolar ATPase subunit C with the peripheral stator stalk subunits E and G. *J Biol Chem*, 285, 24654-24664.

[69] Orgebin-Crist, M.-C. (2003). The Epididymis in the Post-Genome Era. In B. T. Hinton, & T. T. Turner (Eds.), *The Third International Conference on the Epididymis* (pp. 2-22). Charlottesville, VA: The Van Doren Company.

[70] Pastor-Soler, N., Beaulieu, V., Litvin, T. N., Da Silva, N., Chen, Y., Brown, D., Buck, J., Levin, L. R. & Breton, S. (2003). Bicarbonate regulated adenylyl cyclase (sAC) is a sensor that regulates pH-dependent V-ATPase recycling. *J Biol Chem*, 278, 49523-49529.

[71] Pastor-Soler, N., Hallows, K. R., Smolak, C., Gong, F., Brown, D. & Breton, S. (2008). Alkaline pH- and cAMP-induced V-ATPase membrane accumulation is mediated by protein kinase A in epididymal clear cells. *Am J Physiol Cell Physiol*, 294, C488-C494.

[72] Pastor-Soler, N., Pietrement, C. & Breton, S. (2005). Role of acid/base transporters in the male reproductive tract and potential consequences of their malfunction. *Physiology (Bethesda)*, 20, 417-428.

[73] Paunescu, T. G., Russo, L. M., Da Silva, N., Kovacikova, J., Mohebbi, N., Van Hoek, A. N., McKee, M., Wagner, C. A., Breton, S. & Brown, D. (2007). Compensatory membrane expression of the V-ATPase B2 subunit isoform in renal medullary intercalated cells of B1-deficient mice. *Am J Physiol Renal Physiol*, 293, F1915-1926.

[74] Pierucci-Alves, F., Duncan, C. L., Lillich, J. D. & Schultz, B. D. (2010). Porcine vas deferens luminal pH is acutely increased by systemic xylazine administration. *Biol Reprod*, 82, 132-135.

[75] Pierucci-Alves, F. & Schultz, B. D. (2008). Bradykinin-stimulated cyclooxygenase activity stimulates vas deferens epithelial anion secretion *in vitro* in swine and humans. *Biol Reprod*, 79, 501-509.

[76] Pietrement, C., Da Silva, N., Silberstein, C., James, M., Marsolais, M., Van Hoek, A., Brown, D., Pastor-Soler, N., Ameen, N., Laprade, R., Ramesh, V. & Breton, S. (2008). Role of NHERF1, cystic fibrosis transmembrane conductance regulator, and cAMP in the regulation of aquaporin 9. *J Biol Chem*, 283, 2986-2996.

[77] Pietrement, C., Sun-Wada, G. H., Da Silva, N., McKee, M., Marshansky, V., Brown, D., Futai, M. & Breton, S. (2006). Distinct expression patterns of different subunit isoforms of the V-ATPase in the rat epididymis. *Biol Reprod*, 74, 185-194.

[78] Robaire, B., Hinton, B. T. and Orgebin-Crist, M.-C. (2006). The epididymis. In J. D. Neill (Eds.), *Physiology of Reproduction* (pp. 1071-1148). New York, NY: Elsevier.

[79] Ruan, Y. C., Da Silva, N., Belleannee, C., Shum, W. W. C. & Breton, S. (2011). Involvement of CFTR in ATP and HCO_3^- secretion in epididymal principal cells. *FASEB J*, 25, 1039-1011.

[80] Ruz, R., Andonian, S. & Hermo, L. (2004). Immunolocalization and regulation of cystic fibrosis transmembrane conductance regulator in the adult rat epididymis. *J Androl*, 25, 265-273.

[81] Saez, F., Legare, C., Laflamme, J. & Sullivan, R. (2004). Vasectomy-dependent dysregulation of a local renin-angiotensin system in the epididymis of the cynomolgus monkey (Macaca fascicularis). *J Androl*, 25, 784-796.

[82] Saroussi, S. & Nelson, N. (2009). The little we know on the structure and machinery of V-ATPase. *J Exp Biol*, 212, 1604-1610.

[83] Sedlacek, R. L., Carlin, R. W., Singh, A. K. & Schultz, B. D. (2001). Neurotransmitter-stimulated ion transport by cultured porcine vas deferens epithelium. *Am J Physiol Renal Physiol*, 281, F557-570.

[84] Shum, W. W., Da Silva, N., Belleannee, C., McKee, M., Brown, D. & Breton, S. (2011). Regulation of V-ATPase recycling via a RhoA- and ROCKII-dependent pathway in epididymal clear cells. *Am J Physiol Cell Physiol*, 301, C31-43.

[85] Shum, W. W., Da Silva, N., Brown, D. & Breton, S. (2009). Regulation of luminal acidification in the male reproductive tract via cell-cell crosstalk. *J Exp Biol*, 212, 1753-1761.

[86] Shum, W. W., Da Silva, N., McKee, M., Smith, P. J. S., Brown, D. & Breton, S. (2008). Transepithelial projections from basal cells are luminal sensors in pseudostratified epithelia. *Cell*, 135, 1108-1117.

[87] Shum, W. W., Ruan, Y. C., Da Silva, N. & Breton, S. (2011). Establishment of cell-cell cross talk in the epididymis: control of luminal acidification. *J Androl*, 32, 576-586.

[88] Smardon, A. M., Tarsio, M. & Kane, P. M. (2002). The RAVE complex is essential for stable assembly of the yeast V-ATPase. *J Biol Chem*, 277, 13831-13839.

[89] Smardon, A. M. & Kane, P. M. (2007). RAVE is essential for the efficient assembly of the C subunit with the vacuolar H^+-ATPase. *J Biol Chem*, 282, 26185-26194.

[90] Smith, A. N., Jouret, F., Bord, S., Borthwick, K. J., Al-Lamki, R. S., Wagner, C. A., Ireland, D. C., Cormier-Daire, V., Frattini, A., Villa, A., Kornak, U., Devuyst, O. & Karet, F. E. (2005). Vacuolar H^+-ATPase *d2* subunit: molecular characterization, developmental regulation, and localization to specialized proton pumps in kidney and bone. *J Am Soc Nephrol*, 16, 1245-1256.

[91] Stover, E. H., Borthwick, K. J., Bavalia, C., Eady, N., Fritz, D. M., Rungroj, N., Giersch, A. B., Morton, C. C., Axon, P. R., Akil, I., Al-Sabban, E. A., Baguley, D. M., Bianca, S., Bakkaloglu, A., Bircan, Z., Chauveau, D., Clermont, M. J., Guala, A., Hulton, S. A., Kroes, H., Li Volti, G., Mir, S., Mocan, H., Nayir, A., Ozen, S, Rodriguez Soriano, J., Sanjad, S. A., Tasic, V., Taylor, C. M., Topaloglu, R., Smith, A. N. & Karet, F. E. (2002). Novel *ATP6V1B1* and *ATP6V0A4* mutations in autosomal recessive distal renal tubular acidosis with new evidence for hearing loss. *J Med Genet*, 39, 796-803.

[92] Sumner, J.-P., Dow, J. A. T., Earley, F. G. P., Klein, U., Jäger, D. & Wieczorek, H. (1995). Regulation of plasma membrane V-ATPase activity by dissociation of peripheral subunits. *J Biol Chem*, 270, 5649-5653.

[93] Sun-Wada, G.-H., Imai-Senga, Y., Yamamoto, A., Murata, Y., Hirata, T., Wada, Y. & Futai, M. (2002). A proton pump ATPase with testis-specific E1-subunit isoform required for acrosome acidification. *J Biol Chem*, 277, 18098-18105.

[94] Sun-Wada, G.-H., Murata, Y., Namba, M., Yamamoto, A., Wada, Y. & Futai, M. (2003). Mouse proton pump ATPase C subunit isoforms (C2-a and C2-b) specifically expressed in kidney and lung. *J Biol Chem*, 278, 44843-44851.

[95] Sun-Wada, G., Murata, Y., Yamamoto, A., Kanazawa, H., Wada, Y. & Futai, M. (2000). Acidic endomembrane organelles are required for mouse postimplantation development. *Dev Biol*, 228, 315-325.

[96] Sun-Wada, G.-H., Tabata, H., Futai, M. & Wada, Y. (2007). Differential expression of *a* subunit isoforms of the vacuolar-type proton pump ATPase in mouse endocrine tissues. *Cell Tissue Res*, 329, 239-248.

[97] Sun-Wada, G.-H., Wada, Y. & Futai, M. (2003). Lysosome and lysosome-related organelles responsible for specialized functions in higher organisms, with special emphasis on vacuolar-type proton ATPase. *Cell Struct Funct*, 28, 455-463.

[98] Sun-Wada, G.-H., Wada, Y. & Futai, M. (2004). Diverse and essential roles of mammalian vacuolar-type proton pump ATPase: towards the physiological understanding of inside acidic compartments. *Biochim Biophys Acta*, 1658, 106-114.

[99] Sun-Wada, G.-H., Yoshimizu, T., Imai-Senga, Y., Wada, Y. & Futai, M. (2003). Diversity of mouse proton-translocating ATPase: presence of multiple isoforms of the C, *d*, and G subunits. *Gene*, 302, 147-153.

[100] Thimon, V., Metayer, S., Belghazi, M., Dacheux, F., Dacheux, J. L. & Gatti, J. L. (2005). Shedding of the germinal angiotensin I-converting enzyme (gACE) involves a serine protease and is activated by epididymal fluid. *Biol Reprod*, 73, 881-890.

[101] Toei, M., Saum, R. & Forgac, M. (2010). Regulation and isoform function of the V-ATPases. *Biochemistry*, 49, 4715-4723.

[102] Toyomura, T., Mutara, Y., Yamamoto, A., Oka, T., Sun-Wada, G.-H., Wada, Y. & Futai, M. (2003). From lysosome to the plasma membrane: localization of vacuolar-type H^+-ATPase with the *a*3 isoform during osteoclast differentiation. *J Biol Chem*, 278, 22023-22030.

[103] Toyomura, T., Oka, T., Yamaguchi, C., Wada, Y. & Futai, M. (2000). Three subunit *a* isoforms of mouse vacuolar H^+-ATPase. Preferential expression of the *a*3 isoform during osteoclast differentiation. *J Biol Chem*, 275, 8760-8765.

[104] van der Ven, K., Messer L, van der Ven, H., Jeyendran, R. S. & Ober, C. (1996). Cystic fibrosis mutation screening in healthy men with reduced sperm quality. *Hum Reprod*, 11, 513-517.

[105] Vidarsson, H., Westergren, R., Heglind, M., Blomqvist, S. R., Breton, S. & Enerbäck, S. (2009). The forkhead transcription factor Foxi1 is a master regulator of vacuolar H^+-ATPase proton pump subunits in the inner ear, kidney and epididymis. *PLoS One*, 4, e4471.

[106] Vitavska, O., Wieczorek, H. & Merzendorfer, H. (2003). A novel role for subunit C in mediating binding of the H^+-V-ATPase to the actin cytoskeleton. *J Biol Chem*, 278, 18499-18505.

[107] Wagner, C. A., Finberg, K. E., Breton, S., Marshansky, V., Brown, D. & Geibel, J. P. (2004). Renal vacuolar H^+-ATPase. *Physiol Rev*, 84, 1263-1314.

[108] Wong, P. Y. (1998). *CFTR* gene and male fertility. *Mol Hum Reprod*, 4, 107-110.

[109] Wong, P. Y. & Uchendu, C. N. (1990). The role of angiotensin-converting enzyme in the rat epididymis. *J Endocrinol*, 125, 457-465.

[110] Xu, W. M., Shi, Q. X., Chen, W. Y., Zhou, C. X., Ni, Y., Rowlands, D. K., Yi Liu, G., Zhu, H., Ma, Z. G., Wang, X. F., Chen, Z. H., Zhou, S. C., Dong, H. S., Zhang, X. H., Chung, Y. W., Yuan, Y. Y., Yang, W. X. & Chan, H. C. (2007). Cystic fibrosis transmembrane conductance regulator is vital to sperm fertilizing capacity and male fertility. *Proc Natl Acad Sci U S A*, 104, 9816-9821.

[111] Yeung, C.-H., Breton, S., Stetiawan, I., Xu, Y., Lang, F. & Cooper, T. G. (2004). Increase in luminal pH in the epididymis of the infertile c-*ros* knock-out mice: putative role of sodium-hydrogen exchangers and vacuolar H^+-ATPase. *Mol Reprod and Development*, 68, 159-168.

[112] Yeung, C.-H. & Cooper, T. G. (2002). Acquisition and development of sperm motility upon maturation in the epididymis. In B. Robaire, & B. T. Hinton (Eds.), *The Epididymis. From molecules to clinical practice* (pp. 417-434). New York, NY: Kluwer Academic/Plenum Publishers.

[113] Zhang, Z., Zheng, Y., Mazon, H., Milgrom, E., Kitagawa, N., Kish-Trier, E., Heck, A. J. R., Kane, P. M. & Wilkens, S. (2008). Structure of the yeast vacuolar ATPase. *J Biol Chem*, 283, 35983-35995.

[114] Zsembery, A., Fortenberry, J. A., Liang, L., Bebok, Z., Tucker, T. A., Boyce, A. T., Braunstein, G. M., Welty, E. A., Bell, P. D., Sorscher, E. J., Clancy, J. P. & Schwiebert, E. M. (2004). Extracellular zinc and ATP restore chloride secretion across cystic fibrosis airway epithelia by triggering calcium entry. *J Biol Chem*, 279, 10720-10729.

In: Testis: Anatomy, Physiology and Pathology
Editors: Yoichi Nemoto and Norio Inaba

ISBN: 978-1-61942-739-6

Chapter 4

AROMATASE, ESTROGENS AND SPERMATOGENESIS IN MAMMALS SPACE

Serge Carreau*
Biochemistry-EA 2608-USC2006 INRA, France

ABSTRACT

The mammalian testis exerts two main functions in two different compartments: synthesis of steroids and production of spermatozoa. These specific functions are controlled by gonadotropins and numerous locally synthesized factors, among them testosterone, growth factors and more recently estrogens. Indeed since 1993, we know that germ cells in male gonad synthesize estrogens. As a matter of fact aromatase has been demonstrated in numerous mammalian species (review Carreau and Hess, 2010). Aromatase is localized in immature Sertoli cells then in Leydig cells and germ cells in mature rat and it is clear that aromatase transcripts are more expressed in pachytene spermatocytes than in round spermatids but conversely the aromatase activity is reversed (Carreau et al, Current Medical Chemistry 2011). What is interesting is that germ cells not only express aromatase but are also equipped of estrogen receptors (both genomic and non genomic effects; Carreau et al, Life Sciences 2011). In addition from numerous models of mice (either ArKO, or ERαKo or ERβKO) and from men deficient in aromatase we know that estrogens are necessary for a full achievement of spermatogenesis (otherwise the number and motility of spermatozoa are decreased; Carreau et al 2010). In addition looking on the putative effects of endocrine disruptors, it is now clear that they are deleterious since estrogen receptors are everywhere in the male genital tract. Therefore estrogens which are also demonstrated in ejaculated spermatozoa of man are necessary not only on the germ cells renewal, spermatogenesis but also for the final maturation of that sperm cell.

Keywords: Aromatase, Estrogens, Estrogen Receptors, Germ Cell Development, Spermatogenesis, Testis, Mammals

* Address for correspondence: Dr Serge Carreau, University -EA2608, INRA USC2006, Esplanade de la Paix 14032- CAEN Cedex- France; Tel: +33 2 31 56 54 88; E-mail:serge.carreau@unicaen.fr.

INTRODUCTION

Spermatogenesis is the mechanism by which a spermatogonia, is transformed in a spermatozoa, a highly differentiated haploid cell; these events are controlled by numerous factors including gonadotropins and locally produced factors [110]. Among these factors, growing evidences suggest that estrogens, synthesized by the cytochrome P450 aromatase, are concerned in the regulation of spermatogenesis (for reviews [23,28]). More than seventy years ago, Zondek [132] discovers an estrogenic compound in the stallion urine, but it's only 30 years later that evidences have been published showing that human testis synthesize and secrete estrogens [65]which was confirmed later by Hendry et al [58] demonstrating the testicular source of estrogens in men. Indeed in mammals the presence of large quantities of estrogens in the rete testis fluid and the spermatic vein has been reported (reviews [60-61]). Moreover, in mice in which the cytochrome P450 aromatase deficiency is genetically induced (ArKO), failures in spermatogenesis are reported with a decrease of the number and of the quality of spermatids leading to infertility in one year-old animals [107]. Furthermore, studies have enlightened that estrogens could be involved in several aspects of rodent spermatogenesis: proliferation of gonocytes and spermatogonia, control of apoptosis and in some steps of spermiogenesis (for reviews, [28, 92]). Aromatase is encoded by the *Cyp19*gene located on chromosome 15 in human beings with a coding region of 9 exons plus 11 untranslated exons I [42, 112]. According to tissues, aromatase expression is very precisely controlled, but even if there is several mRNAs producedonly one aromatase protein is described in humans [117-118]. In immature rats, Sertoli cells are the major source of estrogens [95,109], while Leydig [95,109] and germ cells produce estrogens in the adults [76]. Moreover from the observations of patients with congenital either estrogen deficiency (ERα) or estrogen resistance (absence of aromatase) a major role for estrogens in spermatogenesis has been demonstrated (review [104]) and animal models such as mice deficient in aromatase (ArKO) [107]. It should be noted that impaired sperm motility and germ cells arrest (at spermatid stage) were observed in both aromatase deficient men and mice (reviews [104-105]). Conversely, exposure of the adult male rat to a high phytoestrogen diet [108] disrupted spermatogenesis or excess of estrogens in man [89]and overexpression of aromatase gene in mice leads to infertility (review [79]).

Human fertility rates are declining all over the world and today, around 15% of couples are confronted with infertility and in half of the cases the cause is of male origin with quantitative and/or qualitative abnormalities of the semen. The causes can be genetic and/or environmental; indeed, several epidemiological studies have shown that decrease sperm counts and increase male reproductive tract disorders (cryptorchidism, hypospadia, testicular cancers) in men can be related to a deleterious effect of endocrine disruptors with either estrogenic or antiandrogenic actions [121-122, 125-126]. In that paper I will focused on aromatase expression in male testicular cells and on the role of estrogens in germ cell development including ejaculated spermatozoa from man.

I. AROMATASE IN MAMMALIAN TESTICULAR CELLS

In testes aromatase is located in the endoplasmic reticulum and transforms irreversibly androgens into estrogens (reviews [23,28, 92]). After being purified, aromatase was cloned and primers made available for checking transcripts together with measurements of aromatase activity and immunohistological studies. The availability of antibodies allowed for immunohistolocalization of aromatase in Leydig cells of young and adult rats [69].

Early in the study of testicular aromatase, it was thought that its expression was in Sertoli cells during development in the rodent species, but then only in Leydig cells in the adult testis (see reviews [24, 62]). In some species such as pig review [37]) and human [63]), a testicular aromatase mRNA was thought to be present only in Leydig cells. Despite the large amount of data published in different species, the precise localization of aromatase has been a subject of debates. As abundantly documented in the literature, it is difficult to find a tissue completely devoid of aromatase gene expression [117-118].

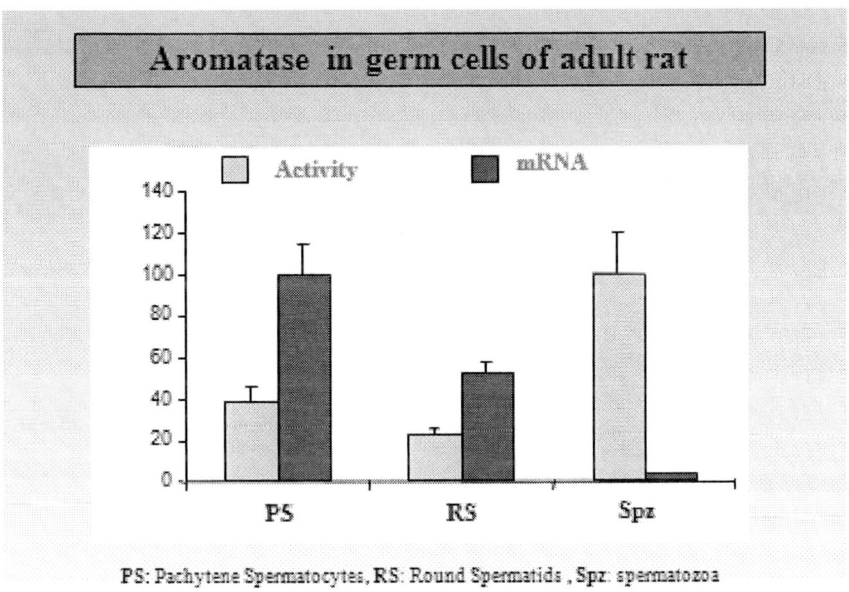

Figure 1. Aromatase transcripts and aromatase activity in purified mature rat germ cells.

Nitta et al [91] were the first and have demonstrated that the adult mouse germ cells express a functional aromatase and that the amount of estradiol produced is equivalent to that of Leydig cells. Cytochrome P450 aromatase has been shown to be expressed in the adult rat testis (Figure 1) at the transcript level [13, 16-17, 75-77, 116] and as a protein [20, 76] biologically active in adult Leydig and germ cells [16-17,76]. Moreover, cytochrome P450 aromatase mRNA levels are regulated according to age, to cell type and to stages of the seminiferous epithelium [13].

In the male rat testis we have described 3 promoters [116] which direct the expression of the aromatase: the promoter PII, the main one promoter used in testicular cells [74], the promoter PI.f, first characterized in the brain [131] and the promoter PI.tr which is specific of the rat testis [116]. In rat germ cells additional promoters have been described (either deleted of exon 9 coding for the heme-binding region or unable to code for a functional aromatase; [77]) and their amounts are high in pachytene spermatocytes (PS). Whatever, these promoters are used very precisely (Figure 2), thus the amount of aromatase RNAm and thus the estrogens produced are strictly controlled [77, review 28].

In somatic cells as well as in germ cells of the bank vole [11] and the protein was more expressed during the breeding season [52]. In the boar a unique Leydig cell source of estrogens has been described [88, 102]. For the stallion aromatase was more expressed in Leydig cells [62], even though recent data are in favor for an additional source in germ cells [44, 120]. In black bear [127], bison [67] and deer [113] aromatase has been demonstrated in somatic and germ cells. In the Rhesus monkey, testis and to a lesser extent, epididymis contains aromatase transcripts [1, 14, 98].

In humans, Leydig cells [96] and Sertoli cells produce estrogens ([47; for reviews [21,29]) but spermatozoa can metabolize pregnenolone into estrogens [29]. Moreover aromatase is expressed in immature germ cells [49] as well as in ejaculated spermatozoa [3-4, 70-71, 73].

In all samples studied individually we have demonstrated the presence of aromatase transcripts ([70]; review [73]) which is in agreement with other reports [3]. In immotile sperm the amount of aromatase transcripts was 30% lower than in motile sample and indeed, the aromatase activity was higher in motile fraction compared to immotile spermatozoa [72]. On western blots we have evidenced the presence of aromatase in both immature germ cells and ejaculated sperm cells, the protein being more abundant in spermatozoa containing cytoplasmic droplets [3,20].

Species	mRNA	Protein	Activity
Mouse	+	+	+
Rat	+	+	+
Bank vole	+	+	+
Squirrel	+	+	+/-
Boar	+	+	+
Ram	ND	ND	+
Stallion	+	+	+
Bear	+	+	+
Monkey	ND	ND	+
Human	+	+	+

Figure 2. Aromatase expression in mammal Leydig cells.

II. ESTROGEN RECEPTORS (ESR1 AND ESR2) AND MEMBRANE RECEPTOR (GPER)

Estrogens interact with estrogen receptors (ERs), a member of the nuclear receptor superfamily (Figure 3), which in turn modulate the expression of target genes (for [57]). The physiological role of estrogens (via the classical genomic pathway) in male reproduction is extensively re-analyzed taking into account the presence of two ERs (ERα and ERβ) in most of the testicular cells and throughout the genital tract (for reviews [26, 36, 92, 111, 115]). In addition a relevant role for estrogens has been recently demonstrated via the rapid membrane interactions leading to new signaling pathways (for reviews [78, 100-101]).

Regarding to spermatozoa eventhough the transcripts of ERα and ERβ were demonstrated we were only able to show the presence of an ERα protein of 46 kDa corresponding to the isoform that lacks exon I ; that variant could be located on the membrane. Aquila et al [4], Solakidi et al. [124] have reported the presence of ERα and ERβ proteins in human ejaculated spermatozoa with some differences on their respective localisation. Moreover numerous spliced variants of ERβ in the human testicular cells have been detected [6]. Therefore in human seminiferous tubules there are controversial data with either the absence or the presence of ER alpha and ER beta [29, 97, 111].

Recently, the existence of estrogen pathways starting at the plasma membrane has been described [78, 100]. As a novel estrogen receptor, GPER has been shown to be implicated in estrogen responses in the mouse spermatogonial cell line GC-1 [119], in rat Sertoli cells [83], in adult rat pachytene spermatocytes [34] and in round spermatids [35]. 17β-estradiol binding to GPER activates MAPK pathway and results in the phosphophorylation of ERK and possibly in the activation of the transcription factors c-Fos or c-Jun [34-35, 82-83]. The activation of GPER and ESR1 inhibits the gene expression of cyclins A1 and B1 and enhanced the gene expression of Bax in purified pachytene spermatocytes [34].

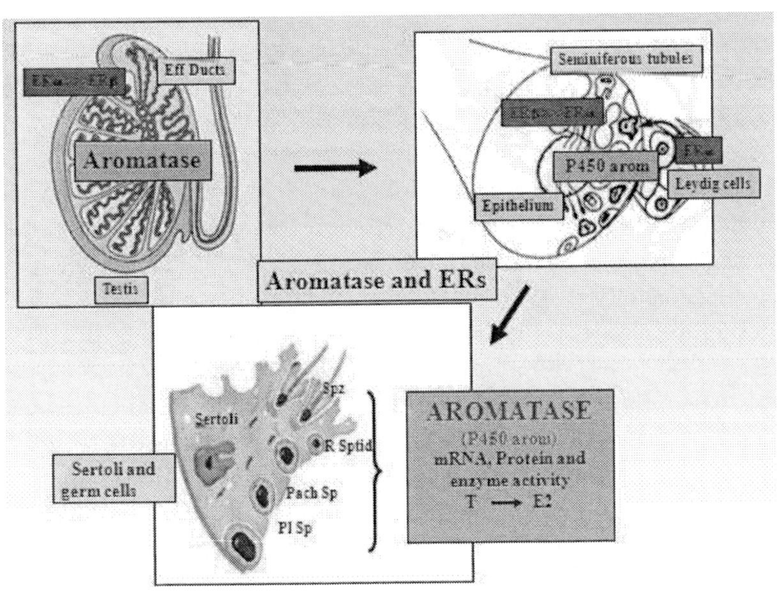

Figure 3. Aromatase expression and estrogen receptors in rat testicular cells.

In addition, the cyclin B1 and Bax genes expression are respectively down- and up-regulated by 17β-estradiol through an activation of MAPK pathway by ESR1 and GPER in purified round spermatids [35]. Thus, 17β-estradiol acts as a regulator of the proliferation/apoptose balance in rat seminiferous tubules, especially in germ cells [99].

Cyclin A1, with CDK2 or CDK1, is involved in G1/S and G2/M transitions respectively [94], which are necessary for the spermatocytes entry in the first meiotic division [80] and is expressed exclusively in germ cells (for review, [130]). Cyclin B1 with CDK1 forms the MPF (mitosis prmoting factor) complex which is involved in the control of G2/M transition. Both cyclin B1 and CDK1 are regulated according to the maturation degree of germ cells with a highest level observed in late spermatocytes, just before the first division of meiosis and they are still present in round spermatids [53-54] suggesting a function in spermatid maturation in addition to its well-known role in the progression of cell cycle.

Moreover from the observations of patients with either estrogen or aromatase deficiencies a major role for estrogens in spermatogenesis has been provided (review [104]). It is noteworthy that impaired sperm motility and germ cells arrest (at spermatid stage) were observed in both aromatase deficient men and mice (reviews [104-105, 107]). Today, around 15% of couples are infertiles and in half of them a male origin with quantitative and/or qualitative abnormalities of the semen is obvious. The causes can be genetic and/or environmental, several epidemiological studies have shown that decrease sperm counts and increase male reproductive tract disorders (cryptorchidism, hypospadia, testicular cancers) in men can be related to a deleterious effect of endocrine disruptors with either estrogenic or antiandrogenic actions [122, 126]. In immature germ cells and spermatozoa of healthy men we have reported the presence of estrogen receptors, not only the full-length but also some variants (see for [73]).

Estrogens and Germ Cell Development

Estrogens play an essential role in controlling the hypothalamus–pituitary–testis axis through a feedback loop(review [92]). It is now well recognized that testicular and germ cellestrogens have a direct role in the regulation of downstream physiology, as the highest concentration of ERα is found in epithelial cells lining the efferent ductules (reviews [60-61]), whose primary function is to reabsorb luminal fluid and increase the concentration of sperm before they enter the epididymis [59]. However, evidence for estrogen having a direct action on the seminiferous epitheliumhas been lacking. Opinions favouring a role for estrogen in spermatogenesis have typically come from indirect evidence (reviews [24-25, 60-62]):(i) prenatal exposure to estrogens, (ii) expression of aromatase in the testis, (iii) expression of ERa and ERb in the testis, (iv) various knockout animal models, and (v) anti-aromatase effects [114]. The original ERα knockout mouse, the neo-ERKO (review [36],[81]), generated by inserting a neo gene into exon 2, produced the first evidence that a classical ER was essential for male fertility.A more detailed study of the neo-ERKO mouse revealed that fluid accumulation was realated to a failure of efferent ductules to reabsorb luminal fluids [59].

The presence of aromatase and of estrogen receptors in most of the testicular cells is demonstrated in several mammals and among them in humans (see reviews [25-26, 29]).

Berensztein et al [10] have immunolocalized aromatase and ER beta in gonocytes and spermatogonia in newborn and infantile testes but the role of estrogens in that developing gonad remain to be clarified (Figure 4). In addition the existence of ERβ isoforms in the human testicular cells have been reported but their specific functions are not fully elucidated even if a putative relationship between ERβ polymorphisms and infertility has been suggested [7].

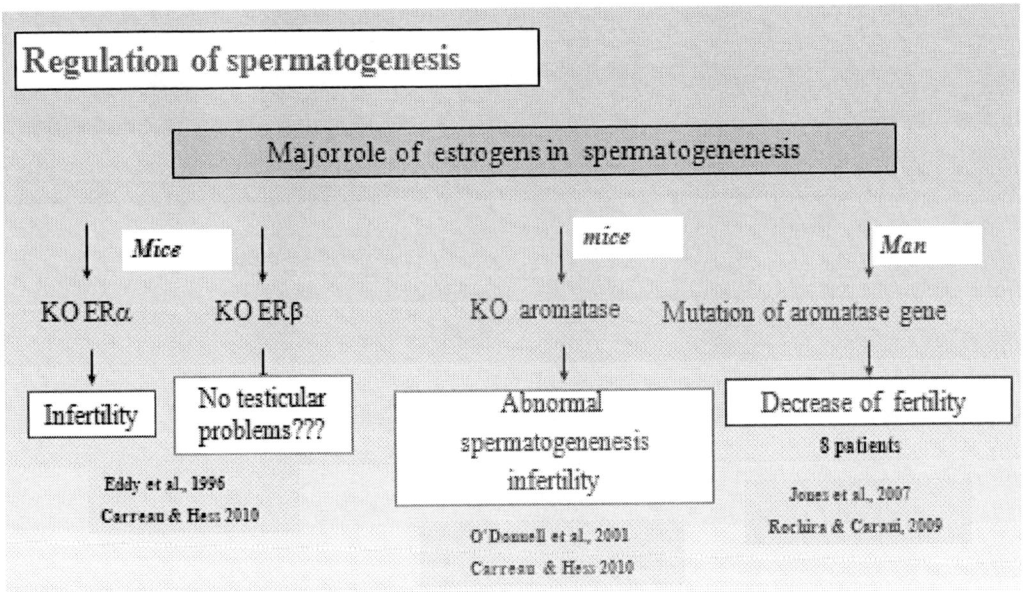

Figure 4. Role (s) of estrogens in spermatogenesis.

What is more interesting is the demonstration of a source and target of estrogens in ejaculated spermatozoa [26, 29]. Eventhough spermatozoa are considered as biologically inert cells which transfer the paternal genome into the oocyte, the presence of mRNAs (for reviews [39-40, 90]) and their potential roles in spermatozoa is still a matter of controversies (for reviews [50, 86-87]). But numerous data suggest that both transcriptional and translational activities could occur in these haploid cells ([55,93], review [40]).

Nevertheless the role of estrogens in man especially in the reproductive function is becoming more obvious after the publication of Smith et al [123] concerning a man with a non-functional ERα and several reports related to men deficient in aromatase (reviews [104-105]). Aromatase deficiency is rather rare in man (8 cases published today) and it occurs following mutations in the Cyp19 gene and then, the protein issued form that gene shows an absence of biological activity and thus very low (or nil) levels of estrogens in the blood (Figure 5).

One of the most dramatic effect recorded on aromatase mutation is on exon IV which is very critical for aromatase function and thus leads to the absence of total enzyme activity [85]. All together 4 exons (IV, V, IX and X) are required for the full biological activity of the protein as also observed in the rat aromatase gene [77].

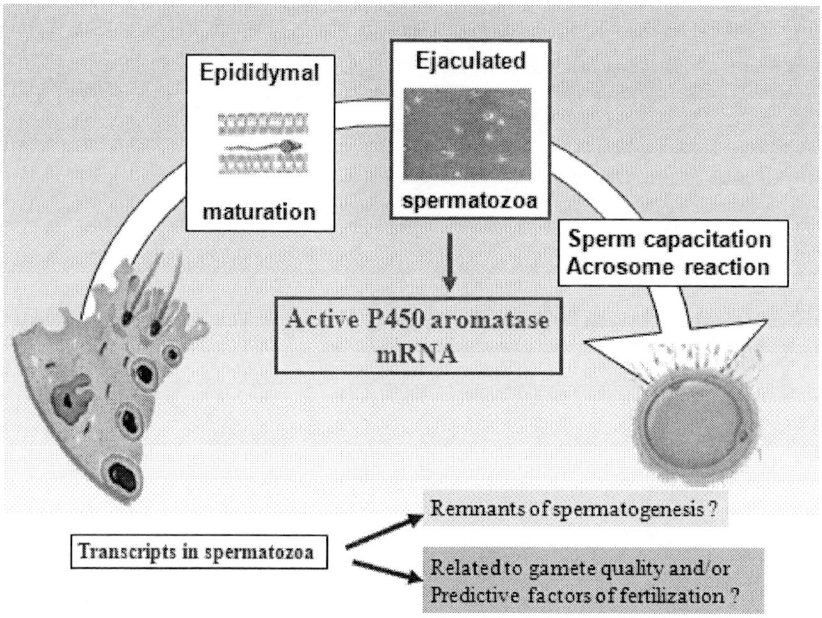

Figure 5. Putative role of aromatase and estrogens, as tools to evaluate man fertility.

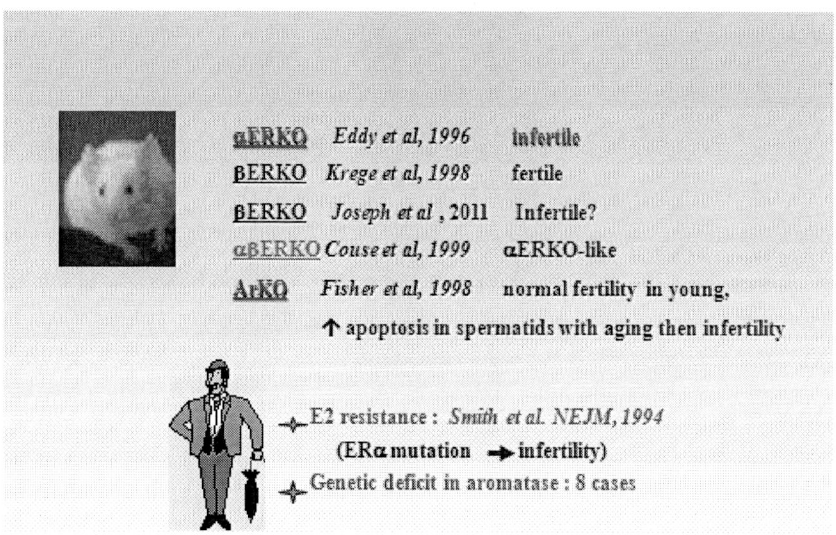

Figure 6. Mice knock out models and human infertility (deficiencies in ERα or aromatase).

From a testicular biopsy of one of these aromatase-deficient men it was reported by Maffei et al [85] that spermatogenesis varied from normal in some seminiferous tubules to highly reduced (hypospermatogenesis) in most of the others therefore suggesting a decrease of germ cell number as observed in ArKO mice leading to infertility at the age of one year (review [92]). The last (8th case) patient described by Carani's group [132] shows moderated alterations of sperm parameters (asthenoteratospermia) which were not back to normal after estradiol treatment but a cryptorchidism history was recorded (reviews [66, 104]. But what is also very interesting is that these aromatase-deficient patients with variable degree of fertility disorder provided additional informations on the roles of estrogens since they have been studied in adulthood age. Carani et al [19] where the first to report a tall stature with linear growth and absence of epiphyseal closure which is the main reason leading these patients to consult a specialized physician. It is of note that these men have normal or subnormal levels of gonadotropins and testosterone [104] and besides these symptoms, most of them have trouble in lipid and glucose metabolisms without clear explanations [66, 132].

What is important to mention is that the human spermatozoa produce estrogens and indeed they express a functional aromatase which is still active after ejaculation [73], and together with the presence of ERs [5, 84, 124], these data open new considerations about the role of estrogens all along the male genital tract and likely also in the sperm mobility and the fertilizing ability. Indeed Fraser et al [49] has demonstrated that either estradiol or a phytoestrogen (genistein) improves the capacitation and acrosome loss of human spermatozoa. It is also relevant to mention that more than 30 years ago it has been reported i) a correlation between the amount of estrogens in the seminal plasma and the fertility and ii) the incubation of spermatozoa with estradiol improves their motility (reviews [23, 29, 51]). Besides the positive effects of estrogens on human spermatogenesis it has also been shown that aromatase inhibitors are powerful to improve the spermocytogram of infertile men with a decreased blood testosterone/estradiol ratio (review [27]). Therefore the effects of estrogens in human ejaculated spermatozoa are more and more obvious: besides the classical genomic effects, membrane estrogen receptors are connected with numerous signal transduction pathways involving quick answers [48,84] and among them, cAMP/PKA/AKAP, nitric oxyde, MEK pathway, calcium channel and a calcium / calmodulin complex, all known to be concerned in sperm mobility and capacitation (for reviews [103]). Aquila et al [4] have also shown a rapid membrane effect of estrogens which in turn activate the PI3K/AKT pathway in human ejaculated spermatozoa.

The mechanisms of action of endocrine disruptors (EDCs) seem to involve divergent pathways including estrogenic, antiandrogenic actions and other nuclear or membrane associated non classical receptors and many other pathways and which can be studied in laboratory *in vitro* and *in vivo* animal models [33, 101].

However, because of the specificity of each species, the real evidence demonstrating the role of a determined chemical pollutant must be established in the human species. Epidemiological studies are the most used approach to reach this aim In humans, the observations of decreased sperm number and motility in men genetically deficient in aromatase, together with our data and those reported in the literature, may suggest a role for aromatase/ estrogens not only during the development and maintenance of spermatogenesis but also in the final maturation of spermatozoa (review [29]).

Conclusion

From the knock out studies in mice and the data reported in aromatase deficient men the estrogen effects on spermatogenesis and spermiogenesis are clearly (reviews [28,29]) but the role of estrogens in male reproduction is becoming more obvious taking into account the existence of specific receptors all along the genital tract (review of [66]). Indeed it is absolutely clear that the estrogen therapy is really beneficial for these man deficient in aromatase [29, 66]. The aromatase is constitutively expressed not only in Leydig cells and Sertoli cells but also in germ cells whatever the stage of development in humans. Besides the gonadotrophin control, it is clear now that neither man with an aromatase deficiency or estrogen resitance has “normal spermatogenesis” [104].

The absence of semen analyses is of course « damaging » for the final conclusion on the sperm number and quality and thus on putative fertility of these patients. Nevertheless in these patients a decreased in sperm motility is recorded and we have a significant decrease of aromatase in immotile spermatozoa which could suggest that aromatase/estrogens are involved in the acquisition of sperm motility. Accordingly two immunoreactive sites for aromatase have been demonstrated [51]: one in the tail plus the midpiece in which an intensive staining was observed as expected, and the second one corresponds to a tight but compact highly fluorescent zone of the head (equatorial region / or upper postacrosomal region). Our preliminary results in teratospermic patients showed a high degree of correlation (r=-0.64) between the aromatase/GAPDH transcripts and the percentage of abnormal spermatozoa. More interesting may be, a negative correlation (r=-0.56) was observed between that ratio and the head malformations (microcephaly or acrosome malformations) than with the tail defects (r=-0.42). From a small group of teratospermic men it appears that the annular aromatase (equatorial localization) is two-fold less than in normospermic men (Galeraud-Denis et al, unpublished results).

Besides a relevant physiological role of that female hormones, it is also well-known that excess of estrogens are very deleterious for testicular functions as for instance Leydig cells tumors in which an enhanced estradiol production is recorded together with presence of ERs lead to excess of cell proliferation [20]. Seminoma cells express aromatase and a rapid membrane estrogen effect as well as genomic ERs have been reported [33, 106]. In addtion it is weell known that testicular germ cell tumors produce high amounts of estrogens which induce a decrease of sperm motility and deep alterations of spermatogenesis [89].

Whatever our knowledge of the role of estrogens in male physiology is increasing and at least, as far as estrogens are concerned in male gamete maturation, not only the existence of estrogen sources but also the presence of ERs in immature germ cells and in ejaculated sperm have been clearly demonstrated therefore suggesting a potential role of estrogens in the latter steps of sperm maturation (capacitation and / or acrosome reaction).

Taking into account that new role of estrogens (even if estrogen-related genes are not yet completely kwnon but cyclins are concerned as also Bax) the presence of aromatase transcripts could be a marker of male gamete quality and the existence of two sites of aromatase could be related to the implication of the estrogens in the motility and the acrosome reaction. In addition since aromatase, ERs and AR recently described [5] are simultaneously present in spermatozoa, a putative autocrine and / or intracrine role of estradiol is suggested.

At least estrogens could play a role if we considered the presence of ERs in the mitochondria [32] an organite tremendosuly important in the midpiece of the spermatozoa. Finally I would also draw attention on the GPR30 (a transmembrane intracellular estrogen receptor) which induces rapid mobilization of calcium in the cytoplasm [100-101], and obviously would be of great interest for sperm activation before acrosome reaction. Male fertility is decreasing in western countries and thus it is a society problem ; consequently, extensive and comparative studies of mRNA maps in ejaculated spermatozoa from fertile and infertile men may contribute to a better understanding of the various aspects of male gamete maturation throughout the genital tract.

ACKNOWLEDGMENTS

I am greatly indebted to my collaborators: Levallet, Bouraima-Lelong, Delalande (and the PhD students: Drs Lambard, de Vienne, Said). All these works have been supported by fundings from the French Ministry of Education and Research, a Polonium grant, and the Région Basse-Normandie during 20 years.

REFERENCES

[1] Albrecht, ED; Lane, MV; Marshall, GR; Merchenthaler, I; Dimorangkir, DR; Pohl, CR; Plant, TM; Pepe, GP. Estrogen promotes germ cell and seminiferous tubule development in the baboon fetal testis. *Biology of Reprod*uction2009,81, 406-414.

[2] Antal, MC; Krust, A; Chambon, P; Mark, M. Sterility and absence of histopathological defects in non reproductive organs of a mouse ERβ-null mutant. *Proceedings National Academy Sciences USA* 2008, 105, 2433-2438.

[3] Aquila, S; Sisci, D; Gentile, M; Middea, E; Siciliano, L; Ando, S. Human ejaculated spermatozoa contain active P450 aromatase. *Journal of Clinical Endocrinology and Metabolism,* 200287, 3385-3390.

[4] Aquila, S; Sisci, D; Gentile, M; Middea, E; Catalano, S; Carpino, A; Rago, V; Ando, S. Estrogen receptor (ER)alpha and ER beta are both expressed in human ejaculated spermatozoa: evidence of their direct interaction with phosphatidylinositol-3-OH kinase/Akt pathway. *Journal of Clinical Endocrinology and Metabolism,* 2004,89, 1443-1451.

[5] Aquila, S;Middea, E; Catalano, S;Marsico, S;Lanzino, M;Casaburi, I;Barone, I;Bruno, R;Zupo, S;Andò, S. Human sperm express a functional androgen receptor: effects on PI3K/AKT pathway. *Human Reproduction*, 2007, 22, 2594-2605.

[6] Aschim, EL; Saether, T; Wiger, R; Grotmol, T; Haugen, TB Differential distribution of splice variants of estrogen receptor beta in human testicular cells suggests specific functions in spermatogenesis. *Journal Steroid Biochemistry* and *Molecular Biology,* 2004, 92, 97-106.

[7] Aschim, EL; Giwercman, A; Stahl, O; Eberhard, J; Cwikiel, M; Nordenskjold, A; Haugen, TB; Grotmol, T; Giwercman Y.L. The Rsal polymorphism inthe estrogen receptor beta gene is associated with maleinfertility. *Journal Clinical Endocrinology and Metabolism*, 2005, 90, 5343–5348.

[8] Assinder, S; Davis, R; Fenwick, M; Glover, A. Adult-only exposure of male rats to a diet of high phytoestrogen content increases apoptosis of meiotic and post-meiotic germ cells. *Reproduction* 2007, 133, 11-19.

[9] Beck, KJ; Herscel, S; Hungershofer, R;Schwinger, E. The effect of steroid hormones on motility and selective migration of X-and Y-bearing human spermatozoa. *Fertility and Sterility,* 1976, 27,407-412.

[10] Berensztein, EB; Baquedano, MS; Gonzalez, CR; Saraco, NI; Rodriguez, J; Ponzio, R; Rivarola, MA; Belgorosky, A. Expression of aromatase, estrogen receptor alpha and beta, androgen receptor, and cytochrome P-450scc in the human early prepubertal testis. *Pediatric Research*, 2006 60, 740-744. Epub 2006 Oct 25.

[11] Bilinska, B; Schmalz-Fraczek, B; Kotula, M; Carreau, S. Photoperiod-dependent capability of androgen aromatization and the role of estrogens in bank vole testis visualized by means of immunohistichemistry. *Molecular and Cellular Endocrinology,*2001, 178, 189-198.

[12] Boitani, C; Ritzen, EM; Parvinen, M. Inhibition of rat Sertoli cell aromatase by factor(s) secreted specifically at spermatogenic stages VII and VIII. *Molecular and Cellular Endocrinology,* 1981, 23,11-22.

[13] Bois, C; Delalande, C; Nurmio, M; Parvinen, M; Zanatta, L; Toppari, J; Carreau, S. Age and cell-related gene expression of aromatase and estrogen receptors in the rat testis. *Journal of Molecular Endocrinology,* 2010, 45, 147-159.

[14] Bonagura, TW; Zhou, H; Babischkin, JS;Pepe, GJ; Albretch, ED. Expression of P-450 aromatase, estrogen receptor α and β and α-inhibin in the fetal baboon testis after estrogen suppression during the second half of gestatiuon. *Endocrine,*2011,39, 75-82.

[15] Bouraïma-Lelong, H; Vanneste, M; Delalande, C; Zanatta, L; Wolczynski, S; Carreau, S. Aromatase gene expression in immature rat Sertoli cells: age-related changes in the FSH signalling pathway. *Reproductive Fertility and Development,* 2010, 22, 508-515.

[16] Bourguiba, S; Chater, S;Delalande, C; Benahmed, M;Carreau, S., Regulation of aromatase gene expression in purified germ cells of adult male rats: effects of transforming growth factor β, tumor necrosis factor α, and cyclic adenosine 3',5'-monophosphate. *Biology of Reproduction,* 2003a,69, 592-601.

[17] Bourguiba, S; Lambard, S;Carreau, S. Steroids control the aromatase gene expression in purified germ cells from the adult male rat. *Journal of Molecular Endocrinology.* 2003b, 31, 83-94.

[18] Bouskine, A; Nebout, M; Mograbi, B; Brucker-Davis, F; Roger, C; Fenichel, P. Estrogens promote human testicular germ cell cancer through a membranemediatedactivation of extracellular regulated kinase and protein kinase A. *Endocrinology,* 2008,149, 565–573.

[19] Carani, C ; Qin, K ; Simoni, M ; Faustini-Fustini, M; Serpente, S ; Boyd, J; Korach, KS ; Simpson ER. Effect of testosterone and estradiol in a man with aromatase deficiency. *New England Journal of Medicine*, 1997 ;337, 91-95.

[20] Carpino, F; Romeo, F; Rago, FV. Aromatase immunolocalization in human ductuli efferentes and proximal ductus epididymis. *Journal of Anatomy,* 2004, 204, 217-220.

[21] Carreau, S. Paracrine control of human Leydig cell and Sertoli cell functions. *Folia Histochemica et Cytobiologica*, 1996, 34 (3), 111-119.

[22] Carreau, S. Leydig cell aromatase: from gene to physiological role. In A.H. Payne and M.P. Hardy. *The Leydig Cell in Health and Disease*. Human Press Inc, Totowa, NJ, USA, 2007, 189-195.

[23] Carreau, S; Genissel, C; Bilinska, B; Levallet, J. Oestrogen sources in the testis and the reproductive tract of the male. *International Journal of Andrology,* 1999, 22, 211- 223.

[24] Carreau, S; Lambard, S; Delalande, C; Galeraud-Denis, I; Bilinska, B; Bourguiba, S. Aromatase expression and role of estrogens in male gonad: a review. *Reproductive Biology and Endocrinology,2003,* 1, 35.

[25] Carreau S, Delalande C, Silandre D, Bourguiba S, Lambard S Aromatase and estrogen receptors in male reproduction. *Molecular and Cellular Endocrinology,* 2006,246, 65-68

[26] Carreau, S; Bourguiba, S; Delalande, C; Silandre, D; Said, L; Galeraud-Denis, I; Lambard, S. Estrogens and Male Reproduction. *Current Medical Chemistry Immunological Endocrinology Metabolic Agents*, 2008, 8, 59-65.

[27] Carreau, S; Delalande, C; Galeraud-Denis, I. Mammalian sperm quality and aromatase expression. *Microscopy Research and Technics,* 2009, 72, 552-557.

[28] Carreau, S; Hess, RA. Oestrogens and spermatogenesis. *Philosophical Transaction Royal Society B,* 2010,365, 1517-1535.

[29] Carreau, S; Wolczynski, S;Galeraud-Denis, I. Aromatase, oestrogens and human male reproduction. Philosophical *Transaction Royal Society* B 2010, 365, 1571-1579.

[30] Carreau, S ; Bois, C ; Zanatta, L ; Silva, FRMB ; Bouraima-Lelong, H ; Delalande, C. Estrogens signaling in testicular cells. *Life Sciences*, 2011, 89, 584-587.

[31] Carreau, S ; Chimento, A ; Bois, C ; Sirianni, R ; Delalande, C ; Pezzi, V. Estrogen rapid signalling in spermatogenesis. *Current Medical Chemistry Immunological Endocrinology Metabolic Agents*, 2011, 11, in press.

[32] Chen, JQ; Yager, JD; Russo J. Regulation of mitochondrialrespiratory chain structure and function byestrogens/estrogen receptors and potential physiological/ pathophysiological implications. *Biochimica Biophysica Acta*, 2005,1746, 1–17.

[33] Chevalier, N., Bouskine, A., Fenichel, P. Bisphenol A promotestesticular seminoma cell proliferation through GPER/GPR30. *International Journal of Cancer*, 2011, doi:10.1002/ijc.25972.

[34] Chimento, A; Sirianni, R; Delalande, C; Silandre, D; Bois, C; Ando, S; Maggiolini, M; Carreau, S; Pezzi, V. 17β-estradiol activates rapid signaling pathways involved in rat pachytene spermatocytes apoptosis through GPR30 and ERα. *Molecular and Cellular Endocrinology,* 2010, 320, 136-144.

[35] Chimento, A;Sirianni, R;Zolea, F; Bois, C; Delalande, C; Ando, S;Maggiolini, M; Aquila, S; Carreau, S; Pezzi, V. GPR30 and ERs are expressed in rat round spermatids and mediate estrogen-dependent rapid pathways modulating expression of cyclin B1 and Bax. *International Journal of Andrology*, 2011, 34, 420-429.

[36] Couse, JF; Korach, KS. Estrogen receptor null mice: what have we learned and where will they lead us? *Endocrine Reviews* 1999, 20, 358-417.

[37] Conley A, Hinshelwood M. Mammalian aromatases. *Reproduction,* 2001, 121, 685-695.

[38] Culty, M. Gonocytes, the forgotten cells of the germ cell lineage. *Birth Defects Research,* 2009, 87, 1-26.

[39] Dadoune JP. Spermatozoal RNAs: what about theirfunctions. *Microscopy Researchand Technics* 2009, 8, 536–551.

[40] Dadoune, JP; Galeraud-Denis, I; Carreau, S. Clinical significance of sperm RNA. In A. Zini and A Agarwal (Eds) "Sperm Chromatin: biological and clinical applications in male infertility and assited reproduction". *Springer Science* 2011, DOI 10.1007/978-1-4419-6857- Chapter 18.

[41] Delbes, G; Levacher, C; Pairault, C; Racine, C; Duquenne, C; Krust, A; Habert, R. Estrogen receptor beta-mediated inhibition of male germ cell line development in mice by endogenous estrogens during perinatal life. *Endocrinology,*2004,145, 3395-3403.

[42] Demura, M; Reierstad, S; Innes, JE; Bulun, SE. Novel promoter I.8 and promoter usage in the CYP19 (Aromatase) gene. *Reproductive Science,* 2008, 15, 1044-1053.
[43] D'Souza, R; Gill-Sharma, M; Pathak, S; Kedia, N; Kumar, R; Balasinor, N. Effect of high intratesticular estrogen on the seminiferous epithelium in adult male rats. *Molecular and Cellular Endocrinology,* 2005, 241, 41-48.
[44] Eisenhauer, KM;McCue, PM; Nayden, DK; Osawa, Y; Roser, JF. Localization of aromatase in equine Leydig cells. *Domestic Animal Endocrinology,* 1994, 11, 291–298.
[45] Fisher, CR; Graves, KH; Parlow, AF; Simpson, ER. Characterization of mice deficient in aromatase (ArKO) because of targeted disruption of the cyp19 gene. *Proceedings National Academy Sciences USA,* 1998, 95, 6965–6970.
[46] Fisher, JS; Millar, MR; Majdic, G; Saunders, PT; Fraser, HM; Sharpe, RM. Immunolocalisation of estrogen receptor-alpha within the testis and excurrent ducts of the rat and marmoset monkey from perinatal life to adulthood. *Journal of Endocrinol*ogy, 1997, 153, 485-495.
[47] Foucault, P; Carreau, S; Kuczynski, W; Guillaumin, JM; Bardos, P; Drosdowsky, MA. The human Sertoli cells in vitro: lactate, estradiol-17ß and transferrin productions. *Journal of Andrology,* 1992, 13, 361–367.
[48] Franco, R; Boscia, F; Gigantino, V; Marra, L; Esposito, F; Ferrara, D; Pariante, P; Botti, G; Caraglia, M; Minucci, S; Chieffi, P. GPR30 is overexpressed in post-puberal testicular germ cell tumors. *Cancer BiologyTherapy*, 2011, *11*, 609-613.
[49] Fraser, LR; Beyret, E; Milligan, SR; Adeoya-Osiguwa, SA. Effects of estrogenic xenobiotics on humanand mouse spermatozoa. *Human Reproduction*, 2006, 21,1184–1193.
[50] Galeraud-Denis, I; Lambard, S; Carreau, S. Relationshipbetween chromatin organization, mRNAs profile and human male gamete quality. *Asian Journal of Andrology*, 2007, 9, 587–592.
[51] Galeraud-Denis, I; de Vienne, CM; Said, L; Chocat, A; Carreau S. Differential expression of aromatase in human spermatozoa from normozoospermic and teratozoospermic patients. *International Journal of Andrology*, 2008, 31, 1.
[52] Gancarczyk, M; Paziewska, A; Carreau, S; Bilinska, B. Dose and photoperiod-dependent effect of 17β-estradiol or ICI 182,780 administration on testicular structure, acceleration of spermatogenesis and aromatase immunoexpression in immature bank voles. *Acta Histochemica,* 2004, 106, 269-278.
[53] Godet, M; Thomas, A; Rudkin, BB; Durand, P. Developmental changes in cyclin B1 and cyclin-dependent kinase 1 (CDK1) levels in the different populations of spermatogenic cells of the post-natal rat testis. *European Journal of Cell Biol*ogy 2000, 79, 816-823.
[54] Gromoll, J; Wessels, J; Rosiepen, G; Brinkworth, MH; Weinbauer, GF. Expression of mitotic cyclin B1 is not confined to proliferating cells in the rat testis. *Biology of Reproduction,* 1997, 57, 1312-1319.
[55] Gur, Y; Breitbart, H. Protein synthesis in sperm: dialogbetween mitochondria and cytoplasm. *Molecular and Cellular Endocrinology*, 2008, 282, 45–55.
[56] Hamden, K; Silandre, D; Delalande, C; El Feki, A; Carreau, S. Protective effects of estrogens and caloric restriction during aging on various rat testis parameters. *Asian Journal of Andrology,* 2008, 10, 837–845.

[57] Heldring, N; Pike, A; Andersson, S; Matthews, J; Cheng, G; Hartman, J; Tujague, M; Ström, A;Treuter, E; Warner, M; Gustafsson, JA. Estrogen receptors: how do they signal and what are their targets. *Physiological Reviews*, 2007, 87, 905-931.

[58] Hendry, WF; Parslow, JM; Stedronska, J. Exploratory scrotomy in 168 azoospermic males. *British Journal of Urology,* 1983, 55, 785-791.

[59] Hess, R.A; Bunick, D; Lee, KH.; Bahr, J; Taylor, J A; Korach, KS; Lubahn, DB.A role for oestrogens in the male reproductive system. *Nature*,1997, 390, 509–51260.

[60] Hess, R.A. The efferent ductules: structure and functions. B. Robaire and B. Hinton. In *"The epididymis: from molecules to clinical practice"*"New York, NJ: Kluwer Academic. 2002, 49–80.

[61] Hess, RA. Estrogen in the adult male reproductive tract: a review. *Reproductive Biology and Endocrinogy,* 2003, 9, 52.

[62] Hess, RA; Carnes, K. The role of estrogen in the testis and the male reproductive tract: a review. *Animal Reproduction*, 2004, 1, 5-30.

[63] Inkster, S; Yue, W; Brodie, A. Human testicular aromatase: immunocytochemical and biochemical studies. *Journal of Clinical Endocrinology and Metabolism*, 1995, 6, 1941-1947.

[64] Isensee, J; Meoli, L; Zazzu, V; Nabzdyk, C; Witt, H; Soewarto, D; Effertz, K; Fuchs, H; Gailus-Durner, V; Busch, D; Adler, T; de Angelis, MH; Irgang, M; Otto, C; Noppinger, PR; Expression pattern of G protein-coupled receptor 30 in LacZ reporter mice. *Endocrinology,* 2009, 150, 1722-1730.

[65] Jayle, MF ; Scholler, RA ; Sfikalis, A ; Héron, M. Excrétion des phénolstéroïdes et des 17 cétostéroïdes après administration de gonadotrophines chorioniques à des hommes. *Clinica Chemica Acta,* 1962, 7, 212-220.

[66] Jones, MEE; Boon, WC; McInnes, K; Maffei, L; Carani, C; Simpson, ER. Recognizing rare disorders: aromatase deficiency. *Nature Clinical Practise Endocrinology and Metabolism,* 2007, 3, 414-421.

[67] Kopera, I; Szczepanowicz, M; Gizejewski, Z; Sadowska, J; Bilinska, B. Immunoexpression of aromatase in immature and adult males of the European bison (Bison bonasus, Linnaeus 1758). *Reproduction Domestic Animal,* 2008, 45, 269-274.

[68] Kotula-Balak, M; Slomczynska, M; Fraczek, B; Bourguiba, S; Tabarowsk, Zi; Carreau, S; Bilinska, B. Complementary approaches demonstrate that cellular aromatization in the bank vole testis is related to photoperiod. *European Journal of Histochemistry,* 2003, 47, 55-62.

[69] Kurosumi, M; Ishimura, K; Fujita, H; Osawa Y. Immunocytochemical localization of aromatase in rat testis. *Histochemistry*, 1985, 83, 401-404.

[70] Lambard, S; Galeraud-Denis, I; Bouraima, H; Bourguiba, S; Chocat, A; Carreau, S. Expression of aromatase in human ejaculated spermatozoa: a putative marker of motility. *Molecular Human* Repro*duction*, 2003, 9, 117-124.

[71] Lambard, S; Galeraud-Denis, I; Saunders, PT; Carreau, S. Human immature germ cells and ejaculated spermatozoa contain aromatase and oestrogen receptors. *Journal of Molecular Endocrinology,* 2004a, 32, 279-289.

[72] Lambard, S, Galeraud-Denis I, Martin, G; Levy, A; Chocat, A; Carreau, S. Analysis and significance of messenger RNAs in human ejaculated spermatozoa from normospermic donors: relation to sperm motility and capacitation. *Molecular Human Reproduction*, 2004b, 10 535-541.

[73] Lambard, S; Carreau, S. Aromatase and oestrogens in human male germ cells *International Journalof Andrology*, 2005, 28, 254-259.

[74] Lanzino, M; Catalano, S; Genissel, C; Ando, S; Carreau, S; Hamra, K; McPhaul, J. Aromatase messenger RNA is derived from the proximal promoter of the aromatase gene in Leydig, Sertoli, and germ cells of the rat testis. *Biology of Reproduction,* 2001,64,1439-1443.

[75] Levallet, J; Carreau, S. Aromatase gene expression in rat testicular cells. *C R Acad Sc Paris*1997, 320,123-129.

[76] Levallet, J; Bilinska, B; Mittre, H; Genissel, C; Fresnel, J; Carreau, S. Expression and immunolocalization of functional cytochrome P450 aromatase in mature rat testicular cells. *Biology of Reproduction*, 1998a, 58, 919-926.

[77] Levallet, J; Delarue, B; Mittre, H; Carreau, S. Alternative splicing events in the coding region of cytochrome P450 aromatase in adult male rat germ cells. *Journal of Molecular Endocrinology,*1998b, 20, 305-312.

[78] Levin, ER. G protein-coupled receptor 30: estrogen receptor or collaborator? *Endocrinology,* 2009, 150, 1563-1565.

[79] Li, X; Rahman, N. Impact of androgen/estrogen ratio: lessons learned from the aromatase over-expression mice. *General and Comparative Endocrinology*, 1998, 159,1-9.

[80] Liu, D; Matzuk, MM; Sung, WK; Guo, Q; Wang, P; Wolgemuth, DJ. Cyclin A1 is required for meiosis in the male mouse. *Nature Genetic,* 1998, 20, 377-380.

[81] Lubahn, DB; Moyer, JS; Golding, TS; Couse, JF; Korach, KS; Smithies, O. Alteration of reproductive function but not prenatal sexual development after insertional disruption of the mouse estrogen receptor gene. *Proceedings National Academy Sciences USA* 1993, 90, 11162–11166.

[82] Lucas, TF; Siu, ER; Esteves, CA; Monteiro, HP; Oliveira, CA; Porto, CS; Lazari, MF. 17 beta-estradiol induces the translocation of the estrogen receptors ERS1 and ERS2 to the cell membrane, MAPK3/1 phosphorylation and proliferation of cultured immature rat Sertoli cells. *Biology of Reproduction,* 2008, 78,101-114.

[83] Lucas, T.F.G, Royer, C., Siu, E.R., Lazari, M.F.M., Porto, C.S., Expression and signaling of G protein-coupled estrogen receptor 1 (GPER) in rat Sertoli cells. *Biology of ReprodUction* 2010, 83, 307-317.

[84] Luconi, M; Francavilla, F; Porazzi, I; Macerola, B; Forti, G; Baldi, E. Human spermatozoa as a model for studying membrane receptors mediating rapid nongenomic effects of progesterone and estrogens. *Steroids*, 2004,69, 553-559.

[85] Maffei, L; Rochira, V; Zirilli, L; Antunez, P; Aranda, C; Fabre, B; Simone, ML; Pignatti, E; Simpson, ER; Houssami, S; Clyne, CD; Carani, C.A novel compound heterozygous mutation of the aromatase gene in an adult man: reinforced evidence on the relationship between congenital oestrogen deficiency, adiposity and the metabolic syndrome. *Clinical Endocrinology (Oxf),* 2007 67, 218-224.

[86] Martins, RP; Krawetz, S.A. RNA in human sperm. *Asian Journal of Andrology*, 2005, 7, 1–4.

[87] Miller, D; Ostermeier, GC. Towards a better understandingof RNA carriage by ejaculate spermatozoa. *Human Reproduction Update*, 2006, 12, 757–767.

[88] Mutembei, H; Pesch, S; Schuler, G; Hoffmann, B. Expression of oestrogen receptors alpha and beta and of aromatase in the testis of immature and mature Boars. *Reproductive Domestic Animimal,* 2005, 40, 228-236.

[89] Nakazumi, H; Sasano, H; Maehara, I; Ozaki, M; Tezukaa, F; Orikasa, S. Estrogen metabolism and impaired spermatogenesis in germ cell tumors of the testis. *Journal of Clinical Endocrinology and Metabolism,*1996, 81, 1289-1295.

[90] Naz, RK. Effect of actinomycine D and cycloheximideon human sperm function. *Archives of Andrology*, 1998, 41,135–142.

[91] Nitta, H; Bunick, D; Hess, RA; Janulis, L; Newton, SC; Milette, CF; Osawa, Y; Shizuta, Y; Toda, K; Bahr, JM. Germ cells of the mouse testis express P450 aromatase. *Endocrinology,*1993, 132,1396-1401.

[92] O'Donnell, L; Robertson, KM; Jones, MEE; Simpson, ER. Estrogen and spermatogenesis. *Endocrine Reviews,* 2001, 22, 289-318.

[93] Oliva, R. Protamines and male infertility. *Human Repoduction Update*,2006,12, 417–435.

[94] Pagano, M; Pepperkok, U; Verde, F ; Ansorge, W ; Draetta, G. Cyclin A1 is required at two points in the human cell cycle. *EMBO Journal* 1992, 11, 961-971.

[95] Papadopoulos, V; Carreau, S; Szerman-Joly, E; Drosdowsky, MA; Dehennin, L; Scholler, R Rat testis 17ß-estradiol: identification by gas-chromatography-mass spectrometry and age-related cellular distribution. *Journal of Steroid Biochemistry,* 1986, 24,1211-1216.

[96] Payne, AH; Kelch, RP; Musich, SS; Halpern, ME. Intratesticular site of aromatization in the human. *Journal of Clinical Endocrinology and Metabolism,* 1976, 42,1081-1087.

[97] Pentikaïnen, V; Erkkilä, K; Suomalainen, L; Otala, M; Pentikaïnen, MO; Parvinen, M; Dunkel, L. Estradiol acts as a germ cell survival factor in the human testsi in vitro. *Journal of Clinical Endocrinology and Metabolism,* 2000, 85, 2057-2067.

[98] Pereyra-Martinez, AC; Roselli, CE; Stadelman, HL; Resko, JA. Cytochrome P450 aromatase in testis and epididymis of male *rhesus* monkeys. *Endocrine,* 2001, 16, 15-19.

[99] Perrard, MH; Durand, P. Redundancy of the effcet of TGFbeta1 and beta-NGF on the second meiotic division of rat spermatocytes. *Microscopy Research and Technics,* 2009, 72, 596-602.

[100] Prossnitz, ER; Aterburn, JB; Smith, HO; Oprea, TI; Sklar, LA; Hathaway, HJ. Estrogen signaling through the transmembrane G protein-coupled receptor GPR30. *Annual Review Physiology*, 2008, 70, 165-190.

[101] Prossnitz, ER; Baton, M. The G-protein-coupled estrpogen receptor GPER in health and disease. *Nature Reviews Endocrinology* 2011, DOI: 10.1038/nrendo.2011.122.

[102] Raeside, JJ; Renaud, RL. Estrogen and andogen production by purified Leydig cells from mature boars. *Biology of Reproduction*, 1983, 28,727-733.

[103] Revelli, A; Massobrio, M, Tesarik, J. Nongenomic actions of steroid hormones in reproductive tissues. *Endocrine Reviews,*1998, 19, 3-17.

[104] Rochira, V; Granata, ARM; Madeo, B; Zirilli, L; Rossi, G; Carani, C. Estrogens in males: what we have learned in last 10 years? *Asian Journal of Andrology,* 2005, 7, 3-20.

[105] Rochira, V; Carani, C. Aromatase deficiency in men: a clinical perspective. *Nature Reviews Endocrinology,* 2009, 5, 559–568.

[106] Roger, C; Lambard, S; Bouskine, A; Mograbi, B; Chevallier, D; Nebout, M; Pointis, G; Carreau, S; Fenichel, P. Estrogen-induced growth inhibition of human seminoma cells expressing estrogen receptor beta and aromatase. *Journal of Molecular Endocrinol*ogy, 2005, 35, 191-199.
[107] Robertson, KM; O'Donnell, L; Jones, MEE; Meachem, SJ; Boon, WC; Fisher, CR; Graves, KH; McLachlan, RI; Simpson, ER Impairment of spermatogenesis in mice lacking a functional aromatase (cyp 19) gene. *Proceedings National Academy Sciences USA,* 1999, 96,7986-7991.
[108] Robertson, K.M., O'Donnell, L., Simpson, E.R., Jones, M.E.E., 2002. The phenotype of the aromatase knockout mouse reveals dietary phytoestrogens impact significantly on testis function. *Endocrinology* 143, 2913-2921.
[109] Rommerts, FF; de Jong, FH; Brinkmann, AO; van der Molen, HJ. Development and cellular localization of rat testicular aromatase activity. *Journal of Reproduction and Fertility* 1982, 65, 281-288.
[110] Saez, JM. Leydig cells: endocrine, paracrine and autocrine regulation. *Endocrine Reviews*, 1994, 15, 574-626.
[111] Saunders, PT; Millar, MR; Macpherson, S;Irvine, DS; Groome, NP; Evans, LR; Sharpe, RM; Scobie, GA. ERbeta1 and the ERbeta2 splice variant (ERbetacx/beta2) are expressed in distinct cell populations in the adult human testis. *Journal of Clinical Endocrinology and Metabolism*, 2002, 87, 2706-2715.
[112] Sebastian, S; Bulun, SE.A highly complex organization of the regulatory region of the human CYP19 (aromatase) gene revealed by the Human genome project. *Journal of Clinical Endocrinology and Metabolism*, 2001, 86, 4600-4602.
[113] Schon, J; Blottner, S. Estrogens are involved in seasonal regulation of spermatogenesis and sperm maturation in roe deer (Capreolus capreolus). *General and Comparative Endocrinology,* 2008, 159, 257-263.
[114] Shetty, G; Krishnamurthy, H; Krishnamurthy, HN;Bhatnagar, AS; Moudgal, NR. Effect of long-term treatment with aromatase inhibitor on testicular function of adult male bonnet monkeys (M. radiata). *Steroids,* 1998, 63, 414-420.
[115] Sierens, JE; Sneddon, SF; Collins, F; Millar, MR; Saunders, PT. Estrogens in Testis Biology. *Annals New York Academy of Sciences,* 2005, 1061, 65-76.
[116] Silandre, D; Delalande, C; Durand, P; Carreau, S. Three promoters PII, PI.f and PI. tr direct the expression of aromatase (cyp19) gene in male rat grem cells. *Journal of Molecular Endocrinology,* 2007, 39, 169-181.
[117] Simpson, ER; Mahendroo, MS; Means, GD; Kilgore, MW; Hinshelwood, MM; Graham-Lorence, S; Amarneh, B; Ito, Y; Fisher, CR; Michael, MD; Mendelson CR; Bulun, SE. Aromatase cytochrome P450, the enzyme responsible for estrogen biosynthesis. *Endocrine Reviews,*1984, 15, 342-355.
[118] Simpson, ER; Zhao, Y; Agarwal, VR; Michael, MD; Bulun, SE; Hinshelwood, MM; Graham-Lorence, S; Sun, T; Fisher, CR; Qin, K; Mendelson, CR. Aromatase expression in health and disease. *Recent Progress in Hormone Research* 1997, 52,185-212.
[119] Sirianni, R; Chimento, A; Ruggiero, C; de Luca, A; Lappano, R; Ando, S; Maggiolini, M; Pezzi, V. The Novel Estrogen Receptor, G Protein-Coupled Receptor 30, Mediates the Proliferative Effects Induced by 17{beta}-Estradiol on Mouse Spermatogonial GC-1 Cell Line. *Endocrinology,* 2008,149, 5043-5051.

[120] Sipahutar, H; Sourdaine, P; Moslemi, S; Plainfossé, B; Seralini, GE. Immunolocalization of aromatase in stallion Leydig cells and seminiferous tubules. *Journal of Histochemistry and Cytochemistry,*2003, 51, 311-318.

[121] Skakkebaek, NE. Male reproductive health and environmental xenoestrogens. *Environmental Health Perspectives,* 1996, 104, 741-803.

[122] Skakkebaek, NE. Testicular dysgenesis syndrome: new epidemiological evidence. *International Journal of Andrology,* 2004, 27, 189–201.

[123] Smith, EP; Boyd, J; Frank, GR; Takahashi, H; Cohen, RM; Specker, B; Williams, TC; Lubahn, DB; Korach, KS. Estrogen resistance caused by a mutation in the estrogen-receptor gene in a man. *New England Journal of Medicine,* 1994, 331, 1056–1061.

[124] Solakidi S, Psarra AMG, Nikolaropoulos S, Sekeris CE. Estrogen receptors alpha and beta (ERalpha and ERbeta) and androgen receptor (AR) in human sperm: localization of ERbeta and AR in mitochondria of the midpiece. *Human Reproduction*, 2005;20, 3481–3485.

[125] Toppari, J; Larsen, JC; Christiansen, P; Giwercman, A; Grandjean, P; Guillette, LJ Jr, Jegou, B; Jensen, TK; Jouannet, P; Keiding, N; Leffers, H; McLachlan, JA; Meyer, O; Muller, J; Rajpert-De Meyts, E; Scheike, T; Sharpe, RM; Sumpter, J; Skakkebaek, NE Male reproductive health and environmental xenoestrogens. *Environmental Health Perspectives* 1996, 104, 741-803.

[126] Toppari, J; Virtanen, HE; Main, KM; Skakkebaek, NE. Cryptorchidism and hypospadias as a sign of testicular dysgenesis syndrome(TDS): environmental connection. *Birth Defects Research A Clinical Molecular Teratology*, 2010, 88, 910-919.

[127] Tsubota, T; Howell-Skalla, L; Nitta, H; Mason, JI; Meiers, PG; Nelson, RA; Bahr, JM. *Journal of Reprouctive. Fertilility,* 1997, 109, 21-27.

[128] van Pelt, AM; de Rooij, DJ; van der Burg, B; van der Saag, PT; Gustafsson, JA; Kuiper, GG. Ontogeny of estrogen receptor-beta expression in rat testis. *Endocrinology,* 1999, 140, 478-483.

[129] Wiszniewska, B. Primary culture of rat epididymal epithelial cells as a source of estrogen. *Andrologia*, 2002, 34, 1-8

[130] Wolgemuth, DJ; Lele, KM; Jobanputra, V; Salazar, G.. The A-type cyclins and the meiotic cell cycle in mammalian male germ cells. *International Journal of Andrology,* 2004, 27, 192-199.

[131] Yamada-Mouri, N; Hirata, S; Kato, J. Existence and expression of the untranslated first exon of aromatase mRNA in the rat brain. *Journal of Steroid Biochemistry and Molecular Biology,* 1996,58,163-166.

[132] Zirilli, L ; Rochira, V; Diazzi, C ; Caffagni, G ; Carani, C. Human models of aromatase deficiency. *Journal of Steroid Biochemistry and Molecular Biology*2008, 109, 212–218.

[133] Zondek, B. Mass excretion of oestrogenic hormone in the urine of the stallion. *Nature (London)*, 1934, 193, 209-210.

In: Testis: Anatomy, Physiology and Pathology
Editors: Yoichi Nemoto and Norio Inaba
ISBN: 978-1-61942-739-6

Chapter 5

BETA ACTIN: ITS IMPLICATION IN THE SEMINIFEROUS TUBULE

A. Losinno[1], L. Lopez[1], F. Capani[2], M. Foscolo[1], J. Ibañez[1], and J.C. Cavicchia[1,*]

[1]Institute of de Histology and Embryology, Medical School, Cuyo National University and CONICET, National Research Council of Argentina, Mendoza, Argentina

[2]Instituto de Investigaciones Cardiológicas "Prof. Dr. Alberto C. Taquini (ININCA), Medical School, Buenos Aires National University, Buenos Aires, Argentina

ABSTRACT

Junctional devices in Sertoli cells play a key role in maturation and differentiation of germ cells. However, the cellular and subcellular organization of these specializations are still not totally understood. By combining light and electron microscopic techniques using β-actin immunolabeling and prosaposin and glutaredoxin antibodies to label Sertoli cytoplasm, we observed the structural (by confocal microscopy) and fine structural (by electron microscopy) organization of tight and adherent junctions, which are the morphological substrate of the blood testis barrier (BTB). The association to the beta actin also characterizes ectoplasmic specializations (ES) found at two different levels of the seminiferous epithelium. We also used freeze fracture to analyze the characteristics of tubular bulbar complexes (TBC), a known component of apical ectoplasmic specializations. These different approaches also allowed us to study the complex arrangement of the actin cytoskeleton of Sertoli cells branches, which surround germ cells in different stages of the spermatogenic cycle. Our results show a consistent labelling for β-actin before, during and after the release of spermatozoa in the tubular lumen (spermiation) suggesting a significant role of the actin network in spermatic cell differentiation. In conclusion, significant interrelations among the β-actin network, the junctional complexes of the BTB and the ectoplasmic specializations were detected at different stages of the seminiferous cycle.

[*] Corresponding author: Juan Carlos Cavicchia, MD. Institute of Histology and Embryology (IHEM), Medical School, Cuyo National University and CONICET (National Research Council of Argentina.) 5500 Mendoza, Argentina. E-mail: jccavic@fcm.uncu.edu.ar.

Keywords: β-actin, ectoplasmic specializations, Sertoli cell, seminiferous epithelium

INTRODUCTION

The network of actin filaments is one of the cytoskeletal structures contributing to the morphological framework of a cell. Actin is a ubiquitous protein that is able to form polar filamentous structure which constitutes the major part of the cytoskeleton of eukaryotic cell. Intracellular actin is present in monomer form (G-actin) or polymerized filament form (F-actin). Once it reaches a critical concentration, G-actin (with the cooperation of ATP) forms F-actin and eventually reaches a steady state. At the steady state, ATP will be hydrolyzed into ADP and the length of filament will become stable [1]. Actin filaments form contractile and protrusive structures that play central roles in many processes such as cell migration, morphogenesis, endocytosis, cytokines [2] and synaptic plasticity [3,4]. During these processes, the dynamics of the actin filaments are tightly regulated by a large array of actin-binding proteins. A number of proteins that regulate actin cytoskeleton have been identified, including cofilin, also named actin depolymerization factor (Arp 2/3) and formins [5,6,7,8,9,10,11]. Arp2/3 complex is active at the leading edge of motile cells, where it produces branches on the sides of existing filaments. Of the known actin isoforms, alfa, beta and gamma actin, alfa integrates the main component of the thin filament of the mioide, peritubular or interlamellar cell and beta actin is located in the cytoplasm cortex, near the plasma membrane in Sertoli cells and also, but in less amount, in germ cells [12,13]. In the seminiferous tubules, beta actin also plays a key role during spermatogenesis, moreover, each component of the cytoskeleton (beta actin, intermediated filaments and microtubules) interact with intercellular junctions. Although Sertoli junctions were previously described, the cellular and subcellular organization of these specializations during the maturation of sperm cells is not totally understood. In this work we focused on the beta actin network, a main component of the cytoskeleton that in Sertoli cells is concentrated in unique structures termed ectoplasmic specializations. By combining light and electron microscopic techniques using β-actin with prosaposin or glutaredoxin antibodies (to stain Sertoli cytoplasm) we observed the structural (confocal microscopy) and ultrastructural (electron microscopy) organization of tight and adherent junctions, which are the morphologic substrate of the blood testis barrier (BTB), their association to ectoplasmic specializations in the seminiferous epithelium and altogether associated to a complex network of beta actin.

The term BTB originated by early physiological studies of Setchell [14] and Setchell and Waites [15] in the mammalian testis. They demonstrated a differential transport of ions and metabolites between the basal area of the seminiferous tubules, the *basal compartment*, in wide contact with body fluids and the apical sector of the seminiferous epithelium, the *adluminal compartment*, close to the tubular lumen and isolated by the barrier. The morphological correlate of such a barrier was found to be located in specialized junctional devices found between the adjacent Sertoli cells, integrated by occluding or tight junctions that seal each inter-Sertoli space near the base of the seminiferous epithelium [16, 17].

Related to the last mentioned topic is the long-time discussed existence of a third compartment in the seminiferous epithelium [18]. The early interpretations of Russell [19,20,21] on the rat BTB were superseded by our observations on monkeys [22,23] as we showed that the impermeable junctions assemble and disassemble simultaneously without forming an actual compartment. Later, in the rat, using intratubular administration of intercellular tracers we arrived at a similar conclusion [24].

The second junctional device found in the seminiferous epithelium is the *zonula adherens*, mainly made by a dense circumferential belt of beta actin filaments near the Sertoli cell membranes and located at two levels: 1) at the BTB level, located in the Sertoli cytoplasm close to tight junctions and surrounding a smooth cistern of the endoplasmic reticulum [16] and 2) higher in the epithelium, in close apposition to germ cells in progressive steps of differentiation (round and elongate spermatids) [25]. These two junctional devices, as a whole, were termed Sertoli cell ectoplasmic specializations (ES) by Russell [20].

Another junctional device found in ES at the two described levels, is the so-called tubular bulbar complexes [26,27]. At the higher place of Sertoli-germ cell contacts, they are elongate processes developed from the spermatid plasma membrane surrounded by a deep invagination of the Sertoli cell membrane and a specialized layer of Sertoli cell cytoplasm. This layer contains abundant bundles of β-actin filaments surrounding the whole extension of the invagination. These tubular bulbar complexes have been found to develop in the regions previously occupied by the ectoplasmic specializations and have been proposed to internalize intact junctions during spermiation [28]. Thus, these complexes are likely significant participants in the mechanism of junctional turnover in the seminiferous epithelium [29].

The cited turnover is related to the well-known endocytic activity of Sertoli cells, residual body formation, their phagocytic activity during spermiation and Sertoli lysosome types including multivesicular bodies (MVB) or multivesicular endosomes (MVE) [30] and secondary lysosomes [31]. Significant progress has been made in the understanding of the mechanisms that regulate multivesicular endosomes transport and the degradation pathway that leads to lysosome formation since the classic study that observed a maximum number of lysosomes marked by acid phosphatase in stages V-VIII of the seminiferous tubules, close to spermiation. [32] (Chemes,1986).

Recently, experimental evidence has been accumulating on the regulation and functional significance of the ectoplasmic specializations (ES) of Sertoli cells [33,34,35]. The simultaneous occurrence of the transit of new germ cells through the BTB and the process of spermiation has been put into a theoretical scheme in which these two cellular events are coordinated by the release of defined protein products, and the presence of an apical ES—BTB—hemidesmosome axis in the Sertoli cell is put forward as a crucial element in the coordination of these events [35].

Although the actin network was previously described in Sertoli junctional devices [31] its role in the subcellular organization of BTB and ectoplasmic specializations at different stages of the seminiferous cycle has not been thoroughly investigated, and its significance in present schemes of spermatogenesis is not well understood.

Then, the main objective of this paper is to report our findings about the cellular and fine structural organization of intercellular junctions rich in beta actin and its possible role in germ cell maturation, differentiation and migration towards the lumen of the seminiferous epithelium.

Animals: all studies involving experimental animals were conducted in accordance with the Ethical Board of the School of Medicine of the National University of Cuyo, Mendoza, Argentina. Animals were handled according to the procedures approved for the UFAW

Handbook on the Care and Management of Laboratory Animals and other Research Animals [36].

Western blot analysis: beta actin was quantified (Western blot technique) in relation to the spermiation period in different segments of the seminiferous tubules visualized by transillumination under stereomicroscopy. These approaches allowed us to study the complex arrangement of beta actin cytoskeleton in Sertoli cells branches that surround germ cells in different tubules.

Rats of the Wister strain of two months of age were used. Testes were removed under Nembutal anesthesia and place in PBS buffer at cold temperature (under ice) to avoid protein degradation. The tunica albuguinea was surgically removed and the seminiferous tubules were carefully separated according to the technique of Christensen and Mason [37] using delicate glass rods. Seminiferous tubule segments were classified according to the criteria of Parvinen and Vanha Perttula [38] and cut using a Zeiss stereomicroscope provided with transillumination. The selected segments correspond to stages II-III of the seminiferous cycle (pre-spermiation stages), stages VII-VIII (spermiation stages) and stages IX-X (post-spermiation stages). A total of 100 mm of seminiferous tubules were required to obtain enough protein for the western blot analysis. The samples were homogenized in the same volume of the lyses buffer containing 0.6 M KCl and a protease inhibitor cocktail. Then, the samples underwent a series of successive liquid nitrogen freezing and de-freezing at room temperature. The material so obtained was centrifuged at 20000 RPM for 20 min at 4°C and frozen and stored at -20°C.

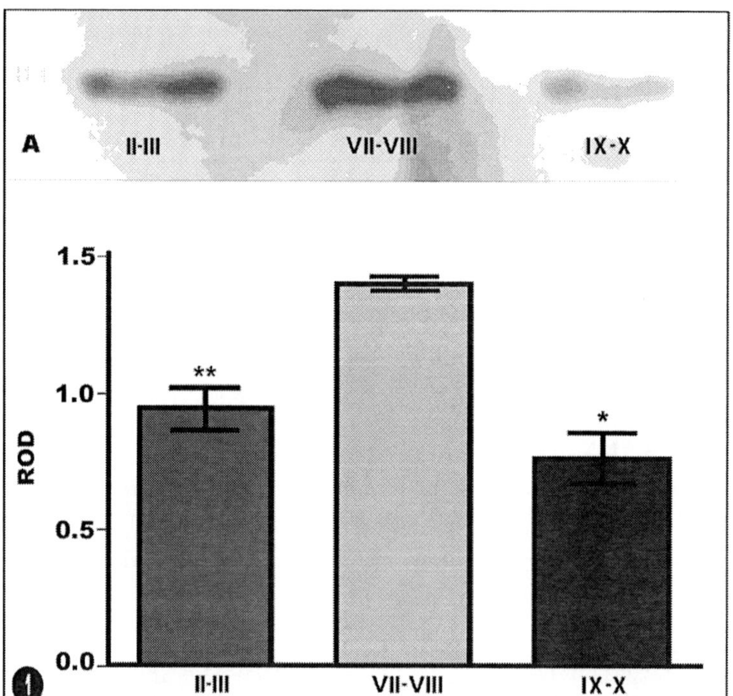

Figure 1. Western blot analysis. Bars indicate (from left to right) stages II-III (pre spermiation), VII-VIII (spermiation) and IX-X (post spermiation). Note the increase of beta actin in the spermiation stages. A: Western blot bands in the tree stage sets normalized for GAPDH expression and quantified by optical densitometry. ROD, relative optical density. $^{*}p \leq 0.05$, $^{**}p \leq 0.01$.

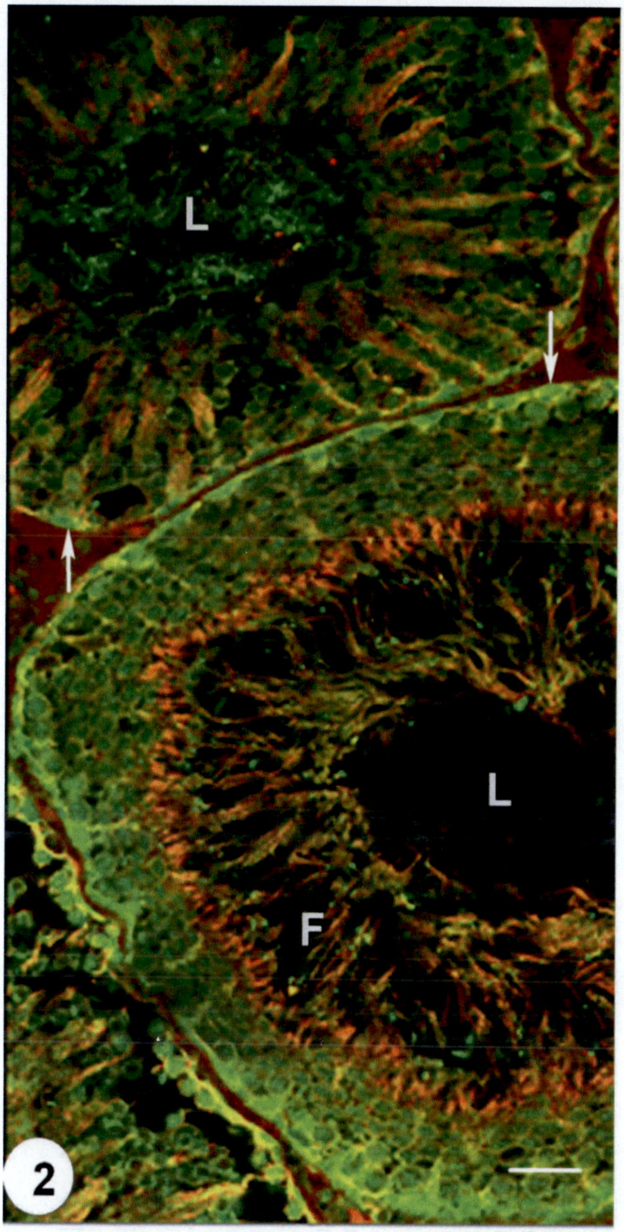

Figure 2. Two seminiferous tubules are shown in cross section at low magnification. The immune stain for β-actin is observed in orange-yellow colour, for prosaposin in green. They clearly exhibit diametrically opposite seminiferous stage situations. The one located below in the figure shows elongate spermatids with flagella (F) that protrude into the lumen. It indicates a pre-spermiation stage very close to spermation. Note the intense beta actin mark in the apical part of the epithelium. The other located above in the figure displays elongate spermatids located in deep infolding of Sertoli cells closer to the basal lamina and thus to the BTB marked with β-actin (which is hardly seen in this low magnification). This indicates a post spermiation stage. Arrows: Basal lamina. L, lumen of the seminiferous tubules. Bar = 25 μm.

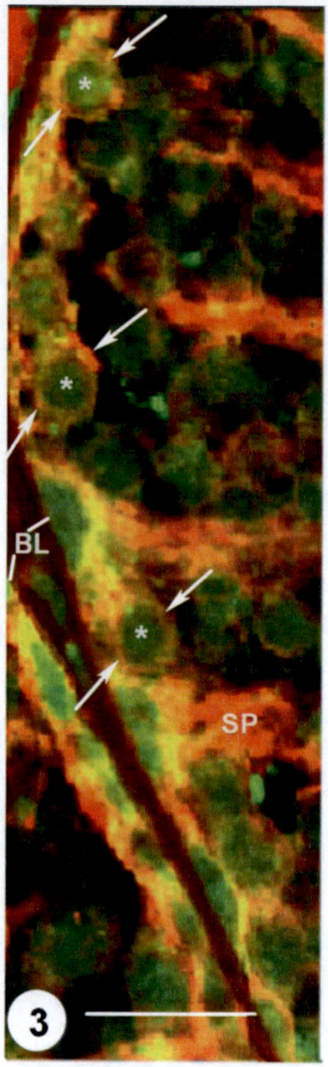

Figure 3. It shows at higher magnification spermatids (SP) located closer to the BTB. In this particular stage beta actin clearly depicts the BTB. Note that the orange-yellow stain (arrows) partly surrounds early spermatocytes (asterisks). Bar = 25 μm.

The proteins of the samples were separated using a 7.5% electrophoresis gel (SDS-PAGE). Each sample (10 μl) was loaded into the well in the gel. Then, they were transferred from within the gel onto a membrane made of nitrocellulose. Beta actin was identified by the monoclonal antibody anti-beta actin (Sigma, 1/500 dilution). For load control anti-GAPDH (glyceraldehyde 3-phosphate dehydrogenase) (Sigma, 1/200 dilution) was employed. Then, the monoclonal antibodies mouse or rabbit anti-IgG label to radish peroxidase (Jackson, 1/2000, dilution) was used to reveal beta actin in the nitrocellulose membrane. Finally, the (Thermo Scientific) Immune-blot kit was used according to the manufactory instructions. The total beta-actin amount in each segment was estimated by quantifying the band optical densities using the Image J software. Results were expressed as media ± SEM for four experiments. The Student-t test was performed and data significance was processed using the Graphad Prism 5 software. A $P \leq 0.05$ was considered to be statistically significant.

Immunohistochemistry and confocal observations: young male rats of the same strain, bred in our laboratory were used throughout this protocol. They were housed under controlled light (lights-on from 07: 00 to 19: 00 h) and temperature (24 □2ºC) conditions, water and food were provided *ad libitum*. They were anesthetized and perfused through the spermatic artery according to the technique of Dym (1973) with 4% paraformaldehyde in 0.1M phosphate buffer, pH 7.4 for the light microscopic studies. Testes were immersed in the same solution for 2 additional hours, included in paraffin and cut into 10-15 μm thick slices using a conventional microtome. The slices were mounted on sylanized slices [39]. They were incubated overnight in β-actin antibody (1:500 dilution) (Sigma, USA). For colocalized studies they were incubated with prosaposin antibody (1:200 dilution) [40] or glutaredoxin antibodies (1:200) [41, 42] for colocalization studies. Sections were washed several times with PBS and incubated with the proper secondary antibody (Alexa Fluor 546 or 488 from Invitrogen, USA). After several washings in PBS, sections were mounted and examined in a Spectral Confocal Olimpus FV-1000. Collected pictures were analyzed and compiled using Adobe Photoshop 8.0 CS3.

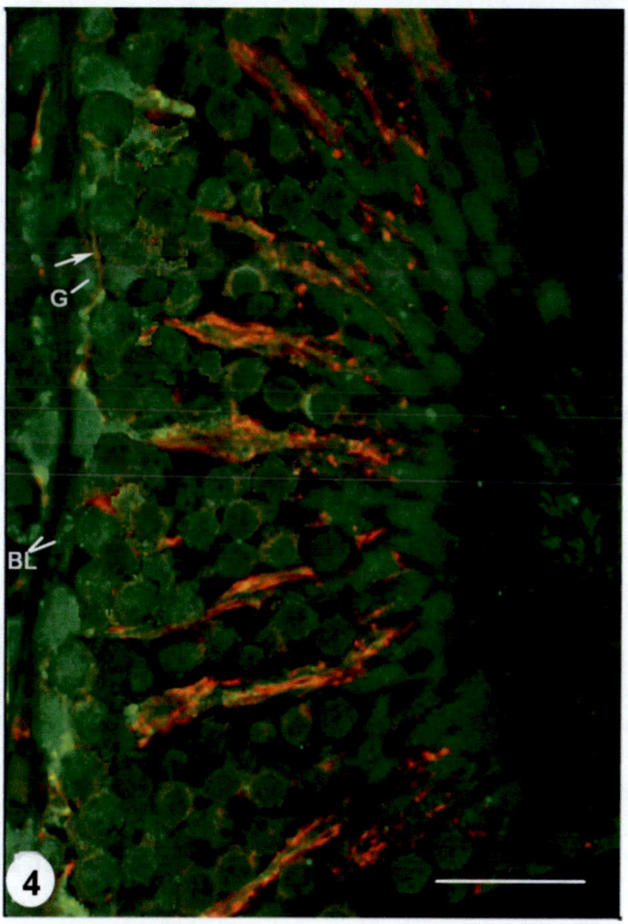

Figure 4. Same immune staining procedure showing a different spermiation stage. In this particular pre-spermiation stage spermatids are located higher in the seminiferous epithelium than in the previous figure. Note that the BTB (arrow) is located above a spermatogonium (G). BL, basal lamina of the seminiferous tubules. Bar = 25 μm.

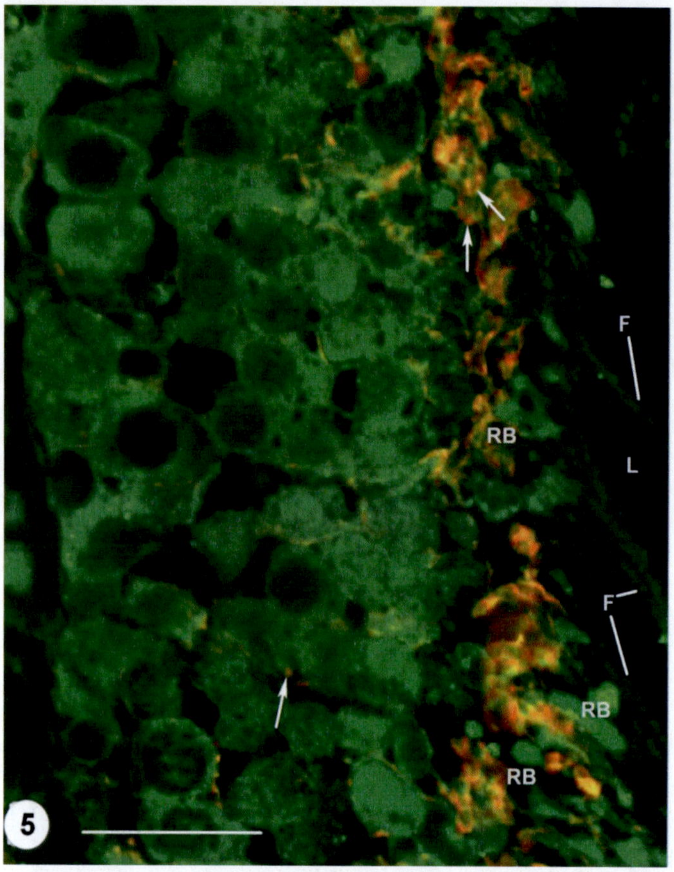

Figure 5. Higher magnification of the colocalization immune staining for β-actin and prosaposin. This figure shows at higher magnification a seminiferous tubule with spermatids located higher in the epithelium in a pre-spermiation stage near spermiation similar to the one shown in the tubule located below in Figure 2. Note the intense actin immune staining surrounding the spermatid heads and numerous spermatid flagella (F) that are protruding into the lumen (L). Residual bodies (RB) are exhibited. Also numerous small dots of β-actin label (arrows), which probably correspond to MVB are clearly depicted. This stage, thus, appears to be VII or VIII (very close to spermiation). Bar = 25 μm.

Epoxy resin sections. electron microscopy: For electron microscopy, after perfusion through the spermatic artery with 4% paraformaldehyde and 0.1% glutaraldehyde in 0.1 M cacodylate buffer, pH 7.4, testes were immersed in the same solution for 2 additional hours and cut using an Oxford vibratome (40 μm thick). The vibratome sections were incubated with the monoclonal anti-beta actin antibody, overnight (same diluted) followed by several wash steps with PBS and incubated with biotinylated anti-mouse secondary antibody for 1 h (Amersham) followed by incubation with ABC complex solution (Vectastain ABC kits, Vector Laboratories Inc., Burlingame, CA, USA) for another 1 h. After washing in PBS, sections were developed with DAB solution until staining was optimal. Then, they were post-fixed in 1% osmium tetroxide in 0.1 M cacodylate buffer for 2h and rinsed in distilled water. Tissue sections were dehydrated in increasing series of ethanol concentrations followed by dry acetone, and embedded in epoxy resin (Durcupan ACM, Fluka, Buchs, Switzerland). Some of the 40 μm sections were mounted and observed with a conventional light microscope. Thin ultra microtome 1μm sections were stained with toluidine blue-sodium borate for light microscopy. Ultrathin sections less than 0.1 µm (silver-gold interference color) were stained with uranyl acetate and lead citrate and examined in a Zeiss EM 900 electron microscope (Carl Zeiss Inc, Berlin, Germany).

Freeze-fracture study: The general procedure followed in this technique was previously reported [43]. In brief, rats were anesthetized and perfused as indicated above for immunohistochemistry. In this case the fixative used was 5% glutaraldehyde in 0.1M sodium cacodylate buffer, pH 7.2-7.4. After perfusion, testes were removed, cut in small pieces and immersed in the same fixative for 2 hr, placed for another 2 hr in 30% glycerol at room temperature (18°C), rapidly frozen in liquid Freon 22 and stored in liquid nitrogen. The material was fractured in a Balzers BAF 301 apparatus at -105°C and shadowed with platinum followed by carbon. Replicas were cleaned with sodium hypochlorite, mounted on copper grids and examined in the same Zeiss electron microscope.

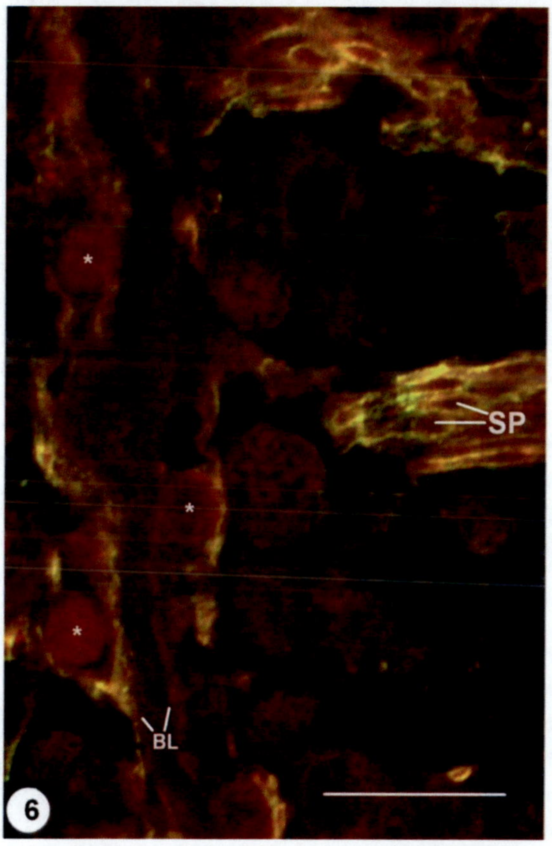

Figure 6. This figure exhibits two seminiferous tubules close to each other and to the basal lamina (BL) of the epithelium in a similar seminiferous stage situation. The immune stain for glutaredoxin is observed in red, the immune stain for β-actin in yellow. In this particular stage the β-actin stain is partially located above or below early spermatocytes (asterisks). For these characteristics these spermatocytes appear to be leptotene-zygotene cells. Also, an intense actin mark surrounds elongated spermatid heads (SP) located deeply into the seminiferous epithelium. The β-actin labelling that surrounds elongate spermatids belongs to adherent junctions of the ectoplasmic specializations and TB complexes located higher than in the BTB. Bar = 25 µm.

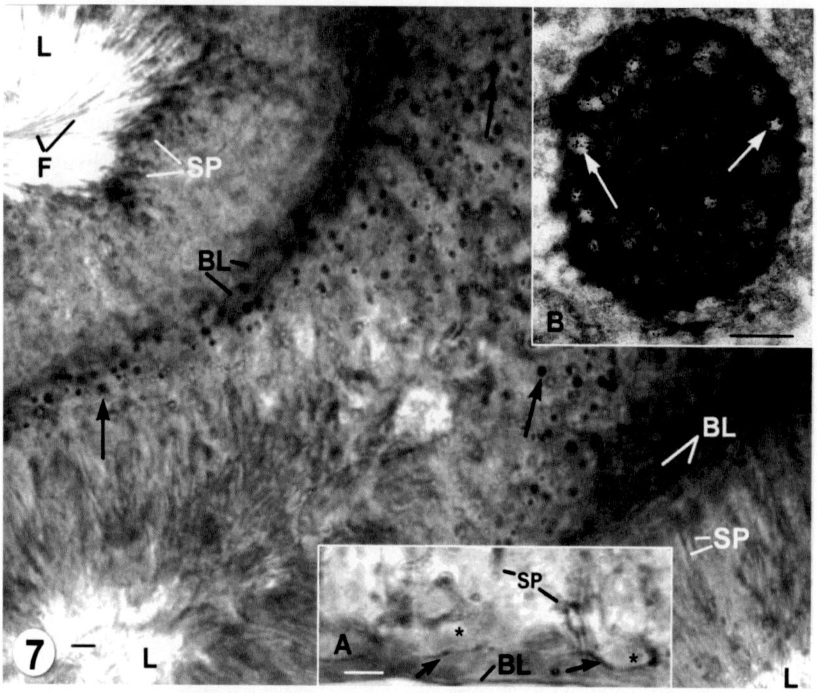

Figure 7. Vibratome 40 micron resin section. It shows at low magnification tree seminiferous tubules. The one to the right exhibits spermatid heads (SP) located in deep infolding of the Sertoli cell similar to the seminiferous tubule in Figure 3. In the central tubule numerous electron dense bodies of beta actin reaction are clearly depicted (arrows). They may correspond to the multivesicular endosomes (MVE). The seminiferous tubule to the left indicates spermatid heads (SP) located higher in the epithelium with their flagella (F) protruding into the lumen (L). Bar = 25 μm. Inset A: It shows at higher magnification a significant area similar to the seminiferous tubule depicted to the right. Spermatids (SP) are also located very close to the BTB (Arrows). The beta actin reaction is clearly observable at this level. Note that the beta actin reaction is located incompletely surrounding early spermatocytes (asterisks). For this features they appear to be leptotene-zygotene cells. Bar = 25 μm. Inset B: It depicts a MVB containing clearly visible β-actin reaction (small dots) Notice that the reaction is mainly located in the MVB vesicles. Bar = 0.5 μm.

The Western blot for beta actin antibody indicates a significant increase during spermiation (Figure 1). The combined immunocytochemistry for β-actin with prosaposin or glutaredoxin antibodies allowed us to observe significant details of the β-actin localization in relation to its height in the seminiferous epithelium using confocal microscopy. Furthermore, the degree of stain, the localization of the BTB in relation to early spermatocytes in pre-spermiation, during spermiation and in post spermiation stages of the seminiferous cycle were determined (Figures 2 to 6). We colocalized β-actin with prosaposin and glutaredoxin since these two last proteins have been well characterized in the seminiferous epithelium and were specially located in the Sertoli cytoplasm [41,42]. In figure 2, in figure 6 and in figure 7, inset A, beta actin staining partially surrounds early spermatocytes at the BHT level; thus, these cells appear to be in the leptotene-zygotene stage of development. When the tubule is observed in a later stage (Figure 4), the mark is observed above the BTB. It clearly stains β-actin associated to Sertoli junctional devices located at this level. In a later stage of development (Figure 5) the immune mark depicts β-actin associated to spermatid-Sertoli ectoplasmic specializations and MVB close to the tubular lumen.

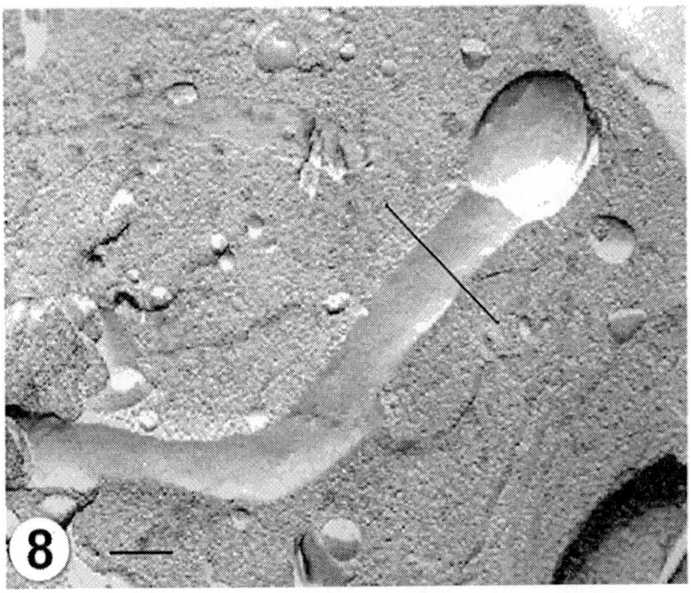

Figure 8. It depicts the freeze fracture image of a tubular bulbar process in longitudinal view. The line that crosses the tubular area corresponds to a similar electron microscopy and a thin section view in cross section is indicated in the next figure. Bar = 0.5 μm.

In forty micron epoxy resin sections of testes immune marked with β-actin, we observed at the light microscopic level, seminiferous tubules in different stages of development. Three seminiferous tubules indicate opposite situations (Figure 7). One tube (right) exhibits spermatid heads located in deep infoldings of the Sertoli cell membrane indicating a post spermiation stage, other (left) shows spermatid heads located higher in the epithelium and spermatid tails protruding into the lumen indicating a pre-spermiation stage. The one in the center exhibits numerous electron dense bodies showing β-actin reaction. They appear to correspond to multivesicular endosomes. By electron microscopy the beta actin localization in the MVE (Figure 7, inset B) is shown into the vesicles.

When tubular bulbar complexes are favorably cleavaged in the testis material they are depicted by freeze fracture exhibiting their characteristic outline (Figure 8) as previously described by scanning electron microscopy [27]. When we compare freeze fracture of this structure with electron microscopy and the beta actin mark, it is clearly shown that the label is seen in the Sertoli cell cytoplasm surrounding the tubular bulbar processes, concentrated between it and the cistern of the smooth reticulum (Figure 9).

Conclusion

Our results show a consistent labelling of β- actin before, during and after the release of spermatozoa in the tubular lumen (spermiation). The Western blot for beta actin antibody indicates a significant increase during spermiation suggesting a significant role of the actin network in spermatic cells differentiation.

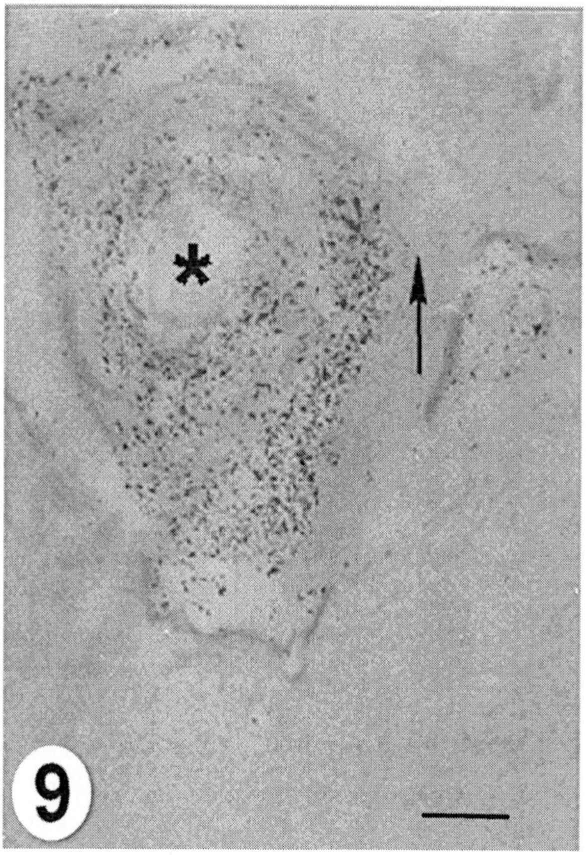

Figure 9. This figure exhibits by electron microscopy and thin sections the immune mark for β-actin surrounding a tubular bulbar process (asterisk) in cross section. Notice that the actin mark is sandwiched between the tubular bulbar process and the smooth cistern of the endoplasmic reticulum (arrow) Bar = 0.5 μm.

Mammalian spermatogenesis is probably the most exquisite example of a spatially organized sequence of cellular associations involving continuous synchronized cell proliferation, differentiation, meiosis, apoptosis, germ translocation, migration and morphogenesis.

Spermatogenesis relies on a population of germ cells capable of self renewal, migration towards the lumen of the seminiferous tubules and differentiation into the male gamete [45]. To maintain close interaction with the surrounded Sertoli cells, both cell lineages possess a well-organized but still poorly understood system of intercellular communications, some of which were explored in the present paper.

The presence of actin in the ectoplasmic specializations in Sertoli cells originally raised the question about its involvement in cell movements related to spermiation, mostly the retraction of Sertoli cell apical cytoplasm. However, accumulated evidence has weakened such a hypothetical role for Sertoli cell actin in these locations. Vogl and Soucy [46]showed that in a glycerinated model of squirrel seminiferous epithelium no evidence of contraction could be shown. Then, Grove and Vogl [47] postulated that actin, in these locations, could have a more structural than mechanical or contractile function since no myosin—based system was detected by immunohistochemistry.

In these two locations, actin consists of the isoform β actin, which forms filament bundles [48]. Actin filaments in each bundle are unipolar and hexagonally packed. The bundles are coupled to the adjacent Sertoli membrane and to each other.

A different kind of function for the actin bundles at ES has emerged from work aimed to elucidate the dynamic state of intercellular junctions. While many studies have been directed towards the identification of adhesion molecules in spermatogenesis studies [35] on the turnover of the elements of cellular junctions have provided evidence about a support role of actin in these junctions. The tubulo-bulbar complexes are known to be the structures following the ES both in the apical locations and in the basal location at the BTB [28]. A immunohistochemical and ultrastructural study has shown that these TBCs contain the integral membrane adhesion molecules nectin 2 (from Sertoli cells) and nectin 3 (from spermatids) as well as the actin-binding protein espin [28]. Furthermore, these and other molecules associated with ES are enriched at the ends of the TBC and in the vesicles associated with these endings, which are also labeled with antibodies for lysosomal and endosomal markers [28]. These observations have led to the proposal that TBCs are structures that internalize intercellular junction materials, both at the apical and at the basal ES [29].

As regards the present work, although tubular bulbar devices were shown by thin sections and by scanning electron microscopy, they were not observed, to our knowledge, in freeze fracture replicas that permit a detailed observation of the involved cell membranes (see Results, Figure 6). Moreover, using immune electron microscopy we detect β-actin surrounding the tubular bulbar complex extending previous observation by Morales and Clermont [31] that described the presence of actin but not of its specific isoform in this Sertoli specialization.

According to the present results, a significant correlation between the special organization of the β-actin filament network and the stages of the spermatogenic cycle of the seminiferous epithelium exists. Moreover, in a given seminiferous epithelium stage, β-actin appears to be modulated in relation to the degree of germ cell maturation and differentiation. We observed a clear correlation between the localization of the β-actin network in the spermiation process and that of the germ cells that appear to ascend from the basal to the adluminal compartment.

Related to the last mentioned topic is the long time discussed existence of a third compartment in the seminiferous epithelium. As already cited (Introduction) in the rat, Russell [19,21] was of the opinion that late leptotene spermatocytes in stages X-XI of the cycle of the seminiferous epithelium are the cells which cross the blood-testis barrier and penetrate into a third or intermediate compartment, which is limited, both below and above, by non-permeable interSertoli junctions as seen by electron-opaque tracers. Simultaneously, in the monkey we observed a similar phenomenon but our interpretation was that these impermeable junctions assemble and disassemble simultaneously without forming a real compartment [22,23]. Later, in the rat, using intratubular administration of intercellular tracers we arrived at a similar conclusion [24].

In the present paper, our results also support the hypothesis of the lack of existence of the so-called third compartment since we never observed leptotene-zygotene spermatocytes totally surrounded by the β-actin mark. Thus, it appears that the dynamic changes of the β-actin polymerization /depolymerization cycle contribute to a fast ascent of spermatocytes avoiding the formation of the postulated intermediate compartment.

Numerous multivesicular bodies were especially in the seminiferous epithelium. Early electron microscopy studies [49] indicated the existence of MVB highlighting the fact that they were somehow related to lysosomes and that contained characteristic accumulations of small vesicles in their lumen or matrix. The existence of β-actin in MVB could be related to the fact that tubular bulbar complexes appear to internalize apical ectoplasmic specializations once the spermatids are released into the lumen of the seminiferous epithelium [31,29]. In relation to our results, we remark that Young et al. [29] postulate that tubulobulbar complexes are intercellular podosome-like structures that internalize intact intercellular junctions during epithelial remodelling events in the rat testis. Thus our observations support the claim that TBCs are actin-related double-membrane projections that form at intercellular junctions in the seminiferous epithelium and internalize intact junctions during sperm release and during the translocation of spermatocytes through basal junction complexes between neighboring Sertoli cells.

The morphological findings, Part of this work, were recently accepted for publication [50]. Bioquimical determinations indicated herein add a crucial, significant demonstration about the impressive dynamic turnover of the beta actin along the cycle of the seminiferous epithelium. Both, morphological observations and actin quantification are centered in the spermiation process. This coincidence is more strong evidence that the testicular organization would be centered upon the species perpetuation

In conclusion, significant interrelations among the β-actin network, the junctional complexes of the BTB and the ectoplasmic specializations were detected at different stages of the seminiferous cycle.

Acknowledgments

Authors thanks the valuable technical assistance of Mrs. Juanita Dávila in preparing the histological slices. This investigation was supported by the grant number 06/J13 from SECYT (Secretaría de Ciencia y Técnica, Universidad Nacional de Cuyo, Argentina) and grant number 6486 from CONICET (National Research Council), Argentina. The prosaposin antibody was generously donated by Prof. Carlos Morales from The Anatomy and Cell Biology Department, Mc Gill University, Montreal, Canada.

References

[1] Korn, E.D., Carlier, M.F.& Pantaloni, D. (1987). Actin polymerization and ATP hydrolysis. *Science, 238*, 638–644.

[2] Poukkula, M., Kremneva, E., Serlachius, M. & Lappalainen, P. (2011). Actin-depolymerizing factor homology domain: a conserved fold performing diverse roles in cytoskeletal dynamics. *Cytoskeleton (Hoboken), 68(9),* 471-490. (Epub 2011)

[3] Capani, F., Martone, M.E., Deerinck, T.J. & Ellisman, M.H. (2001). Selective localization of high concentrations of F-actin in subpopulations of dendritic spines in rat central nervous system: A three-dimensional electron microscopic study. *The Journal of Comparative Neurology, 435*, 156-170.

[4] Ouyang, Y., Wong, M., Capani, F., Rensing, N., Lee, C.S., Liu, Q., Neusch, C., Martone, M.E., Wu, J.Y., Yamada, K., Ellisman, M.H. & Choi, D.W. (2005). Transient decrease in F-actin may be necessary for translocation of proteins into dendritic spines. *The European Journal of Neuroscience, 22,* 2995-3005.

[5] Bamburg, J.R., McGough, A. & Ono, S. (1999). Putting a new twist on actin: ADF / cofilins modulate actin dynamics. *Trends in Cell Biology, 9,* 364-370.

[6] Chen, H., Bernstein, B.W. & Bamburg, J.R. (2000). Regulating actin-filament dynamics in vivo. *Trends in Biochemical Sciences, 25*, 19-23.

[7] Pollard, T.D., Blanchoin, L. & Mullins, R.D. (2000). Molecular mechanisms controlling actin filament dynamics in nonmuscle cells. *Annual Review Biophysics and Biomolecular Structure, 29,* 545-576.

[8] Wear, M.A., Schafer, D.A. & Cooper, J.A. (2000). Actin dynamics: assembly and disassembly of actin networks. *Annual Review Biophysics and Biomolecular Structure, 36,* 451-477.

[9] Condeelis, J. (2001). How is actin polymerization nucleated in vivo?. *Trends in Cell Biology, 11,* 288-293.

[10] Holt, M.R. & Koffer, A. (2001). Cell motility: proline-rich proteins promote protrusions. *Trends in Cell Biology, 11,* 38-46.

[11] Winder, S.J & Ayscough, K.R. (2005). Actin binding proteins. *Journal of Cell Science, 118*, 651-654.

[12] Pollard, T.D.(2007). Regulation of actin filament *Annual Review Biophysics and Biomolecular Structure, 36,* 451-477.

[13] Vogl, A.W., Genereux, K. & Pfeiffer, D.C. (1993). Filamentous actin detected in rat spermatozoa. *Tissue & Cell, 25(1),* 33-48.

[14] Setchell, B.P.(1969). Do Sertoli cells secrete fluid into the seminiferous tubules?. *Journal of Reproduction & Fertility, 19*, 391-392.

[15] Setchell, B.P., & Waites, G.M.H. (1975). The blood-testis barrier. In: Handbook of Physiology, Section7: Endocrinology, Vol.V., Male reproductive System (D.W. Hamilton and R.O. Greep, eds). Washington: *American Physiology Society,* pp143-172.

[16] Dym, M. & Fawcett, D.W.(1970). The blood-testis barrier in the rat and the physiological compartmentation of the seminiferous epithelium. *Biology of Reproduction, 3,* 308-326.

[17] Dym, M.(1973). The fine structure of the monkey (Macaca) Sertoli cell and its role in maintaining the blood-testis barrier. *Anatomical Record, 175*, 636-656.

[18] Yazama, F. (2008). Continual maintenance of the blood-testis barrier during spermatogenesis: the intermediate compartment theory revised. *The Journal of Reproduction and Development, 54*, 299-305.

[19] Russell, L.D. (1977a). Movement of spermatocytes from the basal to the adluminal compartment of the rat testis. *American Journal of Anatomy, 149*, 313-328.

[20] Russell, L.D. (1977b). Observations on rat Sertoli ectoplasmic("junctional") specializations in their association with germ cells of the rat testis. *Tissue & Cell, 9,* 475-498.

[21] Russell, L.D. (1978). The blood-testis barrier and its formation relative to spermatocyte maturation in the adult rat: a lanthanum tracer study. *Anatomical Record, 190,* 99-112.

[22] Dym, M. & Cavicchia, J.C. (1977). Further observations on the blood-testis barrier in monkeys. *Biology of Reproduction, 17*, 390-403.

[23] Dym, M.. & Cavicchia JC (1978). Functional Morphology of the testis. *Biology of Reproduction 18*, 1-15.

[24] Cavicchia, J.C. & Sacerdote, F.L. (1988). Topography of the rat blood-testis barrier after intratubular administration of intercellular tracers. *Tissue & Cell, 20,* 577-586.

[25] Gumbiner, B., Stevenson, B. & Grimaldi, A. (1988). The role of the cell adhesion molecule uvomorulin in the formation and maintenance of the epithelial junctional complex. *The Journal of Cell Biology,107*, 1575-1587.

[26] Russell, L.D.(1979). Spermatid-Sertoli tubular bulbar complexes as devices for elimination of cytoplasm from the head region of late spermatids of the rat. *Anatomical Record, 19,* 233-246.

[27] Russell, L.D. & Griswold, M.D.(1993). The Sertoli Cell. Clearwater FL. Cache *River Press.*

[28] Guttman, J.A., Takai, Y. & Vogl, A.W. (2004). Evidence that tubulobulbar complexes in the seminiferous epithelium are involved with internalization of adhesion junctions. *Biology of Reproduction, 71*, 548-559.

[29] Young, J. S., Guttman, J.A., Vaid, K. S. & Vogl, A.W. (2009). Tubulobulbar complexes are intercellular podosome-like structures that internalize intact intercellular junctions during epithelial remodelling events in the rat testis. *Biology of Reproduction, 80*, 162-174.

[30] Gruenberg, J. & Stenmark, H.(2004). The biogenesis of multivesicular endosomes. *National Review & Molecular Cell Biology, 5*, 317-323.

[31] Morales, C. & Clermont, Y. (1993). Structural changes of the Sertoli cell during the cycle of the seminiferous epithelium. In: Russell LD, Griswold MD, editors. The Sertoli cell. Clearwater FL, Cache *River Press*, pp 305-330.

[32] Chemes, H. (1986). The phagocytic function of Sertoli cells: a morphological, biochemical, and endocrinological study of lysosomes and acid phosphatase localization in the rat testis. *Endocrinology, 119*, 1673-1681.

[33] Wong, C.H., Mruk, D.D., Lui, W.Y. & Cheng, C.Y. (2004). Regulation of blood-testis barrier dymamics: an in vivo study. *Journal of Cell Science, 117*, 383-798.

[34] Wong, E.W., Mruk, D.D. & Cheng, C.Y. (2008). Biology and regulation of ectoplasmic specialization, an atypical adherens junction type, in the testis. *Biochimica et Biophysica Acta, 1778*, 692-708.

[35] [Cheng, C.Y. & Mruk, D.D. (2010). A local autocrine axis in the testes that regulates spermatogenesis. *Nature Reviews Endocrinology, 6*, 380-395.

[36] Hubrecht, R. & Kirkwood, J. (2010). UFAW Handbook on the Care and Management of Laboratory Animals and other Research Animals. Wiley-Blacwell, ed. Universities Federation for Animal Welfare. *Ames, Iowa.*

[37] Christensen, A.K. & Mason, N.R. (1965). Comparative ability of seminiferous tubules and interstitial tissue of rat testes to synthesize androgens from progesterone -4-14 C in vitro. *Endocrinology, 76*, 646-656.

[38] Parvinen, M., & Vanha-Perttula, T. (1972). Identification and enzyme quantification of the stages of the seminiferous epithelial wave in the rat. *Anatomical Record, 174*, 435-450.

[39] Saraceno, G.E., Bertolino, M.L., Galeano, P., Romero, J.I., Garcia-Segura, L.M. & Capani, F. (2010). Estradiol therapy in adulthood reverses glial and neuronal alterations caused by perinatal asphyxia. *Experimental Neurology, 223*, 615-622.

[40] Morales, C.R., Hay, N., El-Alfy, M. & Zhao, Q. (1998). Distribution of mouse sulfated glycoprotein-1 (prosaposin) in the testis and other tissues. *Journal of Andrology, 19*, 156-164.

[41] Lönn, M.E., Hudemann, C., Carsten, B., Cherkasov, V., Capani, F., Holmgren, A., Zeng, J. & Lillig, C.H. (2008). Expression pattern of human glutaredoxin 2 isoforms: identication and characterization of two testis/cancer cell-specific isoforms. *Antioxidants & Redox Signaling, 10*, 547-557.

[42] Godoy, J.R., Funke, M., Ackermann, W., Haunhorst, P., Oesteritz, S., Capani, F., Elsässer, H.P. & Lillig, C.H. (2010). Redox atlas of the mouse. Immunohistochemical detection of glutaredoxin-, peroxiredoxin-, and thioredoxin-family proteins in various tissues of the laboratory mouse. *Biochimica et Biophysica Acta, 1810*, 2-92.

[43] Cavicchia, J.C., Sacerdote, F.L., Morales, A. & Zhu, B.C. (1998). Sertoli cell nuclear porenumber changes in two stage sets of the rat spermatogenic cycle. *Tissue & Cell, 30,* 268-273.

[44] Russell, L.D., Ettlin, R.A., Hikim, A.P.S. & Clegg, E.D.(1990). Histological and histopathological evaluation of the testis. Clearwater, Fl: Cache *River Press.*

[45] Sharpe, R.M.(1994). Regulation of spermatogenesis. In: Knobil E, Neill J D, editors. The physiology of reproduction. New York. *Raven Press,* pp 1363-1434.

[46] Vogl, A.W. & Soucy, L.J. (1985). Arrangement and possible function of actin filament bundles in ectoplasmic specializations of ground squirrel Sertoli cells. *Journal of Cell Biology, 100,* 814- 825.

[47] Grove, B.D. & Vogl, A.W. (1989). Sertoli cell ectoplasmic specialization: a type of actin associated adhesion junction? *Journal of Cell Science, 93*, 309-324.

[48] Pollard, T.D. & Earnshaw, W.C. (2008). Actin and actin-binding Proteins. Saunders Elsevier. Philadelphia. *Cell Biology, 33.* (Second edition).

[49] Trump, B.F., Goldblatt, P.J. & Stowell, R.E.(1965). Studies of necrosis in vitro of mouse hepatic parenchymal cells. Ultrastructural and cytochemical alterations of cytosomes, cytosegresomes, multivesicular bodies, and microbodies and their relation to the lysosome concept. *Laboratory Investigation; a Journal of Technical Methods and Pathology, 14*, 1946-1968.

[50] Cavicchia, J.C., Fóscolo, M., Ibañez, J., Lillig, C. & Capani, F. (2011). Modulation of actin filament network associated to sertoli cell ectoplasmic specializations. *Biocell (in press).*

In: Testis: Anatomy, Physiology and Pathology
Editors: Yoichi Nemoto and Norio Inaba
ISBN: 978-1-61942-739-6

Chapter 6

Comparative Morphology of Anuran Testes

***Classius de Oliveira*[1,*] *and Lilian Franco-Belussi*[2]**
[1]Sao Paulo State University – UNESP, IBILCE – São José do Rio Preto, Department of Biology. Rua Cristóvão Colombo, São José do Rio Preto, SP, Brazil
[2]Animal Biology Post-Graduate Program (UNESP/IBILCE-SJRP), Brazil

Abstract

Testes in anurans are a structure that posses distinct morphology and coloration. Spermatogenesis in these group is a complex and organized process that involves spermatogenic cysts progression through in the seminiferous epithelium. The germ cells are grouped with Sertoli cells and constitute spermatogenic cyst. Germ cells are distinct in species of different families.

Keywords: Anurans; Testis; Reproduction; Spermatogenesis; Spermatocysts; Germ cells

Testicular Morphology of Anurans

The germ tissue in vertebrates is disposed in seminiferous ampoules in the cyclostomes and urodeles, and in seminiferous tubules in amniotes (Hildebrand 1995). The terminology used for the description of this germinative compartment in amphibians is variable. However, the germ epithelium is organized in seminiferous ampoules in salamanders (Hildebrand 1995) or in seminiferous locules in caecilians (Wake 1969) and frogs (Duellman and Trueb 1994), as a general histological architecture of the seminiferous elements. In mammals, the testes have a tunica albuginea with septa. This arrangement of tunica albuginea in teste originates

* Corresponding Author: Dr. Classius de Oliveira; Departamento de Biologia – IBILCE/UNESP; Rua Cristóvão Colombo, 2265 – Jardim Nazareth; CEP 15.054-000 São José do Rio Preto, SP, Brasil; Phone: +55 17 3221 2387; Fax: +55 17 3221 2390; E-mail: classius@ibilce.unesp.br.

the seminiferous tubules. In these animals, the tubules are typically permanent structures that produce spermatozoa during all the reproductive period.

The urogenital system of anurans is formed by gonads and accessory ducts. The anuran testes are paired, rounded, compact, usually yellow structures (Goin and Goin 1962) located in the abdominal cavity, associated ventrally to the kidneys and linked to this organ by the gonadal mesentery or mesorchium. The external appearance of the gonads is granular due to the spherical aspect the seminiferous locules, which can be seen through the transparent tunica albuginea (Figure 1). At the anterior portion of the kidneys and gonads lie the abdominal fatty bodies that have several tiny extensions and coloration varying from whitish to yellowish. Both fatty bodies and gonads may vary in form and weight along the reproductive period, besides other morphofunctional changes related to reproductive seasonality or nutritional status (Santos and Oliveira 2008).

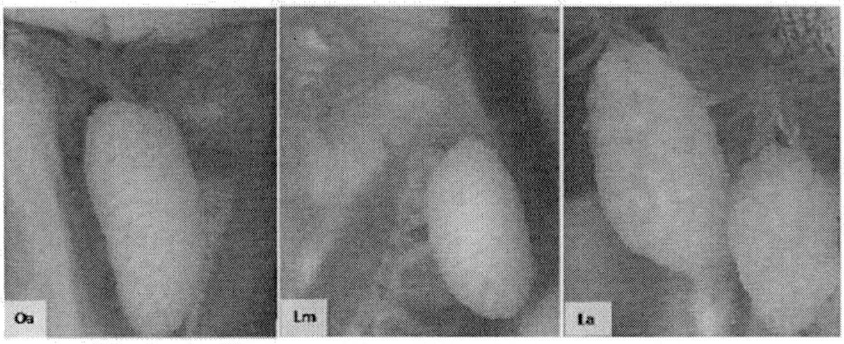

Figure 1. Testes of three anuran species showing the locular morphology. Oa: *Odontophrynus americanus*, Lm: *Leptodactylus mystacinus*, La: *Leptodactylus marmoratus*.

The color, size, and shape of the gonads greatly vary among anuran species from many families, such as *Rhinella ornata* and *R. schneideri* (Bufonidae); *Eupemphix nattereri*, *Physalaemus cuvieri*, *P. centralis*, *P. marmoratus*, and *Pseudopaludicola cf. falcipes* (Leiuperidae); *Leptodactylus fuscus*, *L. podicipinus*, *L. chaquensis*, and *L. latrans* (Leptodacytilidae); *Dendropsophus minutus*, *D. nanus*, *D. sanborni*, *Scinax fuscovarius*, *S. fuscomarginatus*, and *S. similis* (Hylidae); *Hylodes magalhaesi* and *Crossodactylus sp.* (Hylodidae); *Lithobates catesbeianus* (Ranidae); and *Holoaden luederwaldti* (Strabomantidae). *Rhinella ornata* and *R. schineideri* have a cylindric, whitish testis with a pigmented ovarian tissue at its anterior end, called Bidder's organ (Figure 2). On the other hand, *E. nattereri*, *P. cuvieri*, *P. centralis*, *P. marmoratus*, *Crossodactylus sp.*, *Hylodes magalhaesi*, and *S. fuscomarginatus* have ovoid testis with a dark brown external and internal pigmentation; *Leptodactylus podicipinus*, *L. chaquensis*, *L. latrans*, *Holoaden luderwaldti*, *Lithobates catesbeianus*, *D. minutus*, and *S. fuscovarius* have an ovoid, white testis (Figure 3). The testicular pigmentation is due to melanocytes, which are also present in other species (Franco-Belussi et al. 2009, Franco-Belussi et al. in press). These melanin-containing cells are found in different organs (liver, spleen, lung, heart, intestine, and gonads) and tissues (meninges and connective tissues surrounding blood vessels), composing an extracutaneous pigmentary system, whose function is still poorly understood (Zuasti et al. 1998, Gallone et al. 2002).

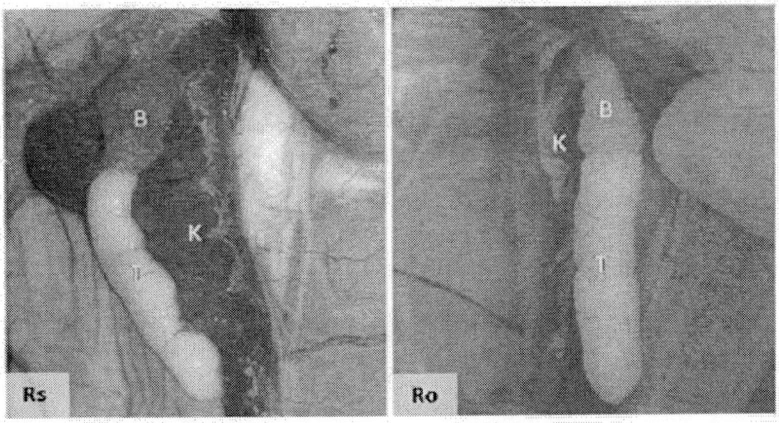

Figure 2. Urogenital system of two bufonid species showing the morphology of testes (T), Bidder's organ (B), and fat bodies (Fb). Rs: *Rhinella schineideri*, Ro: *Rhinella ornata*. K: Kidneys.

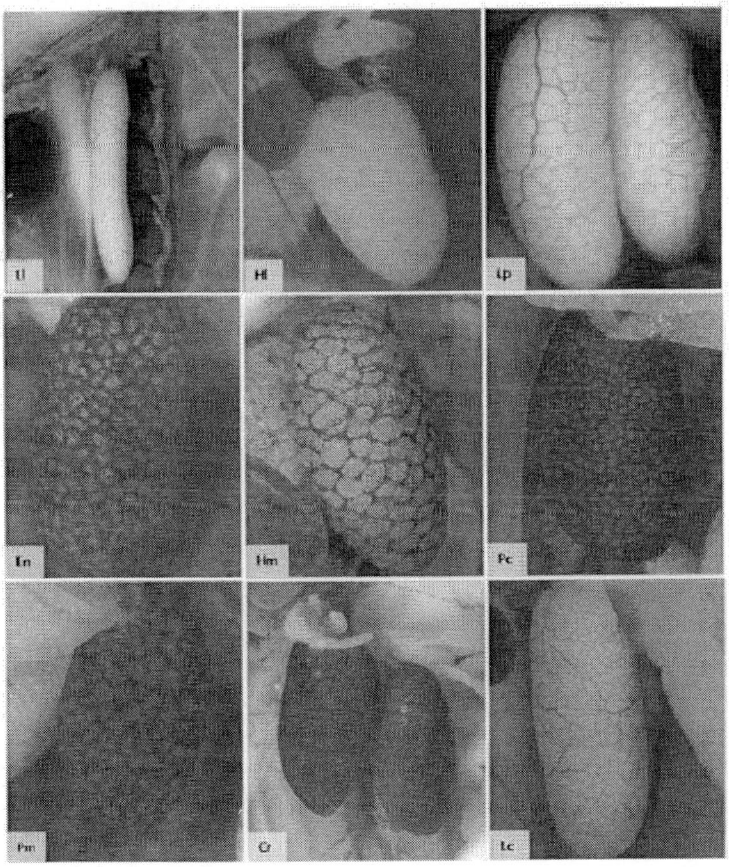

Figure 3. Distinct morphology of anuran testes in different families. Ll: Leptodactylus lattrans, Hl: Holoaden luederwaldti, Lp: Leptodactylus podicipinus, En: Eupemphix nattereri, Hm: Hylodes magalhaesi, Pc: Physalaemus centralis, Pm: Physalaemus marmoratus, Cr: Crossodactylus sp., Lc: Leptodactylus chaquensis.

The extracutaneous pigmentation pattern of *D. nanus*, *P. cuvieri*, and *R. schneideri* was examined during the breeding season. Changes observed in the pigmentary system in some organs during the reproductive period, including the testis may be due to physiological alterations or even represent a species-specific feature (Moresco and Oliveira 2009). A previous work also demonstrated that the pigmentation in testicles of E. nattereri have a protective role against bacteremia that can damage germ cells and influence the reproductive output of the animal (Franco-Belussi and Oliveira 2011).

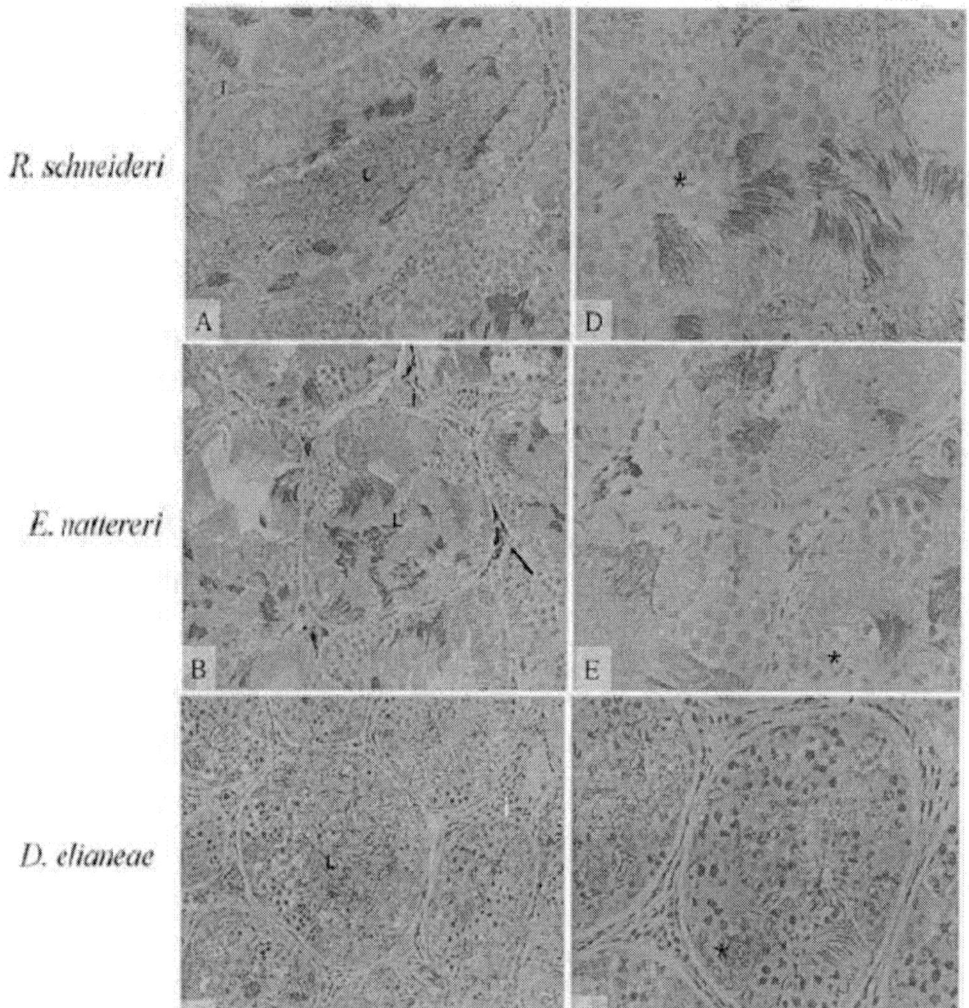

Figure 4. Histological sections of the testes of *Rhinella schneideri, Eupemphix nattereri*, and *Dendropsophus elianeae* showing A-C (20x): L: seminiferous locule, i: intertitial cells. B: arrow: pigmented cells among intertitial cells. D-F (40X): *: spermatogonia. Stained with H-E.

HISTOLOGY

Externaly, the testis has a thin capsule of connective tissue, the testicular capsule or tunica albuginea. This capsule is composed of collagen fibres. Blood vessels in this area run toward the parenchyma. Internally, the germ epithelium has cellular groups (germ cyst or follicles) of spermatogenetic lineage cells arranged in seminiferous tubules. There is an interlocular tissue composed by Leydig cells, fibroblasts, blood vessels, and efferent ductules among the seminiferous area (Figure 4). This cystic arrangement is a characteristic common to all amphibians (Duellman and Trueb 1994, Oliveira et al. 2003a). This arrangement is also found in other anamniotes (Grier 1992). Some cysts seldom have cells with small differences among themselves and, since there is little asynchronism, we consider the cysts as a cellular group in which every sexual cell is at the same developmental stage (Oliveira et al. 2003b).

In anurans, the testis does not have septa and the structures containing the germ epithelium are known as seminiferous locules, because they do not show a typical tubular aspect such as those in mammals. In the germ epithelium, the cystic distribution does not follow a distribution sequence. In this case, the spermatogonia are observed near to the locule wall and the spermatozoon bundles, and near or in the locular lumen (Oliveira et al. 2003b, Santos and Oliveira 2008). According to Hermosilla et al. (1983), thiny extensions of the cytoplasm of the Sertoli cells comprise completely the germ cells, forming a surrounded wall, which also emits cytoplasmatic process between the cells of the cysts. The testes are not lobulated in anurans, but this is observed in urodeles (Sever 1974) and caecilians (Wake 1969). The occurrence of multiple testicular lobes is an important systematic character.

The Sertoli cells rest on the seminiferous basal lamina of the tubule, and continue attached to the wall even in more advanced stages of spermatogenesis. With the formation of cysts, compartments are formed with a fundamental role in the cellular differentiation, providing a structural and functional support to the germ cells (Hermosilla et al. 1983, Rastogi et al. 1988, Báo et al. 1991). The basal membrane resulted in the development of a permanent separation between germinal and interstitial testicular compartment in fish, amphibians, and all amniotes (Grier 1992). The general characteristic of a cyst is the formation of a hematotesticular barrier between its cells. This mechanism may keep the differences between blood composition or hemolymph and the testicular fluid, resulting in the formation of a micro-environment that is appropriate for the development of haploid germ cells (Cavicchia and Moviglia 1983, Bergmann et al. 1983). The same type of spermatogenesis occurs in all anuran species described.

The process starts when the spermatogonia, which are surrounded by follicular or Sertoli cells, forming the cyst wall. This cells located interiorly produces the others cells of spermatogenic lineage. This arrangement will only be altered in the final stages, during the spermiogenesis, when cells will pass through an extraordinary elongation until the formation of the tail and head of the spermatozoon. The Sertoli cells will sustain the bundles with the heads embedded in their cytoplasm, and the free tail turned to the lumen of the seminiferous locule. According to Sprando and Russel (1988), at this moment the lumen of the germ cyst joins the lumen of the seminiferous locule. Thus, the spermatozoa will be released to follow the spermatic production.

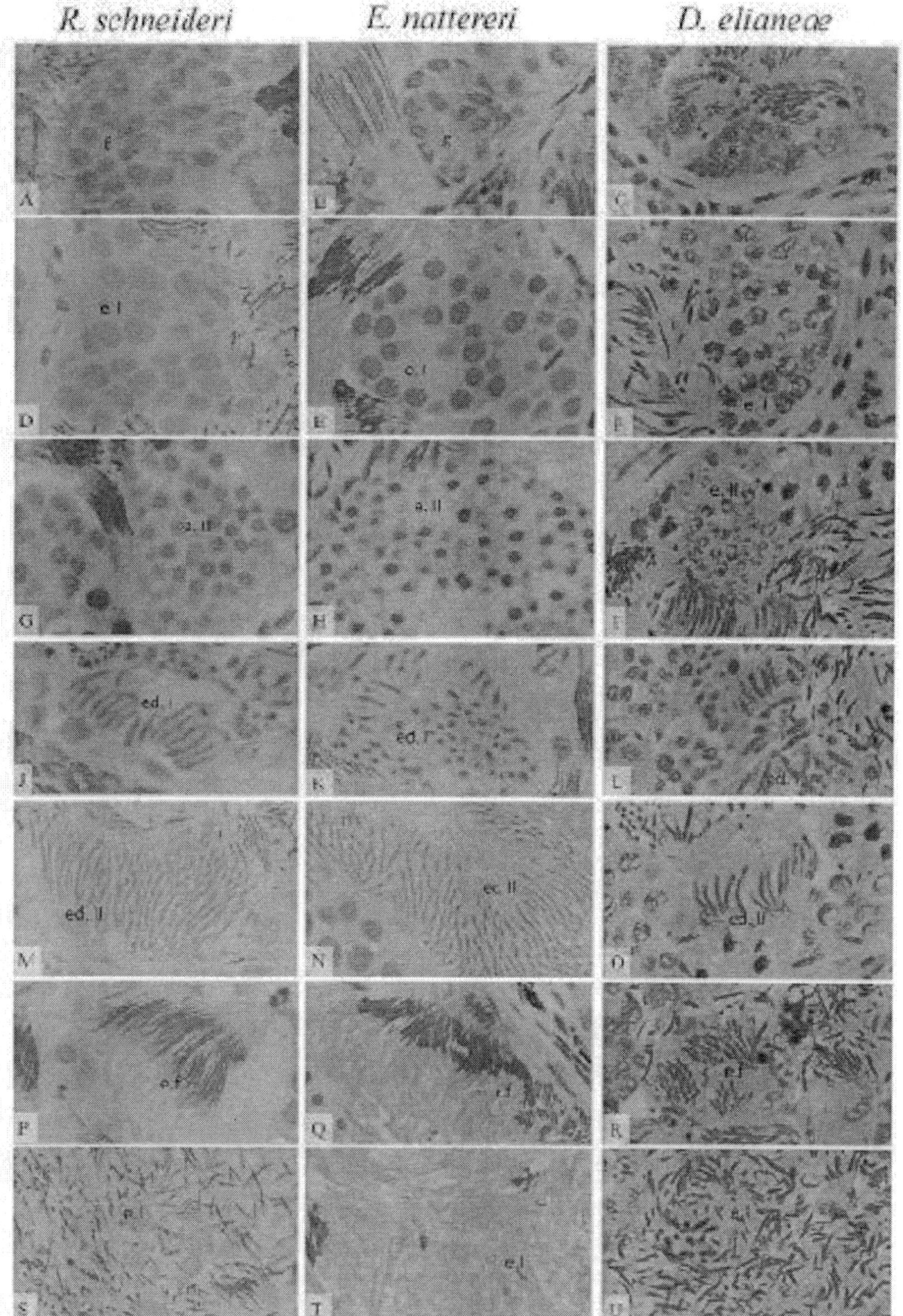

Figure 5. Histological sections of testes of *Rhinella schneideri, Eupemphix nattereri* and *Dendropsophus elianeae* showing A-C: Spermatogonia; D-F: Spermatocyte I; G-I: Spermatocyte II; J-L: Spermatids I; M-O: Spermatids II; P-R: Spermatozoon bundles; S-U: Spermatozoon in lumen. Stained with H-E.

According to Oliveira et al. (2003b), at the basis of the epithelium lie the spermatogonia I, the biggest cells that are always associated with the Sertoli cell. Cysts containing variable number of very small spermatogonia II with loosely distinct cellular boundaries are originated after the mitotic proliferation. After the differentiation and the volumetric growth, the spermatocytes I appear. The nuclei of these cells are spherical and with different degrees of compaction of the nuclear material. Starting the meiotic process, the spermatocytes II are originated, which by means of the second meiotic division become haploid cells, the spermatids I. These two last spermatocysts are very similar. At this phase, the cells undergo a prominent process of differentiation until they form the spermatids II, which are elongated and begin to be organized in bundles supported by prominent Sertoli cells. With the process of spermiogenesis, spermatozoa appear, usually observed in compact bundles with tails turned to the lumen and their heads fitted in their support cells. In more advanced stages, free spermatozoa can be observed in the locular lumen, ready to follow the spermatic production (Figure 5).

Despite the architecture of the germ epithelium of all mentioned species represents general and typical model for the anurans, the final germ cell - the spermatozoon - great varies among species. This can be related to phylogenetic aspects and to reproductive strategies of anurans. Regarding the reproduction, the presence of developed spermatozoa during all reproductive period suggests that reproduction occurs a few times in a single season. Thus, the gametogenic activity occurs simultaneously in all locules. However, while some seminiferous locules shelter mainly free spermatozoa, ready to be spread, others have bigger cellular populations in the previous stages of the cellular differentiation.

Comparative Spermatogenesis in Three Anuran Species

Previous studies about the spermatogenesis in frogs of different families, such as *Rhinella schneideri* (Bufonidae), *Eupemphix nattereri* (Leiuperidae), and *Dendropsophus elianeae* (Hylidae) found the same pattern of germ cell distribution, in which cells were organized in cysts and supported by Sertoli cells (Figure 4). The cysts of the spermatogenic cell line along with Sertoli cells form groups enclosed in a membranous capsule, called germinative cysts or spermatocyst (Lofts 1974, Grier et al. 1980, Grier, 1992) containing germ cells in synchronous developmental stages (Burgos and Fawcett 1956, Burgos and Vitale-Calpe 1967, Vitale-Calpe 1969).

The diameter of the seminiferous locules varies among species (Figures. 4 A, B, and C) and is probably related to species' body size. The locular diameter is wider in *R. schneideri* in relation to other species. This species has also higher body mass than others. *Dendropsophus elianeae* has the smallest locular diameters and also both small size and body mass. On the other hand, *E. nattereri* has intermediate states of those characteristics, and also is the only species that has melanocytes associated with testicular interstitial cells (Figure 4 B). In the other species, these melanin pigments are not observed.

The occurrence of germ cell types in seminiferous locules of *E. nattereri*, *D. elianeae*, and *R. shcneideri* is different. Although there are spermatogonia and sperm in the lumen, there are no morphological differences in cell types in the spermatogenesis of these three species. Lofts (1974) argues that the primary spermatogonia are among the largest cells of the spermatogenic lineage, lying at the basal lamina surrounding the seminiferous structures and associated with follicular cells. There were no major differences in the spermatogonia of the three species. However, in some species the spermatogonia is not well defined, such as in *Dendropsophus elianeae* (Figures 4 A, B and C). Spermatocytes I are large and symmetrically rounded cells (Figures 4 D, E, and F). Smaller cells are derived after the division of the spermatocyte I, denominated spermatocytes II, with half the diameter of its predecessors. This decrease in size is due to the condensation of the genetic material and the cytoplasm (Figures 5 G, H, and I). Spermatids I become slightly elongated (Figures 5 J, K, and L), but with a larger cytoplasmic volume than spermatids II, which make them different from spermatocytes. By its turn, spermatids II are very elongated and cylindrical cells (Figures 5 M, N, and O). At this developmental stage, cells no longer form cysts and begin to be organized into bundles. After differentiation, the nuclear compression of spermatids II increases and cytoplasmic volume decreases, and represents the last developmental stage of the sperm. The sperm has two morphologically distinct regions given the degree of basophilia. The head is highly basophilic, compact and located anteriorly. The flagella are elongated and highly acidophilic. The sperm are firstly arranged in bundles (Figures 5 P, Q and R), but later disintegrate and disperse into the lumen of the seminiferous locules (Figures S, T and U).

Ultrastructural Characteristics of Germ and Sertoli Cells

The ultrastructural analysis of germ cells of *Scinax fuscovarius* reveals the occurrence of spermatogonia, spermatocytes, spermatids, and sperm. The primary spermatogonia are bulky and rounded cells, the largest in the germ line. The nucleus is multilobulated with chromatin without clear compaction, though with some condensed electrondense points. Often, there is a single well-defined eccentric nucleolus, the perinuclear cytoplasm has many indentations, due to the nuclear morphology. The organelles are evenly distributed, with many spherical, relatively large mitochondria. Lipid inclusions are also found (Figure 6 A, B and C). These spermatogonia are completely surrounded by extensions of Sertoli cells, which are identified by their larger electrondense cytoplasm. The nuclei of these Sertoli cells are irregularly small, compact, pyramidal-shaped (multilobulated), in which the peripheral chromatin is in a high degree of condensation. The cytoplasm contains mitochondria, abundant endoplasmic reticulum and some lipid inclusions of various sizes (Figure 6 A, B).

The secondary spermatogonia are small cells and have two well-defined histological types: primary spermatogonia (type I) and secundary spermatogonia (type II). Type I cells are lighter than type II and have an irregular nuclei with much heterochromatin, but without nucleoli. A striking feature is the decrease in cell volume (Figure 6 D).

The spermatocytes are morphologically heterogenous cells, as they undergo two meiotic divisions. We can distinguish at least two cell types: primary and secondary spermatocytes. In a general way, the nucleus is spherical with different degrees of chromatin condensation, according to the stage of differentiation. There is no nucleolus and the cytoplasm undergoes a significant reduction.

Spermatocytes I are only smaller than primary spermatogonia and have spherical nucleus with loosely distributed chromatin and no nucleoli before meiotic division. The cytoplasm has few organelles, mainly mitochondria and cisternae of the Golgi apparatus. Usually this cell type is observed when the first meiotic division starts, which will give rise to secondary spermatocytes. Spermatocytes I have several synaptonemal complexes, which are typical structures of meiotic division, specifically the prophase (Figure 7 A). The spermatocytes I become gradually smaller. The spherical nucleus of these cells becomes progressively compressed. Then, the cell acquires irregular shapes and the intercellular spaces began to appear, apparently without any material. Mitochondria predominate in the cytoplasm and the Golgi apparatus can be observed in some cells. The intercellular bridges, i.e., a continuous membrane that holds the cytoplasm of cells, help to identify the previous cell divisions. The cytoplasmic membrane in these bridges is more electrondense (Figure 7 B).

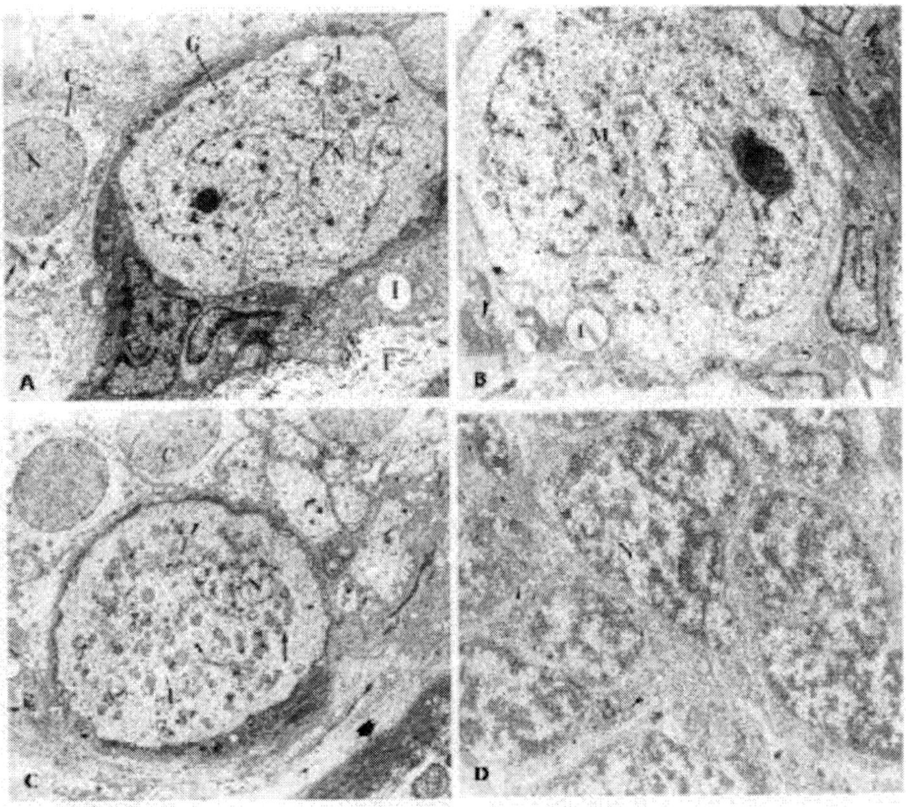

Figure 6. Spermatogonia of *S. fuscovarius*. A, B, and C – primary spermatogonia (G) with the multilobulated nucleus (N), and evident eccentric nucleoli. Many mitochondria (arrowhead) and some lipid inclusions (I) can be seen in the cytoplasm. Notice the lipid inclusions (I) and electron-dense, cytoplasmic extensions involving the primary spermatogonia in Sertoli cells (S). The secondary spermatocyte (C) is smaller, with spherical nucleus (N) with finely distributed chromatin. There is also some mitochondria (arrowhead) and evident Golgi apparatus (arrow). Collagen fibers (F) can be seen in the locular wall. D – Cyst of spermatogonia. A typical feature is the irregular nucleus (N) with scattered heterochromatin. The amount of cytoplasm and organelles is smaller, but with abundant mitochondria (arrowhead), also indicated in the periphery of the seminiferous locule (thick arrow). Magnifications: A and C – 8,000 X; B – 10,000 X; D – 16,500 X.

At this moment, an important change begins to occur in Sertoli cells, which at this stage are more electrondense than germ cells. There is a progressive increase in the number of organelles and lipid inclusions in the cytoplasm. The nucleus still remains irregular in shape and is larger than the preceding stage. The Sertoli cell also changes, following the changes in germ cells. The nuclei of Sertoli cells increase in size, due to a reduction of heterochromatin, which is now uniformly distributed and bears a single and conspicuous nucleolus (Figure 7 C).

The Sertoli cells undergo a dramatic transformation. At the beginning, they are rounded and without nuclear compaction, as the differentiation proceeds, the nucleus starts to compress and extend. There are also cytoplasmic changes, such as the formation of the acrosome, development of a tail filament at the opposite pole and the elimination of cytoplasmic material.

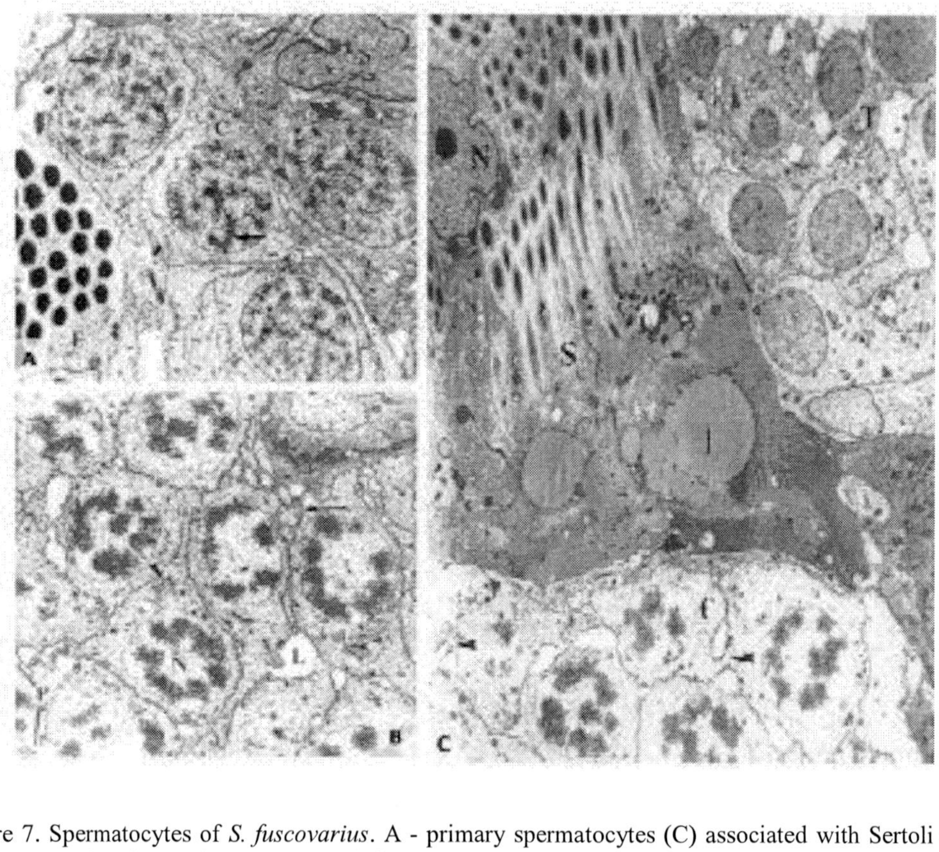

Figure 7. Spermatocytes of *S. fuscovarius*. A - primary spermatocytes (C) associated with Sertoli cell (S). A sperm bundle can be seen on the left (E). Synaptonemal complexes (arrows) are also observed, organized during the pachytene of the first meiotic division. The cytoplasm of these cells is proportionally smaller and irregular. B – Spermatocyte cysts with the nucleus (N) at the beginning of chromatin condensation and Golgi apparatus (arrowhead). Intercellular bridges (P) are observed between nearby spermatocytes. It is also possible to see extensions of the Sertoli cell (arrow) and the lumen of the germinative cyst (L). C - Sertoli cell (S) with a bundle of elongated spermatids. There is a cyst of rounded spermatids on the right side and another cyst of espermatocytes below. The cytoplasm of the Sertoli cell is electrondense and irregular, with large amounts of lipid inclusions (I). The nucleus has regular shape and a central nucleolus. The cyst of spermatocytes (C) has some intercellular bridges (arrowhead). The cyst of rounded spermatids (T) is at the initial stage of cellular elongation, which is evidenced by the irregular aspect of the cytoplasm. Magnifications: A and B – 5,000 X, C – 13,6000 X.

Spermatids I are the first cells of the spermiogenesis, and have a rounded shape. They have an even smaller nucleus than the previous cells and a loosely distributed chromatin. There is probably a single dictyosome of the Golgi complex in the cytoplasm, though we did not record the formation of an acrosome vesicle, as described in other species (Figure 8 A). The cytoplasm of these spermatids often bears two ortogonal centrioles, one of which will give rise to the axoneme. The cytoplasm of the cell decreases in volume and there are also some processes, which are released as vesicles (Figure 8 A) containing cytoplasmic material.

The nucleus of spermatids I undergo condensation of chromatin and a region with nuclear pores originates in the nuclear envelope at the beginning of spermiogenesis. There is a well-developed Golgi complex in this region of the cytoplasm, from which the acrosome will form. In addition, there are often centrioles that give rise to the tail at the opposite pole (Figure 8 B).

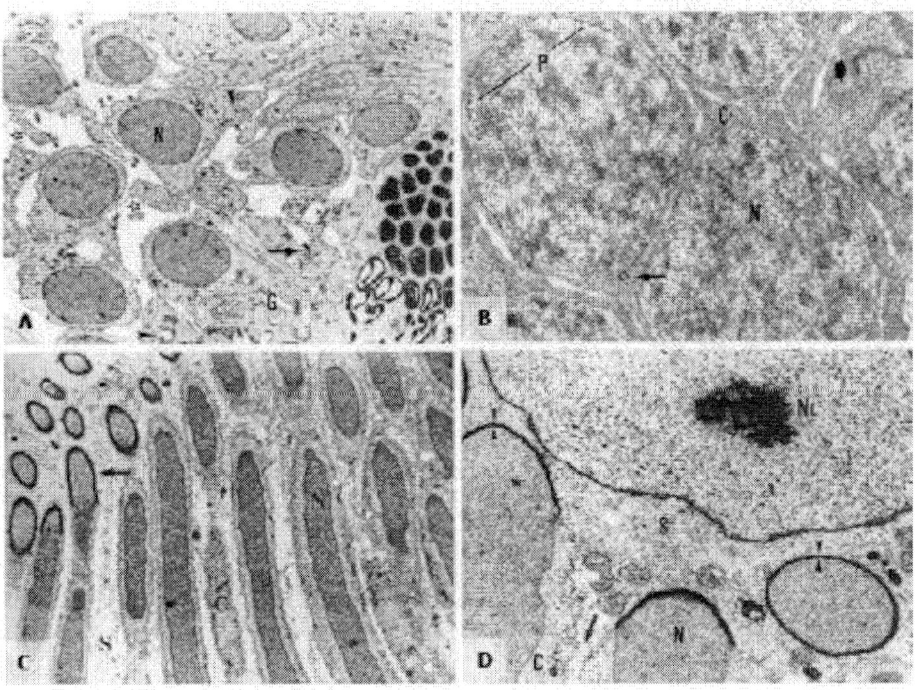

Figure 8. Spermatids of *S. fuscovarius*. A - rounded spermatids showing the spherical nucleus (N) and irregular cytoplasm due to the lost of cytoplasmic portions (star). There is a distinct Golgi apparatus (G) in the cytoplasm and a pair of centrioles (arrow) arranged at right angles, one of which will give rise to a flagellum (arrowhead). A sperm bundle can be senn on the lower right corner. B – Spermatids in early nuclear compression (N), with coarse-grained chromatin and nuclear pores (P) in the nuclear membrane. The cytoplasm (C) is very scarce and generally with a developed Golgi apparatus (thick arrow) that is in general, located near the nuclear surface. Centrioles structures (arrow) can be seen at the opposite pole. C - Long spermatid with nucleus (N) and cytoplasm (C), completely surrounded by extensions of Sertoli cells (S). The arrow indicates the acrosomal cap, an electrondense structure that covers the proximal end of the nucleus of each spermatid. D - Sertoli cells (S) with part of the nucleus showing a conspicuous nucleolus (NL). This cell projects cytoplasmic processes (arrow) that involve the spermatids. Notice the nucleus (N), cytoplasm (C) and the acrosomal cap (arrowhead) of an elongated spermatid (E). Magnification: A – 5,000 X; B and D – 13,000 X; C – 8,000 X.

Like previous cell types, these germ cells are associated with Sertoli cells to form cysts. However, from this stage onwards, these somatic cyst cells acquire large amounts of microtubules that will be sorted into bundles and help to support the sperm (Figure 9 C, D).

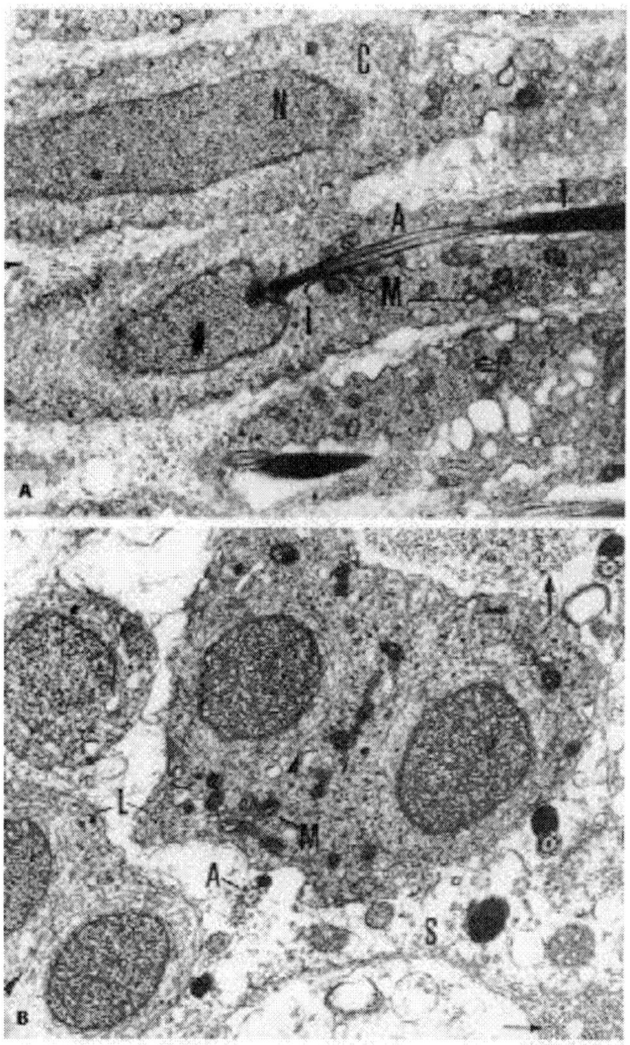

Figure 9. Elongated spermatids of *S. fuscovarius*. A - Longitudinal section of elongated spermatids at the level of the intermediate piece. The nucleus (N) and cytoplasm (C) attached to the elongated spermatid. There is a concentration of mitochondria (M) near the nucleus, known as intermediate piece (I), forming a cytoplasmic sheath. This is where the sperm tail will originate, represented in part by the axoneme (A) and a marginal filament (T). The Sertoli cell is represented by cytoplasmic processes containing microtubules oriented lengthwise (arrowhead). B - elongated spermatids in cross section. The nucleus is well defined and is compacted. Small, electrondense and spherical mitochondria (M) can be observed in the cytoplasm, besides a large amount of concentric microtubules (arrowhead) around the nucleus. Additionaly, longitudinal microtubules (L) can be seen at the cytoplasmic periphery. The Sertoli cell (S) has vesicular cytoplasmic processes and large amounts of microtubules in many orientations (arrows). The final portion of the tail is full of axonemes (A) associated with the marginal filament, the most electrondense structure. Magnification: A – 16,500 X, B – 21,000 X.

The spermatids II are cells with an elongated and compressed nucleus, with increasing levels of electrondensity. The cytoplasm becomes progressively thinner and with few organelles (Figure. 8 A and 9 A). The acrosome is formed from the dictyosome of the spermatid I. The acrosomes are composed of condensed acrosomal membranes and occupy a tiny cytoplasmic layer at the apical region of the spermatid, covering the nucleus with an acrosomal cap (Figure 9 A, B). At this stage, Sertoli cells have a conspicuous nucleus with finely distributed chromatin and a single and evident nucleolus. The cytoplasm has a few mitochondria and numerous processes, including the elongated spermatids that begin to be organized in bundles (Figure 9 A, B).

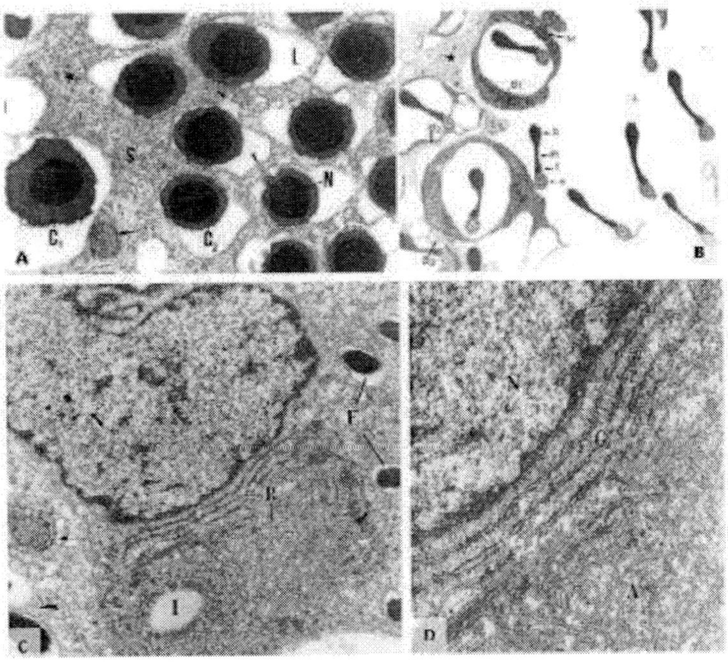

Figure 10. Spermatozoa of *S. fuscovarius*. A - Sperm in cross section: nucleus (N) and cytoplasm (C) of sperm's head. Extensions of the Sertoli cell (S) and lumen (L) of the seminiferous locule. The sperm has a high ratio of nuclear compaction and a decrease in the volume of the cytoplasm, less electrondense than the nucleus, since it no longer has many organelles in this region (compare C1 and C2). The Sertoli cell has a large amount of transverse (arrowhead) and longitudinal (star) microtubules and eventually mitochondria (arrow). B - sperm tails sectioned at different levels. Notice the large amount of longitudinal microtubules (star) in Sertoli cell's extensions. Sections in the middle portion are represented by cytoplasmic sheaths surrounding the tail. The sheath is progressively thicker (B1) towards the intermediate piece, and contains more mitochondria (M). As the section moves away from this portion, the sheath becomes thinner (B2) and without organelles, until not involve the tail (B3). The tail filament moves towards the locular lumen (L) and is represented by the axoneme (a), marginal filament (t), undulating membrane (m), and axial stick (b). C - Sertoli cell: the nucleus (N) and the cell itself is larger in all associations of these cells with those of the germ cell line. A large amount of endoplasmic reticulum (R) is found in the cytoplasm, as well as lipid inclusions (I) and a mitochondrium closely associated with a segment of the granular reticulum (arrow). In addition, a few sperm (E) are associated to the cytoplasm of the cell, that are oriented by many microtubules (arrowheads). D – Detail of part of the previous figure. The nucleus (N) has little heterochromatin, attached primarily to the nuclear envelope. A granular endoplasmic reticulum (G) is found at the perinuclear cytoplasm and a large amount of smooth reticulum externally (A). Magnifications: A and B – 27,500 X; C – 21,000 X; D – 50,000 X.

When spermatids reach an advanced degree of differentiation, the nucleus becomes compressed and the cytoplasm increasingly reduces, shifting the organelles, especially mitochondria, to the intermediate piece. We can also identify the cytoplasmic sheath that covers the beginning of the tail and some of its structures, such as axoneme and marginal filament (Figure 9 C).

The spermatids have a well-defined nucleus in cross section (Figure 10 D) with increasing nuclear compaction. At this stage, there are only small electrondense mitochondria and a large number of microtubules in the cytoplasm, which are oriented concentrically along the main axis of the nucleus. The cytoplasm of the Sertoli cell has an extraordinary amount of microtubules and a few organelles, especially mitochondria.

The sperm of *Scinax fuscovarius* have three main parts: head, intermediate piece, and tail. The acrosome cap is located at the apical portion of the head and the elongated nucleus is right below. The cytoplasm is scarce and without organelles in the remainig of the head not covered by the acrosome. The nucleus undergoes a compression and stretching, turning it strongly electrondense. The extensions of Sertoli cells that surround the sperm are filled with microtubules that organize the sperm in bundles (Figure 10 A). The intermediate piece is where the axoneme of the tail begins, and extends as a sheath surrounding the proximal and the free part of the tail. There is a concentration of organelles in this cytoplasmic sheath, especially mitochondria, which are mostly small, spherical and electrondense (Figure 10 B).

The tail is composed of the axoneme closely associated with the marginal filament, which is continuous to the axial stick, among which the undulating membrane. The axoneme has a typical arrangement, i.e., nine pairs of peripheral and one central pair of microtubules. An axial stick, continuous to the marginal filament, develops in parallel to the axoneme, with which it merges at the tail end and does not reach the extreme point in the telomeric region. The undulating membrane is formed between the axoneme and the axial stick (Figure 10 B).

The Sertoli cells have voluminous nuclei in these bundles, with finely distributed chromatin and few heterochromatin masses. The cytoplasm has a large amount of endoplasmic reticulum, besides some mitochondria, lipid inclusions, and many microtubules (Figure 10 C). An organized granular endoplasmic reticulum is often observed near the nucleus of these cells. A large amount of smooth endoplasmic reticulum is found externally (Figure 10 D).

Acknowledgments

The authors are indebted to FAPESP (Sao Paulo Research Fundation – Grant numbers: 02/08016-9, 05/02919-5, 09/13925-7, 06/57990-9, 08/52389-0 and 2011/01840-7) and CNPq (Brazilian Research Council – Grant numbers: 475248/2007-4 and 473499/2010-0) for financial support and fellowships. We also thank Dr. Carlos Alberto Vicentini, Dr. Rodrigo Zieri, Dr. Lia Raquel de Souza Santos, Juliane Silberschmitd Freitas, and Gabriela Baroni Leite for their many contributions to our laboratory that allowed to gather the data that make up this paper.

REFERENCES

Báo, S.N.; Dalton, G.C.; Oliveira, S.F. 1991. Spermiogenesis in *Odontophrynus cultripes* (Amphibia, Anura, Leptodactylidae): ultrastructural and cytochemical studies of proteins using E-PTA. *J. Morphol.,* 207 (3): 303-314.

Bergmann, M.; Greven, H.; Schindelmeiser, J. 1983. Observations on the blood testis barrier in a frog and salamander. *Cell. Tissue Res.,* 232(1): 189-200.

Burgos, M.H. and Fawcett, D.W. 1956. An electron microscope study o spermatid differentiation in the toad Bufo arenarum Hensel. *J. Biophys. Biochem. Cytol.,* 2, 223–239.

Burgos, M. H. and Vitale-Calpe, R. 1967. The fine structure of the Sertoli cell-spermatozoan relation-ship in toad. *J. Ultrast Res.,* 19, 221-237.

Cavicchia, J.C. and Moviglia, G.A. 1983. The blood-testis barrier in the toad (*Bufo arenarum* Hensel): a freeze-fracture and lanthanum tracer study. *Anat. Rec.,* 205(4): 387- 396.

Duellman, W.E. and Trueb, L. 1994. *Biology of amphibians*. New York: McGraw-Hill,670p.

Franco-Belussi, L.; Zieri, R.; Santos, L.R.S.; Moresco, R.M.; Oliveira, C. 2009. Pigmentation in anuran testes: anatomical pattern and variation. *Anat. Rec.* 292, 178-182.

Franco-Belussi, L.; Santos, L.R.S.; Zieri, R.; Oliveira, C. Visceral pigmentation in three species of the genus *Scinax* (Anura: Hylidae): distinct morphological pattern. *Anat. Rec. in press.*

Franco-Belussi, L. and Oliveira, C. 2011. Lipopolysaccharides induce changes in the visceral pigmentation of *Eupemphix nattereri* (Anura: Leiuperidae). Zoology. 114, 298-305.

Gallone, A.; Guida, G.; Maida, I.; Cicero, R. 2002. Spleen and liver pigmented macrophages of *Rana esculenta* L. A new melanogenic system? *Pig. Cell Res.* 15, 32-40.

Goin, C.J. and Goin, O.B. 1962. *Introduction to herpetology.* San Francisco: W. H. Freeman, 341p.

Grier, H. J.; Linton, R. L; Leatherland, J. F.; De Vlaming, V. L. 1980. Structural evidence for two different testicular types in teleost fishes. *Am. J. Anat.,* 159, 331-345.

Grier, H.J. 1992. Chordate testis: the extracellular matrix hypothesis. *J. Exp. Zool.* 261, 151–160.

Hermosilla, B.I.; Urbina, P.A.; Cabrera, P.J.C. 1983. Espermatogenesis en la Rana chilena *Caudiverbera caudiverbera.* (Linne, 1758) (Anura, Leptodactilidae). *Bol. Soc. Biol.* Concepción, Chile, Tomo, 54: 103-115.

Hildebrand, M. 1995. *Análise da estrutura dos vertebrados.* São Paulo: Atheneu, 700p.

Lofts, B. 1974. Reproduction. *Physiology of the amphibia.* New York: Academic Press, 2:107-218.

Moresco, R.M. and Oliveira, C. 2009. A comparative study of the extracutaneous pigmentary system in three anuran amphibian species evaluated during the breeding season. *S. Am. J. Herpetol.* 4, 1-8.

Oliveira, C, Santanna, A.C., Omena, P.M., Santos, L.R.S., Zieri, R. 2003a. Morphological considerations on the seminiferous structures and testes of anuran amphibians: *Bufo crucifer, Physalaemus cuvieri* and *Scinax fuscovarius*. *Biociências.* 11: 39-46.

Oliveira, C., Vicentini, C. A., Taboga, S. R. 2003. Structural characterization of nuclear phenotypes during *Scinax fuscovarius* spermatogenesis (Anura, Hylidae). *Caryologia.* 56(1): 75 - 83.

Rastogi, R.K.; Bagnara, J.T.; IELA, L.; Krasovich, M.A. 1988. Reproduction in the mexican leaf frog, *Pachymedusa dacnicolor*. IV. Spermatogenesis: a light and ultrasonic study. *J. Morphol.,* 197(3), 277-302.

Santos, L.R.S., Oliveira, C. 2008. Histological aspects and structural characteristics of the testes of *Dendropsophus minutus* (Anura, Hylidae). *Micron.* 39, 1266–1270.

Server, D. 1974. The occurrence of multiple testes in the genus *Eurycea* (Amphibia: Plethodontidae). *Herpetol.* 30, 187-193.

Sprando, R. L. and Russel, L. D. 1988. Spermiogenesis in the bull frog (*Rana catesbeiana*): a study of cytoplasmic events including cell volume changes and cytoplasmic elimination. *J. Morphol.* 198, 303-319

Vitale-Calpe R. 1969. The fine structure of the organ of Bidder in newly differentiate male of *Bufo arenarun. Zeit Anat. Entwicklungsgeschi.* 129, 1-13.

Wake, M.H. 1969. Evolutionary morphology of the caecilian urogenital system. I. The gonads and the fat bodies. *J. Morph.,* 126(3): 291-331.

Zuasti, A.; Jiménez-Cervantes, C.; Garcia-Borrón, J.C.; Ferrer, C. 1998. The melanogenic system of *Xenopus laevis. Arch. Histol. Cytol.* 61, 305-316.

In: Testis: Anatomy, Physiology and Pathology
Editors: Yoichi Nemoto and Norio Inaba
ISBN: 978-1-61942-739-6

Chapter 7

MOLECULAR BASIS OF HEAT STRESS DAMAGE IN MAMMALIAN TESTIS*

Ricardo D. Moreno[1,4,†], Raúl Lagos-Cabré[1], Julio Buñay[1], Natalia Urzúa[2] and Ximena Bustamante-Marín[3]

[1]Facultad de Ciencias Biológicas, Santiago, Chile
[2]Facultad de Agronomía e Ingeniería Forestal, Santiago, Chile
[3]Pontificia Universidad Católica de Chile, Faculty of Health Sciences, Universidad de Antofagasta, Antofagasta, Chile
[4]Centro de Ciencia e Innovación en Biotecnología Vegetal (ceCIBUC), Santiago, Chile

ABSTRACT

Germ cell apoptosis have been recognized as an important event in order to regulate daily sperm production in humans and in animal models as well. Several studies in rat, mouse and monkeys have shown that testicular mild heat stress (43°C for 15 min) induces a massive increase in germ cell apoptosis along with oxidative damage and activation of diverse signaling pathways. In addition, heat stress produces a decrease in sperm viability, increase sperm damage and decrease embryo quality. In human, testis exposure to heat stress may result from occupational exposure, life style or clinical disorders including cryptorchidism or varicocele. Thus, in the past years researchers have focused on two major areas; the first is to find the molecular signaling pathway trigger by heat stress, and 2) to seek for new molecules with antioxidant abilities which may prevent germ cell apoptosis and/or to improve sperm performance. However, the link between heat stress and male infertility in humans still remains controversial. Here we critically review the available literature in human and animal models, and we propose a new model

---

* A version of this chapter also appears in *Heat Stress: Causes, Treatment and Prevention*, edited by Stanislas Josipovic and Elias Ludwig, published by Nova Science Publishers, Inc. It was submitted for appropriate modifications in an effort to encourage wider dissemination of research.

† To whom correspondence should be addressed: Dr. Ricardo D. Moreno, Departamento de Fisiología, Facultad de Ciencias Biológicas, Pontificia Universidad Católica de Chile. Alameda 340, Santiago, Chile. E-mail: rmoreno@bio.puc.cl.

which explain the elevate apoptosis rate and sperm damage observed after heat stress. Finally we review the available data in pharmacological therapies to protect testicular damage from heat stress.

Keywords: Testis, apoptosis, oxidative damage, infertility, germ cell

INTRODUCTION

Infertility defined as "a failure to conceive after 12 months of unprotected sexual intercourse", it is a complex and multifactorial pathology involving emotional, social, psychological and physical factors (WHO, 2010). Male factor is responsible for 30-50% of cases of infertility, and as many as 20% of infertile men totally lack spermatozoa in their ejaculated (azoospermic) (Bhasin et al., 1994; Lee et al., 2011). Spermatozoa are generated in the testis by a process named spermatogenesis, which could be defined as the process by which germ cells proliferate and differentiate in a mature spermatozoon (Clermont and Lebond, 1955; de Kretser and Kerr, 1988; Moreno and Alvarado, 2006). Spermatogenesis is an orderly and highly complex process at the interior of seminiferous tubules. Interestingly, just to give an idea of the complexity of this process, about 4% of mice genome is uniquely expressed in the testis and about 175 transcripts are postmeiotically expressed (Schultz et al., 2003). Thus, making a spermatozoa require a coordinate expression of many genes along with para/juxtacrine signaling between germ cells and with the Sertoli cell (Hermo et al., 2010).

Body temperature regulation is critical to ensure optimal organ function and proper regulation of different physiological functions (Waites and Setchell, 1990; Setchell, 1993). In many mammals, including men, testes are in the scrotum, which is a dual chamber protuberance of skin and muscle, divided by a septum. In most of mammals, the onset of spermatogenesis is preceded by the descent of the testis from its original position in the abdominal cavity, through the inguinal canal, into the scrotum. In many species, the testis descent takes place at an early age and is permanent. In others (most rodents, insectivores and bats), the testes descend into the scrotum at the beginning of the breeding season and they are withdrawn into the abdominal cavity at the end of the season (Kleisner et al., 2010). On the other hand, in monotremes, edentates, cetaceans and prosboscideans, the testis remains permanently within the abdomen (Hansen, 2009). Several hypotheses have been put forward to explain the testes descent and origin of the scrotum. (Werdelin and Nilsonne, 1999; Skandhan and Rajahariprasad, 2007; Hansen, 2009; Kleisner et al., 2010). One of the widest known, but not yet fully accepted, hypothesis is that the positioning of the testes in the scrotum helps to cool them down, because their temperature is slightly lower than the rest of the body (1-2 °C less than body temperature). However other explanations may be related to place the epididymis in a cooler environment, "to train" spermatozoa in a hostile environment or to signal a sexual pole in male animals (Bedford, 1978).

Whatever the explanation for the descent of the testes, outside the abdominal cavity, the organ finds itself in a cooler environment (Bedford et al., 1982; Foldesy and Bedford, 1982; Wong et al., 1982; Bedford, 1991). The scrotal skin has a great number of sweat glands to keep the temperature down by evaporative heat loss, even in those animals like the sheep, in which sweating is not an important mechanism in general thermoregulation (Setchell, 1993). As the testis descent, the testicular artery becomes elongated and it may reach up to 7 m long in a structure only about 10 cm long. This artery is surrounded by a complex system of veins forming the plexus pampiniform, these veins will eventually rejoin into a single vein near the inguinal canal (Waites and Setchell, 1990). This complex vascular system constitutes a highly efficient countercurrent heat exchanger in which the arterial blood is precooled before it reaches the testis to the temperature of the scrotal skin, and the venous blood is warmed to body temperature before return to the abdomen (Mariotti et al., 2011). Interestingly, a similar mechanism of countercurrent has been described in animal lacking scrotum such as the hedgehog and armadillo. Thus it is possible that other functions, besides thermoregulation, are fulfilled by the plexus pampiniform (Waites and Setchell, 1990; Setchell, 1993).

The idea that hyperthermia is harmful for spermatogenesis, at least for animals with scrotal testes, comes from observations where the failure in testes descent into the scrotal cavity impair sperm production (Griffiths, 1893; Bedford et al., 1982; Foldesy and Bedford, 1982; Jung and Schuppe, 2007). In addition, application of heat to the normal scrotum or its transfer into the abdominal cavity induces germ cells death, exfoliation in many mammals, including human (Cameron and Blackshaw, 1980; Socher et al., 1997; Jannes et al., 1998; Lue et al., 1999; Hjollund et al., 2000; Yin et al., 2002; Ohta et al., 2003; Johnson et al., 2008; Paul et al., 2008). On the contrary, the increase of nocturnal scrotal temperature significant decrease sperm concentration and total sperm count (Jung et al., 2005; Jung et al., 2005), but if the changes are not too severe, spermatogenesis can be gradually restored.

In the past decades the scientific and medical community has realized that environmental insults such as pollutants, plasticizers, genotoxics and temperature play an adverse role in male fertility. Regarding temperature, it has been documented and speculated that modern lifestyle (use of underwear) and occupational exposure (e.g. car divers) may adversely influence sperm production, and contribute to male infertility (Jung et al., 2005; Jung and Schuppe, 2007). Even more, it is believed that, among other factors, an undescended testis (cryptochidism) is one of the risk factor in the etiology of testicular cancer. Therefore, heat stress, defined here as any increase in environmental temperature which could lead to histological and functional damage in testis physiology, is a risk factor for male infertility.

Mammalian Spermatogenesis

The making of mammalian spermatozoa starts with the engagement into a differentiation pathway of a diploid cell named spermatogonium, which sits down at the basal lamina of seminiferous tubules (de Rooij and Russell, 2000; Oatley and Brinster, 2008). Through several mitotic divisions, type A spermatogonial stem cells either renew themselves or differentiate into later-stage spermatogonia to eventually initiate meiosis (Oatley and Brinster, 2008). Germ cells in meiosis, spermatocytes, will undergo two successive divisions, without a S phase, and will become haploid round spermatids, which eventually transform into mature spermatozoa (Hermo et al., 2010). Mingled among germ cells are the Sertoli cells, which are the somatic component of seminiferous epithelium and they provide mechanical and nutritional support to germ cell (Figure 1). Germ cells, in adult rat testis, are grouped in 14 cell association or stages (numbered I-XIV) and six in humans (I-VI). Each stage can be distinguish according to acrosome development of spermatids, localization of elongated spermatids and meiosis steps (Clermont and Lebond, 1955; Clermont, 1963; Heller and

Clermont, 1963; Nikkanen et al., 1978; Hermo et al., 2010). Adjacent Sertoli cells bind to each other through tight junctions (TJs) constituting blood–testis barrier (BTB) between 10 and 16 days of age in mice, and 20-25 days in rats, providing a protected environment for germ cell development named the adluminal compartment (Dym and Fawcett, 1970; Sharpe et al., 2003; Yan et al., 2008). The TJs, which are the only known examples of occluding junctions, consist of three classes of integral membrane proteins, namely occludins, claudins and junctional adhesion molecules (Mruk and Cheng, 2004). In this way only spermatogonia and pre-leptotene spermatocytes are attached to the basal lamina and outside from the adluminal compartment (Figure 1).

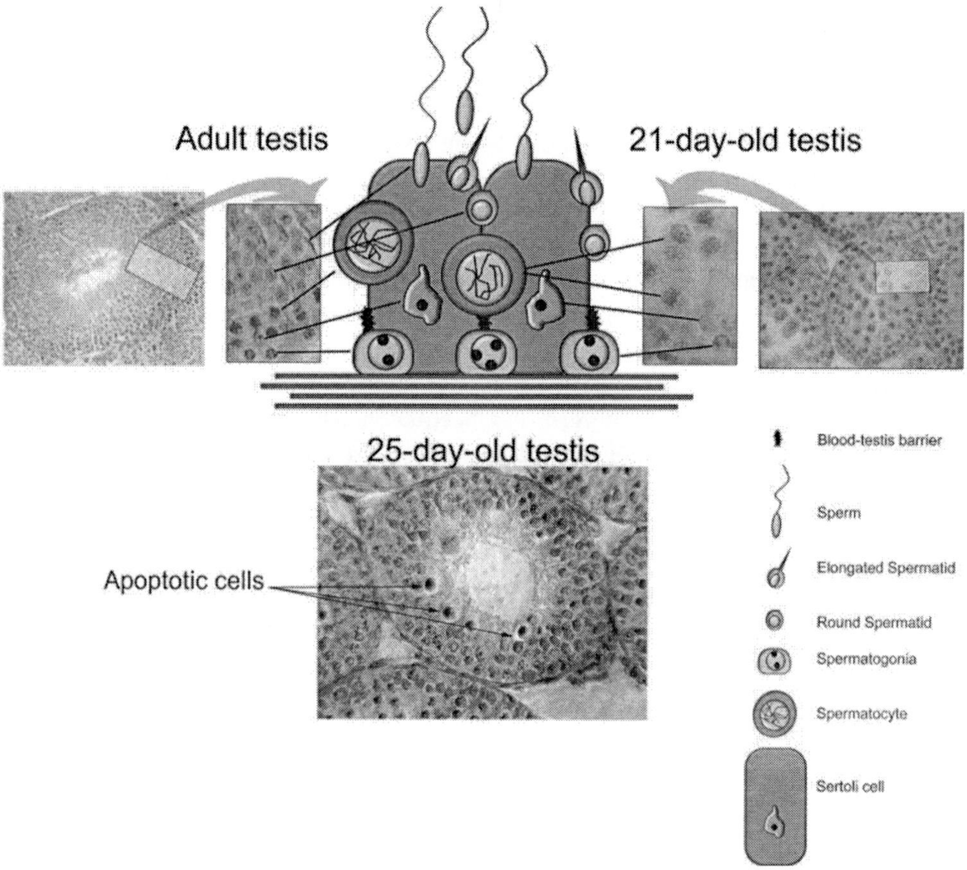

Figure 1. Adult and pubertal rat testis seminiferous tubule histology and organization. The central cartoon represents the general organization of germ and Sertoli cells in a seminiferous tubule. The right hand side pictures show adult seminiferous tubules, and the arrows indicate the corresponding cell type depicted in the cartoon. Note that pubertal seminiferous tubules (21 day old) have a simpler histological organization, and they lack round or elongating spermatids. Many tubules in 25 day old rats show several apoptotic germ cells, which can be easily visualized as condensed pycnotic cells, as indicate by the arrows in the lower picture.

Adult testis histology is different from prepuberal individuals. In the rat, at postnatal days 6–7, the testis contains somatic cells and spermatogonia cells only. By Days 13–14, leptotene spermatocytes are formed; which will become zygotene spermatocyte by Days 17–18; early and late pachytene spermatocytes appeared between 19–20 and 22–23 days, respectively.

Haploid round spermatids first appear at days 24–25 and elongating spermatids by days 30–31; later by day 36, elongated spermatozoa can be found (Malkov et al., 1998). This differentiation cycle will continues throughout all the fertile life of the male, because spermatogonial stem cells enter spermatogenesis at relative short periodic time intervals for example every 13 days in the Wistar rat, 11.6 days in the monkey (*Macaca arctoides*), 8,6 days in mouse, and 16 days in humans (Dadoune and Demeoulin, 1993; Hogarth and Griswold, 2010). Numerous studies indicate that Sertoli cells are involved in the progression of spermatogenesis through a variety of paracrine signals regulating gene expression and metabolism of germ cells (Skinner, 2005). Sertoli cells regulate survival of germ cells via paracrine secretion of trophic factors such as insulin growth factor (IGF), nerve growth factor (NGF), growth factor derived from glia (GDNF) and stem cell factor (SCF). Moreover, it has been shown that apoptosis of germ cells is somehow controlled by hormonal levels including testosterone, estrogen and FSH (Shetty et al., 1996; Yan et al., 2000; Tesarik et al., 2002). Testosterone is essential for meiosis and subsequent differentiation of spermatids (De Gendt et al., 2004). Testosterone exerts its action through the Sertoli cell, which expresses the androgen receptor, and stimulates the synthesis of various proteins and trophic factors in specific periods of spermatogenesis (Wang et al., 2009). Therefore, germ cell development is a complex differentiation process controlled by juxta/paracine, and endocrine interactions.

Apoptosis and the Control of Sperm Production

Apoptosis is a programmed cell dead characterized by several hallmarks such as: internucleosomal DNA fragmentation, caspases activation and externalization of phophatidyl serine (Degterev and Yuan, 2008; Fadeel et al., 2008). Caspases are a family of serine-proteases with around 14 members, which are synthesized as inactive zymogens and become active upon specific death stimuli. The extrinsic pathway is characterized by activation of dead receptors such as Fas (CD95/Apo-1) or tumor necrosis factor receptor 1 (TNFR1). Activation, by trimerization of dead receptors in response to ligand binding it, induces the formation of a multimeric complex named dead induced complex (DISC), which allows activation of procaspase-8 in mice and capsase-10 in humans (Scaffidi et al., 1998; Scaffidi et al., 1999; Salvesen, 2002; Henkler et al., 2005). Caspase-8 and/or 10 initiate apoptosis by inducing proteolytic processing of caspases-3, -6 and -7. Among them, caspase-3 is the main executioner caspase involved in the Golgi apparatus, nuclear lamina fragmentation, DNA fragmentation (due in part to proteolysis of a DNAse inhibitor) and decrease of the mitochondrial membrane potential (Sato et al., 2004; Kuribayashi et al., 2006).

The intrinsic pathway is activated by stimuli such as radiation, DNA fragmentation or cell stress and metabolic alterations (Degterev and Yuan, 2008). This pathway is characterized by a decrease in mitochondria membrane potential and release of cytochrome C, which along with dATP, the cytosolic protein Apaf-1 and procaspase-9 assemble a complex named apoptosome. Within this complex, procaspase-9 becomes active and then it activates caspase-3, connecting the intrinsic and the extrinsic pathways (Shi, 2002; Shi, 2006). Mitochondria membrane permeabilization is carry out by proapoptotic proteins belonging to the Bcl-2 family. The B-cell lymphoma-2 (BCL-2) family members encompass proteins that promote apoptosis whereas others prevent apoptosis (Youle and Strasser, 2008).

BCL-2, BCL-x and BCL-w are three anti-apoptotic proteins that interact with and repress the activity of pro-apoptotic proteins. Two general classes of proapoptotic family proteins exist: (1) those that share three homology regions (BH1, BH2 and BH3), and that are termed multidomain proteins; and (2) those that share little sequence homology except for the conserved BH3 domain, also termed "BH3-only" proteins (Chen et al., 2005; Zhai et al., 2008; Ku et al., 2010; Young et al., 2010). The multidomain protein is also known as Bcl-2/Bax-family in honor of Bax (Bcl-2 Antagonist X), the first Bcl-2 antagonist discovered by Korsmeyer. Other members of this group are Bcl-2 Antagonist/Killer (BAK) and Bcl-2 Ovarian Killer (BOK) (Hsu and Hsueh, 1998; Hsu et al., 1998). Among the "BH3-only" group we can find Bcl-2 Antagonist of cell Death (BAD) and p53 upstream modulator (PUMA) (Villunger et al., 2003). It appears that the pro-apoptotic family members BAX and BAK are crucial for the induction of permeabilization of the outer mitochondrial membrane (OMM) and the subsequent release of apoptogenic molecules, such as cytochrome-c and DIABLO (also known as SMAC), which leads to caspase-9 activation (Riedl and Shi, 2004; Westphal et al., 2010).

Thus apoptosis is a complex process involving activation of several independent, but convergent, pathways in order to induce cell death avoiding an inflammatory response. However, many of these elements such as caspase activation or phosphatydilserine externalization are involved in non-apoptotic events like sperm capacitation or embryo development (Sugimura et al., 1999; de Vries et al., 2003; Wang et al., 2004; Busso et al., 2010). Even more, other cell death pathways such as necrosis or autophagy share many common elements with apoptosis, making difficult to elucidate the exact death pathway taken by cell after a specific stimulus.

Apoptosis During Mammalian Spermatogenesis

Sperm production relies on physiological and environmental factors, which may attenuate or even totally suppress testicular function. Germ cell apoptosis has been show to play an important role in controlling sperm output in many species, and in humans it has been related to infertility (Feng et al., 1999; Weikert et al., 2004; Ji et al., 2009). Even more, it is believed that a substantial worldwide decline in human sperm production is caused by environmental toxicants that induce germ cell apoptosis (Sinawat, 2000). In the same way, modern lifestyle and use of underwear has been proposed to produce an elevated scrotal temperature that may cause germ cell apoptosis, akin to transient (43°C for 15 min) heat stress in testis (Jung and Schuppe, 2007; Paul et al., 2008; Hansen, 2009). Germ cells undergoing meiosis (spermatocytes) are highly sensitive to heat shock, ionizing radiation, growth factor deprivation and chemotherapeutic agents (Russell et al., 2004; Meachem et al., 2005; Bieber et al., 2006; Lizama et al., 2009). Many studies have shown the relevance of apoptosis in regulating spermatozoa output and eliminating damaged germ cells, particularly spermatocytes (Knudson et al., 1995; Beumer et al., 1998; Yin et al., 1998; Allemand et al., 1999; Feng et al., 1999; Honarpour et al., 2000; Yan et al., 2000; Russell et al., 2002; Moreno et al., 2006). In this way, it has been reported that a massive germ cell death occurs in physiological conditions (constitutive apoptosis) during the first round of spermatogenesis (Oakberg, 1956; Rodriguez et al., 1997; Moreno et al., 2006). Different experimental approaches have pointed out that spermatocytes are the main cell type undergoing apoptosis, and a smaller fraction of spermatogonia (Jahnukainen et al., 2004; Moreno et al., 2006). The importance of apoptosis in spermatogenesis is evident when apoptotic genes are deleted (BAX, Bim or Bik) or anti-apoptotic genes are over-expressed (such as BCL-2), both conditions are associated to infertility due to arrest of spermatogenesis at the onset of meiosis (Knudson et al., 1995; Feng et al., 1999; Yamamoto et al., 2001; Russell et al., 2002; Yan et al., 2003; Coultas et al., 2005). Furthermore, inhibition of apoptotic bodies engulfment by Sertoli cells results in a reduction of sperm production and sub fertility (Shiratsuchi et al., 1997; Maeda et al., 2002; Elliott et al., 2010).

Results from our laboratory indicate an increase in levels of Fas receptor, the transcription factor p53 and activation of caspases 8, 9, 3 2 and 6, in apoptotic germ cells (Lizama et al., 2007; Codelia et al., 2008). In this way, pharmacological inhibition of caspase-8 reduces by more than 50% the number of apoptotic germ cells, suggesting an important role of the extrinsic pathway in this process. Nevertheless, this data do not rule out the involvement of other death receptors, which are found in testes (Pentikainen et al., 2001; Giammona et al., 2002). We have also shown that etoposide, a DNA damage agent, induces apoptosis mainly of spermatocytes (Ortiz et al., 2009; Codelia et al., 2010; Lizama et al., 2011; Lizama et al., 2011), and germ cell apoptosis in this condition seems to rely more in the intrinsic than in the extrinsic pathway (Codelia et al., 2010). Thus, the mechanism involving constitutive (physiological) and externally induced apoptosis are far from being understood.

Germ cell death can be induced by different external stimuli among which temperature has been extensively studied. In the next section we will review the data concerning germ cell death induced by heat stress, and we will discuss whether or not the experimental evidence supports a bona fide apoptosis mechanism. This knowledge may help to define pharmacological approaches to prevent germ cell apoptosis induced by heat stress without side effect in physiological germ cell apoptosis, which might interfere with the normal progress of spermatogenesis.

Effects of Heat Stress in Male Fertility

Mice and rats have been the most used animal models to study the effect of hyperthermia in spermatogenesis, although other species such as boars, sheeps and monkeys as been studied in this same regard. A widely used model is to immerse the lower third of the animal (mouse or rat) in a warm bath (normally at 43°C) for a period of time ranging 15-30 min (hence heat stress). The incidence of germ cell apoptosis is normally quite low, in control animals, showing the highest rate in early zygotene and ending pachytene spermatocytes (stage I and XII for rats and mice; stage 5 and 2 for rabbits; and stage Ia and VIIa for cats) and spermatocytes at the zygotene–pachytene transition (stage XIV for rats; stage XII for mice; stage 4 for rabbits; and stage VIII for cats) (Blanco-Rodriguez et al., 2003). Heat stress, after 1 or 2 days, induces germ cell apoptosis predominantly at early (I–IV) and late (XII–XIV) stages. Pachytene spermatocytes at stages I–IV and IX–XII, diplotene and dividing spermatocytes at stages XIII–XIV, and early (steps 1–4) spermatids, are the most frequently cell types observed to die after heat stress (Lue et al., 1999). This increase in germ cell apoptosis leads to a reduction in testis size (Jannes et al., 1998). Eventually, spermatogenesis is recovered to levels similar to non treated animals, because spermatogonia are relatively resistant to heat, with the exception of B-type spermatogonia of rams (Waites and Setchell, 1990; Lue et al., 1999) and bulls. Interestingly, isolated haploid germ cells, but not somatic testicular undergo apoptosis at 37°C under the same culture conditions, which indicates that heat stress activate the apoptotic pathway only in germ cells (Yin et al., 1998). After heat stress there is a gradually lost in sperm viability and concentration (Jannes et al., 1998; Setchell et al., 1998; Rockett et al., 2001; Paul et al., 2008; Perez-Crespo et al., 2008). In monkeys, scrotal heat stress induces azoospermia or oligozoospermia 6 or 8 weeks after the first heat treatment (Lue et al., 2002). Similarly, in a stallion model it has been observed an increased susceptibility of spermatozoa DNA to denaturation in the absence of protamine changes (Love and Kenney, 1999). In rats, spermatocytes damage at the time of heat stress results into a lower concentration of spermatozoa 23-28 days after treatment, which have a highly reduced DNA integrity, as compared to not treated animals, but the higher degree of DNA damage is found in spermatozoa resulting from spermatids present within the testis at the time of heat stress (Perez-Crespo et al., 2008). Moreover, after mating of normal females to heat exposed males, there is a reduction in pregnancy rate and an increase of embryo reabsorption, and those surviving embryos experience a reduction in weight during intrauterine development. *In vitro* fertilization with sperms recovered 16 h or 23 d after scrotal stress at 42 °C produces embryos experiencing a block at 4-cell and blastocyts stage, suggesting a pre-implantational effect of heat stress in development and/or deficient egg activation (Paul et al., 2008; Paul et al., 2008). The reduce weight and number of embryo sired by heat stressed males, could be explain by the high levels of DNA damage which promotes abnormal embryo, yolk sac, trophoblast and placenta development. The pattern of weight reduction is thus different from that seen in gynogenetic embryos or when the gene for insulin-like growth factor (IGF)-II is disrupted, and suggests a reduction in embryo growth at the earlier stages, with compensatory growth occurring later in pregnancy (Setchell, 1993; Setchell et al., 1998). Interestingly, there is a sex ratio distortion when spermatozoa present in the epididymis at the time of thermal stress produce embryos after mating (Perez-Crespo et al., 2008). Therefore, the available evidence clearly indicated that heat stress has a profound impact in spermatogenesis, with an increase in germ cell apoptosis and DNA damage in those spermatozoa produced by germ cells present at the time of injury. Thus, it is possible that in humans, low embryo weight may also be related to damage DNA sperm, which, in turn, might be rise from environmental and/or pathological conditions.

Germ Cell Apoptosis in Heat Stress

Cell cycle progression and differentiation relays upon a strict control at different steps, especially those including DNA replication and integrity. In this way, it has been shown that heat stress reduces the levels of poly(ADPR)polymerase (PARP), a chromatin-associated enzyme with a role in DNA repair during replication and recovery from strand breaks (Tramontano et al., 2000). Low PARP levels could promote poor DNA repair, which in turn will promote apoptosis. Another signal to promote apoptosis is cell cycle arrest, which has been observed in experimental unilateral cryptorchidism testis in rabbits, with reduced levels of Cdc2 and Cyclin B1. The pachytene/diplotene primary spermatocytes are unable to form the Cdc2/CyclinB1 complex, and they arrest at the G2/M transition (Kong et al., 2000). Similarly, it has been observed a reduction of Cdc2 levels in mice testes after heat stress (Zhang et al 2008). Therefore, increase DNA fragmentation and cell cycle arrest are two important molecular signals involved in triggering germ cell apoptosis during heat stress.

Heat stress induces relocation of Bax along with cytosolic translocation of cytochrome-C in rats and monkey (Lue et al., 2002; Hikim et al., 2003; Matsuki et al., 2003; Vera et al., 2004; Jia et al., 2009). Interestingly, genomic studies have shown a dowregulation of several apoptotic genes including BAX (alpha isoform), BAK and caspase-2 (Rockett et al., 2001). Caspase-9 and 3 activation, two hallmarks of apoptosis, have been described in rat germ cell after heat stress, and their pharmacological inhibition prevent germ cell death (67%), suggesting that caspases are responsible for germ cell death after heat stress (Hikim et al., 2003; Matsuki et al., 2003; Vera et al., 2005). In this way, pharmacological and genetic evidence indicates that, contrary to physiological apoptosis, heat stress induces the intrinsic pathway of apoptosis, because using the FasL-defective *gld* mice, heat-induced germ cell apoptosis is not blocked (Hikim et al., 2003; Vera et al., 2004). However, germ cell apoptosis in experimental cryptorchidism is delay by 3 days in Fas-deficient mouse testes (Yin et al., 2002). Thus contradictory results have been reported using cryptorchidism or a warm bath to induce heat stress in mice and/or rat testis, suggesting that probably those models do not share exactly the same executioner apoptotic pathway. In the same token, germ cells undergoing constitutive or etoposide-induced apoptosis upregulate matrix metalloproteases of the ADAM family and pharmacological inhibition of these enzymes prevent apoptosis (Lizama et al., 2010; Lizama et al., 2011; Lizama et al., 2011). However, heat stress does not induces upregulation of ADAM17, ADAM10 or ADAM9, suggesting that this treatment trigger apoptosis in a different way than etoposide or physiological conditions. Calpains constitute a super family of intracellular calcium-dependent neutral cysteine proteases whose members are widely expressed in a variety of cells and tissues (Squier and Cohen, 1996; Saez et al., 2006; Saez et al., 2008). Calpains have been shown to be activated in caspase-dependent and caspase-independent (necrosis) cell death. In fact, over-expression of calpastain, an endogenous calpain inhibitor, or pre-treatment with synthetic inhibitors, germ cell apoptosis is prevented after experimental cryptorchidism or heat stress, suggesting activation of these enzymes in these models (Somwaru et al., 2004; Coureuil et al., 2006; Lizama et al., 2009). Therefore apoptosis seems to be the major cell death pathway trigger by heat stress in germ cells, but necrosis, or at least some elements of the necrotic pathway are activated by heat stress. Interestingly, caspase-2, the most evolutionary conserved caspase, is activated in spermatocytes and spermatids after heat stress in monkey testes. Even more, it seems that caspase-2 is upstream of caspase-9 and caspase-3 activation (Johnson et al., 2008). Upstream of apoptosis execution, it is possible that activation of transcription factors is involved in pro/anti-apoptotic factor gene regulation, such as p53 and p73 (Dobbelstein et al., 2005; Murray-Zmijewski et al., 2006). In this way, using a mouse model of experimental unilateral cryptorchidism, testicular weight reduction, germ cell loss, and DNA fragmentation are delayed by 3 days in $p53^{-/-}$ mice, suggesting that cryptorchidism induces germ cell loss through two apoptotic pathways: a p53-dependent pathway responsible for the initial phase of germ cell apoptosis, and a p53-independent pathway that accounts for subsequent apoptosis (Yin et al., 1998; Yin et al., 2002). Normally, at scrotal temperature, Heat Shock Protein 105 (HSP105) forms a complex with p53, and dissociate from it during heat stress. This mechanism contributes to the stabilization of p53 protein in the cytoplasm of the germ cells, preventing the potential induction of apoptosis by p53 (Kumagai et al., 2000). The Heat Shock Factor 1 (HSF1) induces germ cell apoptosis when is over expressed in mice testes, but heat-induced apoptosis of spermatocytes is prevented in mice lacking HSF1 (Nakai et al., 2000; Widlak et al., 2003; Hayashida et al., 2006). Interestingly, germ cell apoptosis induced with doxorubicin (DOXO; 5 mg/kg), increases significantly after two days of treatment. Later, by 21 days, meiotic cells were depleted in controls but not in *Hsf1* deficient testes. Thus, heat stress and acute response to genotoxic stress in the testis involves HSF1-dependent mechanisms that induce apoptotic cell death in a TRP53-independent manner (Salmand et al., 2008). Therefore a complex gene regulation network is established in mammalian testes in order to control germ cell apoptosis induced by heat stress.

In addition to transcription factor, the generation of reactive oxygen species (ROS) in the initiation of apoptosis seems to be of paramount importance in germ cell apoptosis and DNA damage (Makker et al., 2009). ROS are molecules that have at least one unpaired electron, rendering them highly unstable and highly reactive in the presence of lipids, amino acids and nucleic acids (Franco et al., 2008; Hirano, 2008; Tuteja et al., 2009). At physiologic levels, ROS are essential for normal reproductive function, acting as metabolic intermediates, regulating vascular tone, gene expression, and sperm capacitation (Sikka, 2001; Franco et al., 2008; Hirano, 2008; Makker et al., 2009; Tuteja et al., 2009). The experimental evidence point out that heat stress induces oxidative stress which in turn triggers a number of cell responses including cell survival and apoptosis, depending upon the cell type and the extent of the insult. Currently, the mechanisms by which oxidative stress occurs is not yet fully understood. A major focus of studying oxidative stress involves exploring the ROS-generating enzymes that produce ROS as by-products of their enzymatic activity. Xanthine oxidase (XO) catalyzes the conversion of hypoxanthine and xanthine to uric acid and generates hydrogen peroxide as a by-product. Interestingly, XO inhibitors suppress testicular germ cell apoptosis induced by experimental cryptorchidism, suggesting a role of this enzyme in this model (Kumagai et al., 2002). However, there is a lack of information whether other ROS-generating enzymes such as cyclooxygenase (COX), lipoxygenase (LOX) and NADPH oxidase (NOX) are activated after testicular heat stress. Additionally, it has been shown that major source of non-enzymatic ROS generation in aerobic cells comes from mitochondrial sources, specifically complex I and complex III. Under normal conditions, 1-2% of all oxygen consumed during respiration undergoes a single electron reduction by leakage of electrons from quinone pools to form the superoxide radical (Raha and Robinson, 2000; Raha et al., 2002; Ott et al., 2007). Then, mitochondrial superoxide dismutase (SOD) converts superoxide into hydrogen peroxide which is then converted to water and oxygen by catalase and glutathione peroxidase (GPx). Under stress conditions, the amount of electrons leaking out is enhanced, leading to an increase and accumulation of superoxide in mitochondria. It has been shown in fungi and skin cells that mitochondrial dysfunction and XO are the major sources of ROS production (Davidson and Schiestl, 2001; Shin et al., 2008). The enzyme GPx produces water using glutathione (GSH) as electron donor (Meister and Anderson, 1983). The levels of GSH are maintained by the action of glutathione reductase (GR), which recycles oxidized glutathione (GSSG) to GSH using NADPH as the electron donor. It has been reported that GR activity is affected by ROS and that Ascorbic Acid is capable of preventing this effect (El-Missiry, 1999). Nitric oxide (NO) is synthesized intracellularly through the action of a family of Nitric oxide synthethase (NOS) enzymes. NOS enzymes catalyze the NADPH- and O2-dependent oxidation of L-arginine to L-citrulline producing NO (Hill et al., 2010). This molecule is a free radical and chemically more stable and less reactive than other ROS such as superoxide anion or hydrogen peroxide (Pacher et al., 2007). In monkey testes, endothelial nitric oxide syntethase (eNOS) and inducible NOS (iNOS) are expressed in Sertoli and germ cells. No obvious alteration in eNOS levels is detected after heat stress but iNOS increases 3 days after treatment compared with that of controls. Immunocytochemistry shows a robust increase of iNOS expression in germ cells (Guo et al., 2009). Thus, heat stress induces NO production and it may contribute to germ cells oxidative damage. However, it is unknown the molecular targets modified by NO production and their consequences in testis physiology.

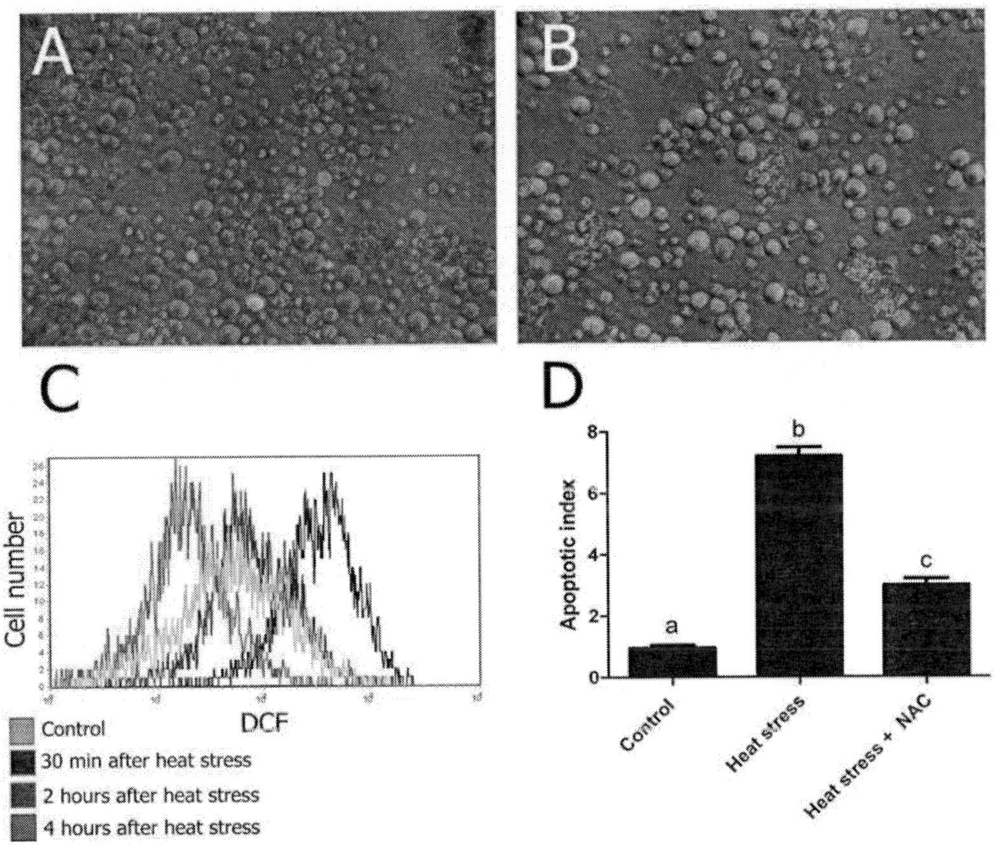

Figure 2. Heat stress induces ROS and germ cell apoptosis. A) Control and B) heat stress treated germ cells and labeled with a fluorescent probe to detect ROS in live cells. C) Flow cytometry shows that ROS levels dramatically increase after 30 min of treatment (compare grey line with black line). Then, 2 hrs later, ROS levels stars to decrease (blue line) and 4 hrs later they reach basal levels (green line). D) In vivo, heat stress induces a significant increase in the number of apoptotic cells 24 hrs after treatment. Interestingly, a ROS sacavenger (L-NAC), prevent germ cell apoptosis. n=3, different letters indicate a significant difference, $p<0.05$.

Under different conditions, the production of ROS exceeds the antioxidant capacity resulting in oxidative stress which elicits degenerative responses such as DNA damage, necrosis, and apoptosis (Figure 2). Heat stress results in an increase of apoptosis and ROS levels in isolate germ cells (Ikeda et al., 1999). Interestingly, oxidative damage, along with increased apoptosis, is also a hallmark of other pathologies involved in male infertility, such as varicocele and testicular torsion (Turner et al., 2004; Turner et al., 2005; Shiraishi and

Naito, 2007; Shiraishi et al., 2010). Heat stress cause upregulation of heme oxygenase 1 (Hmox1) and the antioxidant enzymes glutathione peroxidase 1, glutathione S-transferase alpha and SOD1, consistent with a robust oxidative stress response (Table 1). Consistent with the hypothesis that these enzymes participates in the antioxidant response, germ cells isolated from SOD1-knockout mice are more vulnerable to apoptosis induced by heat stress than wild type animals, suggesting a protective role of this enzyme in the oxidative stress insult induced by heat stress (Ishii et al., 2005). However, other studies have reported a downregulation of mRNAs encoding for Glutathione reductase 1, Glutathione S-transferase alpha 2, Manganese superoxide dismutase 2 (SOD2), Extracellular superoxide dismutase Cu-Zn (SOD3) (Rockett et al., 2001).

Thus, it is seems that heat stress induces upregulation of specific isoforms of stress response enzymes (SOD1 but not SOD2 or SOD3), indicating the activation of specific genetic response program. Peroxiredoxin-4 (Prx4) belongs to a new antioxidant family protein and it plays a role regulating NF-κB (nuclear factor κB). Prx4-knockout male mice are fertile, except for testicular atrophy and an increase in germ cell apoptosis (Iuchi et al., 2009).

Interestingly, Prx-4 knockout germ cells show elevated oxidation of lipids and protein thiols, and male mice display an increase apoptosis (TUNEL-positive cells) after heat stress, suggesting that Prx4 is important in the oxidative stress response in germ cells.

Table 1. Proteins and enzyme upregulated after heat stress

Protein/Enzyme	Localization	References
Superoxide Dismutase	Sertoli cell	(Ahotupa and Huhtaniemi, 1992)
Glutation Peroxidase	Sertoli cell	(Ahotupa and Huhtaniemi, 1992; Ikeda et al., 1999; Paul et al., 2008)
Glutation S-transferase	Sertoli cell	(Paul et al., 2008)
Hsp70.2 (heat shock protein)	Spermatocytes	(Widlak et al., 1994; Widlak, 2006)
Heat shock factor 1 and 2 (19,20)	Spermatocytes	(Nakai et al., 2000; Hayashida et al., 2006)
High temperature requirement A2 (HtrA2)	spermatocytes and some spermatids,	(Hayashi et al., 2006)
Peroxiredoxin 4	Germ cell	(Matsuki et al., 2002; Iuchi et al., 2009)
heme oxygenases (HO-1 and HO-2)	Sertoli cell, spermatocytes and spermatids	(Ewing and Maines, 1995)
Thiol specific antioxidant protein	Sertoli cell	(Ishii et al., 2005)
PARP	Sertoli and germ cells	(Tramontano et al., 2000; Scarabelli et al., 2010)

Downstream ROS production different intracellular pathways are activated among which the ASK1/p38MAPK has been shown to be important in germ cell apoptosis after heat stress (Ueda et al., 2002; Matsuzawa and Ichijo, 2008). ROS are able to oxidize Thioredoxine (Trx) reactive thiol groups and, respectively, to mediate activation of apoptosis signal-regulating kinase 1 (ASK1)/MKKK5ASK1, a ubiquitously expressed enzyme that activates JNK and p38 MAP kinase pathways (Hsieh and Papaconstantinou, 2006; Matsuzawa and Ichijo, 2008; Hsieh et al., 2010). In rats and monkeys, heats stress induces sustained activation of both mitogen-activated protein kinase (MAPK) 1/3 and MAPK14 (p38MAPK) (Johnson et al., 2008; Jia et al., 2009; Lizama et al., 2009). Interestingly, the protection offered by caspase-2 or calpain inhibitors prevents MAPK14 (p38MAPK) activation, suggesting that caspase and calpain activation is upstream of MAPK activation (Johnson et al., 2008; Lizama et al., 2009).

Functional genomics studies have shown that About 416 transcripts are differentially expressed between normal C57BL/6 testisand normal MRL/MpJ-+/+ testis (a heat stress resistant mouse strain). The biological functions of 185 out of these 416 transcripts are unknown, and 36 are involved in transport, 24 in DNA-dependent regulation of transcription, 15 in metabolic processes, 13 in protein amino acid phosphorylation, and 5 in apoptosis (Li et al., 2009). In this same study the authors identified a total of 67 transcripts as being heat-regulated in C57BL/6. In another study using ICR mice with a heat stress protocol of 35°C for 24 h, it was shown that 225 genes are differentially expressed (Cammack et al., 2009). Proteomic analysis of human testicular biopsies before and at 2 and 9 wk after heat treatment shows that 31 and 36 known proteins are differentially expressed at 2 and 9 wk after heat treatment, respectively (Zhu et al., 2010).

The available evidence strongly suggests that heat stress induce a strong REDOX state imbalance. Despite to upregulate many enzymes involved in antioxidant response, some germ cells cannot cope with the elevate ROS levels and they die by apoptosis. However, other group of germ cells can overcame this oxidative stress and accomplishes differentiation, but the sperms produced by this way bear high levels of DNA fragmentation, and probably other yet unknown harmful modifications, which could explain embryo developmental abnormalities observed after heat stress.

A Model to Germ Cell Apoptosis Induced by Heat Stress

Our model is based in basically two types of oxidative stress environments. One is where germ cells can cope most of the oxidative damage and they did not enter into apoptosis (Figure 3, right handside). In the second scenario, the antioxidant defense mechanism is overcome by the elevated ROS production and then it induces germ cell demise, probably because it accelerates apoptosis in cells prone to undergo this process. In our model, heat stress induces an elevate ROS production probably due to an increase in iNOS expression (Figure 3). An interesting, but yet unexplored possibility is that other elements, such XO upregulation or mitochondrial dysfunction might contribute at this early step. Enhanced ROS levels will induce expression of antioxidant defense enzymes such as GPx, SOD glutathione S-transferase alpha (GSTA) and HMOX1 that will lower ROS levels and they preserve germ cell viability by preventing oxidative damage in spermatocytes and spermatids (Figure 3, cell survival pathway). In our model, those germ cells will produce sperm bearing chromatin abnormalities product of that early and severe oxidative damage (as evaluated by 8-oxo-dG and histone modifications) experienced during spermatogenesis. On the other side, if the antioxidant defense mechanism is overwhelmed by the levels of ROS, oxidative stress will induce activation of caspase-2 and/or calpains, which in turn will activate p38 MAPK/MAPK14. In this way, it has been shown that p38 MAPK induces phosphorylation and activation of p53 (Huang et al., 1999), a major transcription factor that targets different proapoptotic genes such as *bax* and *Fas*, which have been shown to be upregulated after testis heat stress or experimental cryptochidism (Figure 3). Then, BAX, and probably other yet unidentified proapoptotic protein such as BAD, BAK or BIM will translocate to the mitochondria and induce its permeabilization and promotes released of cytochrome-C and other proapoptotic proteins after testis heat stress. Then, the apoptosome formation will activate caspase-3 that ultimately dismantles the germ cell (Figure 3). In addition, studies in somatic cells have shown that p38 MAPK increases mitochondrial permeability and promotes BAX translocation to the mitochondria, but this mechanism has not been studied in germ cells (Wang et al., 2008; Lu et al., 2010). Alternatively, oxidative damage leads to DNA damage by down-regulation of genes involved in DNA repair such as *Ogg1* (involved in base excision repair), *Xpg* (involved in nucleotide excision repair) and *Rad54* (involved in double-strand break repair) were all down-regulated (Rockett et al., 2001). DNA damage is a strong apoptotic signal that induces activation of p53 and p73, which is expressed in germ cells, but its role in apoptosis induced by heat stress have not yet been studied. Activation of p53 and/or p73 could lead to cyclinB1 degradation and arrest of germ cell cycle. Therefore, an elevate levels of apoptosis will lead to a decrease in sperm production and to contribute to male infertility (Figure 3). Therefore, in our model low sperm count is due to increased levels of germ cell apoptosis, and embryo miscarriage is explained by those spermatozoa produced by germ cell that despite to have been under oxidative stress they did not underwent apoptosis, but they carry DNA abnormalities. This models is based on the available literature on testis heat stress, but it also may apply to other insults and/or pathologies involving oxidative damage such as varicocele, testicular torsion or hypoxia (Turner et al., 2005; Jung and Schuppe, 2007; Farias et al., 2010; Shiraishi et al., 2010).

This model is center on changes and modification in observed germ cells and it does not take account other modifications such as hormone production or the contribution of Sertoli cell to germ cell apoptosis. In this regard, there is no data concerning the role of Sertoli cell to germ cell apoptosis. Thus, this is an open field to study the contribution of para/juxtacrine interactions between germ and Sertoli cells after heat stress.

Therapeutical Approaches to Reduce Apoptosis and Oxidative Stress Induced by Heat Stress

Since oxidative stress is the major source of damage after testicular heat stress, it seems logical that antioxidant supplement have been chosen has the primary treatment in order to prevent germ cell apoptosis and sperm damage in several animal models. In recent decades, Chinese clinical studies have shown that *Lycium barbarum* polysaccharides prevent germ cell apoptosis after in vitro heat shock (Wang et al., 2002). They reported that polysacarides of *L.barbarum* could inhibit time-and hypertermia-induced structural damage in murine seminiferous epithelium and delay apoptosis in this system. They also found that polysacarides of *L. barbarum* has a strong antioxidant activity which may explain its protective effect; it is possible that polysacarides of L. barbarum could inhibit apoptosis in cultured seminiferous tubules by protecting them from the reactivity of free radicals (Table 1). In another study, the treatment with polysacarides of L. barbarum prevent testis weight reduction after heat stress all four concentrations (10, 50, 100, and 200mg/kg per day), along with increase SOD activity and reduced malondialdehyde MDA levels (Luo et al., 2006). They also observed that the morphological structure of seminiferous tubules was close to that normal control show intact structure and spermatogonia arrangements (Table 2). Ghrelin is an endogenous ligand for growth hormone secretagogue receptor that regulates growth hormone secretion, increases appetite and contributes to energy homeostasis. Some reports propose the potential involvement of ghrelin regulating the reproductive axis by suppression LH secretion and decrease LH responsiveness to GnRH (Fernandez-Fernandez et al., 2004). Recently, it was proposed that ghrelin may act as an antioxidant and/or antiinflammatory agent increasing the activity of antioxidant enzymes such as superoxide dismutase, catalase and glutathione peroxidase and decreasing the level of malondialdehyde (Zwirska-Korczala et al., 2007). Oral administration of ghrelin for 60 days in daily basis, after heat stress, shows a rapid recovery of seminiferous tubule damage. The protective effect of ghrelin also have been shown in spermatozoa since it enhances viability of rat sperm during incubation al 37°C (Kheradmand et al., 2011).

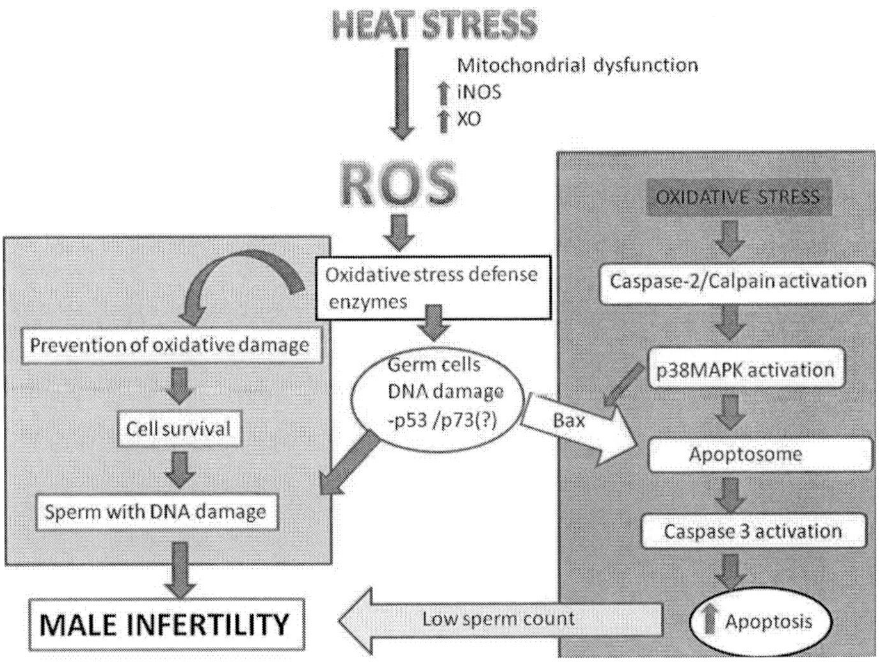

Figure 3. A model of germ cell apoptosis induced by heat stress. Our model is based in basically two types of oxidative stress environments. One is where germ cells can cope most of the oxidative damage and they survive and achieve differentiation (left hand side). However, the spermatozoa produced by these germ cells bear high levels of DNA damage giving rise to abnormalities during embryo development. On the other hand, the antioxidant defense mechanism is overcome by the elevated ROS production and germ cells enter into apoptosis (right hand side). Central in this model is the DNA damage in testicular germ cells (spermatocytes and spermatids), produced by ROS production, regardless they survive or die by apoptosis. In addition, the low sperm count after heat stress can be explained by the high apoptosis.

Table 2. Therapeutical approaches to prevent testicular damage after oxidative damage

Molecule	Biological function	Dosis / Administration	Insult	Reference
Calpain synthetic inhibitors	Calpain inhibitor	intratesticular	Heat stress	(Lizama et al., 2009)
Ghrelin	Anti-oxidant	2 nmol/100 µl saline Subcutaneus	Heat stress	(Kheradmand et al., 2011)
Tetrahydrobiopterin (BH4)	Tetrahydrobiopterin (BH4)	Gavage	Heat stress	(Kondo et al., 2008)
Lycium barbarum	Anti-oxidant	Oral	Heat stress	(Luo et al., 2006)
Ferula hermonis	Anti-oxidant	0.025 ml/ 100 g 50% Oral	Heat stress	(Hanafi, 2010)
α- Tocopherol	Anti-oxidant	30 mg/kg i.p.	Cryptorchidism	(Vigueras-Villasenor et al., 2010)
Alopurinol	Xanthine oxidase Inhibitor	≥ 1 mg/kg/dia i.p.	Cryptorchidism	(Kumagai et al., 2002)
BOF 2472	Xantine oxidase Inhibitor	300 µg/dia i.p.	Cryptorchidism	(Kumagai et al., 2002)
Prunus armeniaca L (apricot)	Anti-oxidant	Gavage + 20% Apricot	Radiation	(Ugras et al.)
Granulocyte colony-stimulating factor (GCSF)	Growth Factor	100 µg/kg/day Subcutaneous	Radiation	(Kim et al., 2011)
Licopeno	Anti-oxidant	4 mg kg–Oral	Cisplatin	(Luo et al., 2006)
Curcumin (CMN)	Anti-oxidant	7 mg/kg i.p.	Cisplatin	(Ilbey et al., 2009)
Melatonin	Hormone	25 mg/kg i.p.	Formaldehyde	(Ozen et al., 2008)
L-carnitine	Anti-oxidant	(500 m g/kg/d)	Ischemia-reperfusion	(Gurocak et al., 2011)
Meloxicam	AINES	3 mg/kg/d i.p.	Ischemia-reperfusion	(Gurocak et al., 2011)
Rosiglitazone	Thiazolidinediones	4 mg/kg i.v.	Ischemia-reperfusion	(Inan et al., 2007)
Anandamide	Cannabinoid	10 mg/kg i.p.	Ischemia-reperfusion	(Rabani, 2006)
Sivelestat	Elastase inhibidor	15 mg/kg - 60 mg/kg i.ab.	Ischemia-reperfusion	(Tsounapi et al., 2011)
anax ginseng (P. ginseng)	Anti-oxidant	100 mg/kg/day Oral	Ischemia-reperfusion	(Kim et al., 2010)

Dietary administration of tetrahydrobiopterin (BH4), an essential cofactor of NOS, prevent the increase of GTP cyclohydrolase I (GTPCH I) activity, nitrotyrosine levels, and NO production, in a cryptorchid model mice. In addition, BH4 administration prevents testis weight reduction and testicular histological damage in crytorchid mice. Allopurinol and BOF-4272, two xanthine oxidade inhibitors have been shown to decrease germ cell apoptosis after unilateral cryptorchidism with i.p. injection of inhibitor on daily bases for 7 days after treatment (Table 2). In this way, α-Tocopherol has been shown to have similar results than xanthine oxidase inhibitors after experimental cryptorchidism (Vigueras-Villasenor et al., 2010). Thus, a number of putative therapies, not always based in antioxidant compounds, may be useful to prevent testicular damage induced by heat stress (Table 2).

Interestingly, infertile patients treated oral with α-tocopherol (vitamin E) significantly decreased spermatozoa MDA concentration and increased motility. Vitamin E treatment greatly decreased the MDA concentration in spermatozoa down to normospermic levels, and this change in levels seemed to be a good predictor of pregnancy (Makker et al., 2009). Thus, antioxidant therapy does not only include benefits to testicular damage by heats stress, but other pathologies involving elevate ROS production may also benefit. In this way, germ cell apoptosis and testicular damage after ischemia-reperfusion, radiation and anti-cancer drugs, reduce significantly if an antioxidant is supplemented before or during the insult (Table 2).

Conclusion

Testicular heat stress involves oxidative damage at the levels of germ cell, Leydig cells, and probably Sertoli cells. It is clear that heat stress is related to some pathological conditions such as varicocele or cryptorchidism. Thus, pharmaceutically approaches could be focus to decrease oxidative damage, probably by dietary supplement with natural-derive antioxidant (such as plant extracts) or chemical defined compounds. By this approach it is possible to find a good therapeutical protocol in order to decrease sperm DNA damage and germ cell apoptosis and in this way prevent and/or decrease male infertility.

Acknowledgments

Part of this work was financed by FONDECYT (1110778) to RDM.

References

Ahotupa, M. and I. Huhtaniemi. Impaired detoxification of reactive oxygen and consequent oxidative stress in experimentally cryptorchid rat testis. *Biol. Reprod.* 1992, 46, 1114-1118.

Allemand, I.; A. Anglo; A. Y. Jeantet; I. Cerutti and E. May. Testicular wild-type p53 expression in transgenic mice induces spermiogenesis alterations ranging from differentiation defects to apoptosis. *Oncogene.* 1999, 18, 6521-6530.

Bedford, J. M. Anatomical evidence for the epididymis as the prime mover in the evolution of the scrotum. *Am. J. Anat.* 1978, 152, 483-507.

Bedford, J. M. Effects of elevated temperature on the epididymis and testis: experimental studies. *Adv. Exp. Med. Biol.* 1991, 286, 19-32.

Bedford, J. M.; M. Berrios and G. L. Dryden. Biology of the scrotum. IV. Testis location and temperature sensitivity. *J. Exp. Zool.* 1982, 224, 379-388.

Beumer, T. L.; H. L. Roepers-Gajadien; I. S. Gademan; P. P. van Buul; G. Gil-Gomez; D. H. Rutgers and D. G. de Rooij. The role of the tumor suppressor p53 in spermatogenesis. *Cell Death Differ.* 1998, 5, 669-677.

Bhasin, S.; D. M. de Kretser and H. W. Baker. Clinical review 64: Pathophysiology and natural history of male infertility. *J. Clin. Endocrinol. Metab.* 1994, 79, 1525-1529.

Bieber, A. M.; L. Marcon; B. F. Hales and B. Robaire. Effects of chemotherapeutic agents for testicular cancer on the male rat reproductive system, spermatozoa, and fertility. *J. Androl.* 2006, 27, 189-200.

Blanco-Rodriguez, J.; C. Martinez-Garcia and A. Porras. Correlation between DNA synthesis in the second, third and fourth generations of spermatogonia and the occurrence of apoptosis in both spermatogonia and spermatocytes. *Reproduction.* 2003, 126, 661-668.

Busso, D.; C. Dominguez; T. Perez-Acle and R. D. Moreno. Life-giving caspases: revealing new roles during mouse embryo preimplantation development. *Int. J. Dev. Biol.* 2010, 54, 857-865.

Cameron, R. D. and A. W. Blackshaw. The effect of elevated ambient temperature on spermatogenesis in the boar. *J. Reprod. Fertil.* 1980, 59, 173-179.

Cammack, K. M.; E. Antoniou; L. Hearne and W. R. Lamberson. Testicular gene expression in male mice divergent for fertility after heat stress. *Theriogenology.* 2009, 71, 651-661.

Clermont, Y. The cycle of the seminiferous epithelium in man. *Am. J. Anat.* 1963, 112, 35-51.

Clermont, Y. and C. P. Lebond. Spermiogenesis of man, monkey, ram and other mammals as shown by the "periodic acid-schiff" technique. *Am. J. Anat.* 1955, 96, 22-50.

Codelia, V. A.; M. Cisterna; A. R. Alvarez and R. D. Moreno. p73 participates in male germ cells apoptosis induced by etoposide. *Mol. Hum. Reprod.* 2010, 16, 734-742.

Codelia, V. A.; P. Cisternas and R. D. Moreno. Relevance of caspase activity during apoptosis in pubertal rat spermatogenesis. *Mol. Reprod. Dev.* 2008, 75, 881-889.

Coultas, L.; P. Bouillet; K. L. Loveland; S. Meachem; H. Perlman; J. M. Adams and A. Strasser. Concomitant loss of proapoptotic BH3-only Bcl-2 antagonists Bik and Bim arrests spermatogenesis. *Embo J.* 2005, 24, 3963-3973.

Coureuil, M.; P. Fouchet; M. Prat; B. Letallec; V. Barroca; C. Dos Santos; C. Racine and I. Allemand. Caspase-independent death of meiotic and postmeiotic cells overexpressing p53: calpain involvement. *Cell Death Differ.* 2006, 13, 1927-1937.

Chen, L.; S. N. Willis, et al. Differential targeting of prosurvival Bcl-2 proteins by their BH3-only ligands allows complementary apoptotic function. *Mol. Cell.* 2005, 17, 393-403.

Dadoune, J. P. and A. Demeoulin. Structure anf function of the testis. In: Thibault, C., M. C. Levasseur and R. H. F. Hunter (Eds), *Reproduction in Mammals and Man.* Paris: Ellipses; 1993.

Davidson, J. F. and R. H. Schiestl. Mitochondrial respiratory electron carriers are involved in oxidative stress during heat stress in Saccharomyces cerevisiae. *Mol. Cell Biol.* 2001, 21, 8483-8489.

De Gendt, K.; J. V. Swinnen, et al. A Sertoli cell-selective knockout of the androgen receptor causes spermatogenic arrest in meiosis. *Proc. Natl. Acad. Sci. U. S. A.* 2004, 101, 1327-1332.

de Kretser, D. and J. Kerr. The cytology of the testis. In: Knobil, E. and J. Neil (Eds), *The Physiology of Reproduction.* New York: Raven Press; 1988; 837-919.

de Rooij, D. G. and L. D. Russell. All you wanted to know about spermatogonia but were afraid to ask. *J. Androl.* 2000, 21, 776-798.

de Vries, K. J.; T. Wiedmer; P. J. Sims and B. M. Gadella. Caspase-independent exposure of aminophospholipids and tyrosine phosphorylation in bicarbonate responsive human sperm cells. *Biol. Reprod.* 2003, 68, 2122-2134.

Degterev, A. and J. Yuan. Expansion and evolution of cell death programmes. *Nat. Rev. Mol. Cell Biol.* 2008, 9, 378-390.

Dobbelstein, M.; S. Strano; J. Roth and G. Blandino. p73-induced apoptosis: a question of compartments and cooperation. *Biochem. Biophys. Res. Commun.* 2005, 331, 688-693.

Dym, M. and D. W. Fawcett. The blood-testis barrier in the rat and the physiological compartmentation of the seminiferous epithelium. *Biol. Reprod.* 1970, 3, 308-326.

El-Missiry, M. A. Enhanced testicular antioxidant system by ascorbic acid in alloxan diabetic rats. *Comp. Biochem. Physiol. C Pharmacol. Toxicol. Endocrinol.* 1999, 124, 233-237.

Elliott, M. R.; S. Zheng, et al. Unexpected requirement for ELMO1 in clearance of apoptotic germ cells in vivo. *Nature.* 2010, 467, 333-337.

Ewing, J. F. and M. D. Maines. Distribution of constitutive (HO-2) and heat-inducible (HO-1) heme oxygenase isozymes in rat testes: HO-2 displays stage-specific expression in germ cells. *Endocrinology.* 1995, 136, 2294-2302.

Fadeel, B.; A. Ottosson and S. Pervaiz. Big wheel keeps on turning: apoptosome regulation and its role in chemoresistance. *Cell Death Differ.* 2008, 15, 443-452.

Farias, J. G.; M. Puebla; A. Acevedo; P. J. Tapia; E. Gutierrez; A. Zepeda; G. Calaf; C. Juantok and J. G. Reyes. Oxidative stress in rat testis and epididymis under intermittent hypobaric hypoxia: protective role of ascorbate supplementation. *J. Androl.* 2010, 31, 314-321.

Feng, H. L.; J. I. Sandlow; A. E. Sparks; A. Sandra and L. J. Zheng. Decreased expression of the c-kit receptor is associated with increased apoptosis in subfertile human testes. *Fertil. Steril.* 1999, 71, 85-89.

Fernandez-Fernandez, R.; M. Tena-Sempere; E. Aguilar and L. Pinilla. Ghrelin effects on gonadotropin secretion in male and female rats. *Neurosci. Lett.* 2004, 362, 103-107.

Foldesy, R. G. and J. M. Bedford. Biology of the scrotum. I. Temperature and androgen as determinants of the sperm storage capacity of the rat cauda epididymidis. *Biol. Reprod.* 1982, 26, 673-682.

Franco, R.; O. Schoneveld; A. G. Georgakilas and M. I. Panayiotidis. Oxidative stress, DNA methylation and carcinogenesis. *Cancer Lett.* 2008, 266, 6-11.

Giammona, C. J.; P. Sawhney; Y. Chandrasekaran and J. H. Richburg. Death receptor response in rodent testis after mono-(2-ethylhexyl) phthalate exposure. *Toxicol. Appl. Pharmacol.* 2002, 185, 119-127.

Griffiths, J. The Structural Changes in the Testicle of the Dog when it is Replaced within the Abdominal Cavity. *J. Anat. Physiol.* 1893, 27, 482 481-500.

Guo, J.; Y. Jia, et al. Expression of nitric oxide synthase during germ cell apoptosis in testis of cynomolgus monkey after testosterone and heat treatment. *J. Androl.* 2009, 30, 190-199.

Gurocak, S.; A. Yilmaz; E. Alp; I. Ure; S. Sozen; S. Menevse; A. Menevse and I. Bozkirli. Inflammation and Oxidative Stress in Testicular Torsion: Do They Deserve Intensive Treatment to Save Both Guilty and Innocent Testes? *Urology*. 2011.

Hanafi, E. M. A Novel Herbal Remedy to Alleviate Drawbacks of Heat Stress in Rats with Special References to Some Reproductive and Molecular Alterations. *Global Journal of Biotech. & Biochem.* 2010, 5, 145-152.

Hansen, P. J. Effects of heat stress on mammalian reproduction. *Philos. Trans. R Soc. Lond. B Biol. Sci.* 2009, 364, 3341-3350.

Hayashi, T.; S. Yoshida; A. Yoshinaga; R. Ohno; N. Ishii and T. Yamada. HtrA2 is up-regulated in the rat testis after experimental cryptorchidism. *Int. J. Urol.* 2006, 13, 157-164.

Hayashida, N.; S. Inouye; M. Fujimoto; Y. Tanaka; H. Izu; E. Takaki; H. Ichikawa; J. Rho and A. Nakai. A novel HSF1-mediated death pathway that is suppressed by heat shock proteins. *Embo J.* 2006, 25, 4773-4783.

Heller, C. G. and Y. Clermont. Spermatogenesis in man: an estimate of its duration. *Science*. 1963, 140, 184-186.

Henkler, F.; E. Behrle; K. M. Dennehy; A. Wicovsky; N. Peters; C. Warnke; K. Pfizenmaier and H. Wajant. The extracellular domains of FasL and Fas are sufficient for the formation of supramolecular FasL-Fas clusters of high stability. *J. Cell Biol.* 2005, 168, 1087-1098.

Hermo, L.; R. M. Pelletier; D. G. Cyr and C. E. Smith. Surfing the wave, cycle, life history, and genes/proteins expressed by testicular germ cells. Part 1: background to spermatogenesis, spermatogonia, and spermatocytes. *Microsc. Res. Tech.* 2010, 73, 241-278.

Hikim, A. P.; Y. Lue; C. M. Yamamoto; Y. Vera; S. Rodriguez; P. H. Yen; K. Soeng; C. Wang and R. S. Swerdloff. Key apoptotic pathways for heat-induced programmed germ cell death in the testis. *Endocrinology*. 2003, 144, 3167-3175.

Hill, B. G.; B. P. Dranka; S. M. Bailey; J. R. Lancaster, Jr. and V. M. Darley-Usmar. What part of NO don't you understand? Some answers to the cardinal questions in nitric oxide biology. *J. Biol. Chem.* 2010, 285, 19699-19704.

Hirano, T. Repair system of 7, 8-dihydro-8-oxoguanine as a defense line against carcinogenesis. *J. Radiat. Res. (Tokyo)*, 2008, 49, 329-340.

Hjollund, N. H.; J. P. Bonde; T. K. Jensen and J. Olsen. Diurnal scrotal skin temperature and semen quality. The Danish First Pregnancy Planner Study Team. *Int. J. Androl.* 2000, 23, 309-318.

Hogarth, C. A. and M. D. Griswold. The key role of vitamin A in spermatogenesis. *J. Clin. Invest.* 2010, 120, 956-962.

Honarpour, N.; C. Du; J. A. Richardson; R. E. Hammer; X. Wang and J. Herz. Adult Apaf-1-deficient mice exhibit male infertility. *Dev. Biol.* 2000, 218, 248-258.

Hsieh, C. C.; M. Kuro-o; K. P. Rosenblatt; R. Brobey and J. Papaconstantinou. The ASK1-Signalosome regulates p38 MAPK activity in response to levels of endogenous oxidative stress in the Klotho mouse models of aging. *Aging. (Albany NY)*, 2010, 2, 597-611.

Hsieh, C. C. and J. Papaconstantinou. Thioredoxin-ASK1 complex levels regulate ROS-mediated p38 MAPK pathway activity in livers of aged and long-lived Snell dwarf mice. *Faseb. J.* 2006, 20, 259-268.

Hsu, S. Y. and A. J. Hsueh. A splicing variant of the Bcl-2 member Bok with a truncated BH3 domain induces apoptosis but does not dimerize with antiapoptotic Bcl-2 proteins in vitro. *J. Biol. Chem.* 1998, 273, 30139-30146.

Hsu, S. Y.; P. Lin and A. J. Hsueh. BOD (Bcl-2-related ovarian death gene) is an ovarian BH3 domain-containing proapoptotic Bcl-2 protein capable of dimerization with diverse antiapoptotic Bcl-2 members. *Mol. Endocrinol.* 1998, 12, 1432-1440.

Huang, C.; W. Y. Ma; A. Maxiner; Y. Sun and Z. Dong. p38 kinase mediates UV-induced phosphorylation of p53 protein at serine 389. *J. Biol. Chem.* 1999, 274, 12229-12235.

Ikeda, M.; H. Kodama; J. Fukuda; Y. Shimizu; M. Murata; J. Kumagai and T. Tanaka. Role of radical oxygen species in rat testicular germ cell apoptosis induced by heat stress. *Biol. Reprod.* 1999, 61, 393-399.

Ilbey, Y. O.; E. Ozbek; M. Cekmen; A. Simsek; A. Otunctemur and A. Somay. Protective effect of curcumin in cisplatin-induced oxidative injury in rat testis: mitogen-activated protein kinase and nuclear factor-kappa B signaling pathways. *Hum. Reprod.* 2009, 24, 1717-1725.

Inan, M.; U. Basaran; D. Dokmeci; M. Kanter; O. Yalcin; N. Aydogdu and N. Turan. Rosiglitazone, an agonist of peroxisome proliferator-activated receptor-gamma, prevents contralateral testicular ischaemia-reperfusion injury in prepubertal rats. *Clin. Exp. Pharmacol. Physiol.* 2007, 34, 457-461.

Ishii, T.; S. Matsuki; Y. Iuchi; F. Okada; S. Toyosaki; Y. Tomita; Y. Ikeda and J. Fujii. Accelerated impairment of spermatogenic cells in SOD1-knockout mice under heat stress. *Free Radic Res.* 2005, 39, 697-705.

Iuchi, Y.; F. Okada; S. Tsunoda; N. Kibe; N. Shirasawa; M. Ikawa; M. Okabe; Y. Ikeda and J. Fujii. Peroxiredoxin 4 knockout results in elevated spermatogenic cell death via oxidative stress. *Biochem. J.* 2009, 419, 149-158.

Jahnukainen, K.; D. Chrysis; M. Hou; M. Parvinen; S. Eksborg and O. Soder. Increased apoptosis occurring during the first wave of spermatogenesis is stage-specific and primarily affects midpachytene spermatocytes in the rat testis. *Biol. Reprod.* 2004, 70, 290-296.

Jannes, P.; C. Spiessens; I. Van der Auwera; T. D'Hooghe; G. Verhoeven and D. Vanderschueren. Male subfertility induced by acute scrotal heating affects embryo quality in normal female mice. *Hum. Reprod.* 1998, 13, 372-375.

Ji, G.; A. Gu, et al. Polymorphisms in cell death pathway genes are associated with altered sperm apoptosis and poor semen quality. *Hum. Reprod.* 2009, 24, 2439-2446.

Jia, Y.; J. Castellanos; C. Wang; I. Sinha-Hikim; Y. Lue; R. S. Swerdloff and A. P. Sinha-Hikim. Mitogen-activated protein kinase signaling in male germ cell apoptosis in the rat. *Biol. Reprod.* 2009, 80, 771-780.

Johnson, C.; Y. Jia, et al. Role of caspase 2 in apoptotic signaling in primate and murine germ cells. *Biol. Reprod.* 2008, 79, 806-814.

Jung, A.; F. Leonhardt; W. B. Schill and H. C. Schuppe. Influence of the type of undertrousers and physical activity on scrotal temperature. *Hum. Reprod.* 2005, 20, 1022-1027.

Jung, A.; W. B. Schill and H. C. Schuppe. Improvement of semen quality by nocturnal scrotal cooling in oligozoospermic men with a history of testicular maldescent. *Int. J. Androl.* 2005, 28, 93-98.

Jung, A. and H. C. Schuppe. Influence of genital heat stress on semen quality in humans. *Andrologia*. 2007, 39, 203-215.

Kheradmand, A.; O. Dezfoulian and M. J. Tarrahi. Ghrelin attenuates heat-induced degenerative effects in the rat testis. *Regul. Pept.* 2011, 167, 97-104.

Kim, J.; S. Lee; B. Jeon; W. Jang; C. Moon and S. Kim. Protection of spermatogenesis against gamma ray-induced damage by granulocyte colony-stimulating factor in mice. *Andrologia*. 2011, 43, 87-93.

Kim, Y. H.; G. H. Kim; J. H. Shin; K. S. Kim and J. S. Lim. Effect of korean red ginseng on testicular tissue injury after torsion and detorsion. *Korean J. Urol.* 2010, 51, 794-799.

Kleisner, K.; R. Ivell and J. Flegr. The evolutionary history of testicular externalization and the origin of the scrotum. *J. Biosci.* 2010, 35, 27-37.

Knudson, C. M.; K. S. Tung; W. G. Tourtellotte; G. A. Brown and S. J. Korsmeyer. Bax-deficient mice with lymphoid hyperplasia and male germ cell death. *Science*. 1995, 270, 96-99.

Kondo, Y.; T. Ishikawa; K. Yamaguchi; T. Yada and M. Fujisawa. Oral administration of tetrahydrobiopterin attenuates testicular damage by reducing nitric oxide synthase activity in a cryptorchid mouse model. *J. Androl.* 2008, 29, 153-163.

Kong, W. H.; G. Zheng; J. N. Lu and J. K. Tso. Temperature dependent expression of cdc2 and cyclin B1 in spermatogenic cells during spermatogenesis. *Cell Res.* 2000, 10, 289-302.

Ku, B.; C. Liang; J. U. Jung and B. H. Oh. Evidence that inhibition of BAX activation by BCL-2 involves its tight and preferential interaction with the BH3 domain of BAX. *Cell Res*. 2010, 21, 627-641.

Kumagai, A.; H. Kodama; J. Kumagai; J. Fukuda; K. Kawamura; H. Tanikawa; N. Sato and T. Tanaka. Xanthine oxidase inhibitors suppress testicular germ cell apoptosis induced by experimental cryptorchidism. *Mol. Hum. Reprod.* 2002, 8, 118-123.

Kumagai, J.; J. Fukuda; H. Kodama; M. Murata; K. Kawamura; H. Itoh and T. Tanaka. Germ cell-specific heat shock protein 105 binds to p53 in a temperature-sensitive manner in rat testis. *Eur. J. Biochem*. 2000, 267, 3073-3078.

Kuribayashi, K.; P. A. Mayes and W. S. El-Deiry. What are caspases 3 and 7 doing upstream of the mitochondria? *Cancer Biol. Ther*. 2006, 5, 763-765.

Lee, J. Y.; R. Dada; E. Sabanegh; A. Carpi and A. Agarwal. Role of genetics in azoospermia. *Urology*. 2011, 77, 598-601.

Li, Y.; Q. Zhou; R. Hively; L. Yang; C. Small and M. D. Griswold. Differential gene expression in the testes of different murine strains under normal and hyperthermic conditions. *J. Androl.* 2009, 30, 325-337.

Lizama, C.; I. Alfaro; J. G. Reyes and R. D. Moreno. Up-regulation of CD95 (Apo-1/Fas) is associated with spermatocyte apoptosis during the first round of spermatogenesis in the rat. *Apoptosis*. 2007, 12, 499-512.

Lizama, C.; C. F. Lagos; R. Lagos-Cabre; L. Cantuarias; F. Rivera; P. Huenchunir; T. Perez-Acle; F. Carrion and R. D. Moreno. Calpain inhibitors prevent p38 MAPK activation and germ cell apoptosis after heat stress in pubertal rat testes. *J. Cell Physiol.* 2009, 221, 296-305.

Lizama, C.; A. Ludwig and R. D. Moreno. Etoposide induces apoptosis and upregulation of TACE/ADAM17 and ADAM10 in an in vitro male germ cell line model. *Biochim. Biophys. Acta*. 2011, 1813, 120-128.

Lizama, C.; D. Rojas-Benitez; M. Antonelli; A. Ludwig; X. Bustamante-Marin; J. Brouwer-Visser and R. D. Moreno. TACE/ADAM17 is involved in germ cell apoptosis during rat spermatogenesis. *Reproduction*. 2010, 140, 305-317.

Lizama, C.; D. Rojas-Benitez; M. Antonelli; A. Ludwig and R. D. Moreno. Involvement of TACE/ADAM17 and ADAM10 in etoposide-induced apoptosis of germ cells in rat spermatogenesis. *J. Cell Physiol*. 2011, 2011.

Love, C. C. and R. M. Kenney. Scrotal heat stress induces altered sperm chromatin structure associated with a decrease in protamine disulfide bonding in the stallion. *Biol. Reprod*. 1999, 60, 615-620.

Lu, T. H.; S. Y. Hsieh, et al. Involvement of oxidative stress-mediated ERK1/2 and p38 activation regulated mitochondria-dependent apoptotic signals in methylmercury-induced neuronal cell injury. *Toxicol. Lett*. 2010.

Lue, Y. H.; A. P. Hikim; R. S. Swerdloff; P. Im; K. S. Taing; T. Bui; A. Leung and C. Wang. Single exposure to heat induces stage-specific germ cell apoptosis in rats: role of intratesticular testosterone on stage specificity. *Endocrinology*. 1999, 140, 1709-1717.

Lue, Y. H.; B. L. Lasley; L. S. Laughlin; R. S. Swerdloff; A. P. Hikim; A. Leung; J. W. Overstreet and C. Wang. Mild testicular hyperthermia induces profound transitional spermatogenic suppression through increased germ cell apoptosis in adult cynomolgus monkeys (Macaca fascicularis). *J. Androl*. 2002, 23, 799-805.

Luo, Q.; Z. Li; X. Huang; J. Yan; S. Zhang and Y. Z. Cai. Lycium barbarum polysaccharides: Protective effects against heat-induced damage of rat testes and H2O2-induced DNA damage in mouse testicular cells and beneficial effect on sexual behavior and reproductive function of hemicastrated rats. *Life Sci*. 2006, 79, 613-621.

Maeda, Y.; A. Shiratsuchi; M. Namiki and Y. Nakanishi. Inhibition of sperm production in mice by annexin V microinjected into seminiferous tubules: possible etiology of phagocytic clearance of apoptotic spermatogenic cells and male infertility. *Cell Death Differ*. 2002, 9, 742-749.

Makker, K.; A. Agarwal and R. Sharma. Oxidative stress & male infertility. *Indian J. Med. Res*. 2009, 129, 357-367.

Malkov, M.; Y. Fisher and J. Don. Developmental schedule of the postnatal rat testis determined by flow cytometry. *Biol. Reprod*. 1998, 59, 84-92.

Mariotti, A.; L. Di Carlo, et al. Scrotal thermoregulatory model and assessment of the impairment of scrotal temperature control in varicocele. *Ann. Biomed. Eng*. 2011, 39, 664-673.

Matsuki, S.; Y. Iuchi; Y. Ikeda; I. Sasagawa; Y. Tomita and J. Fujii. Suppression of cytochrome c release and apoptosis in testes with heat stress by minocycline. *Biochem. Biophys. Res. Commun*. 2003, 312, 843-849.

Matsuki, S.; I. Sasagawa; Y. Iuchi and J. Fujii. Impaired expression of peroxiredoxin 4 in damaged testes by artificial cryptorchidism. *Redox. Rep*. 2002, 7, 276-278.

Matsuzawa, A. and H. Ichijo. Redox control of cell fate by MAP kinase: physiological roles of ASK1-MAP kinase pathway in stress signaling. *Biochim. Biophys. Acta*. 2008, 1780, 1325-1336.

Meachem, S. J.; S. M. Ruwanpura; J. Ziolkowski; J. M. Ague; M. K. Skinner and K. L. Loveland. Developmentally distinct in vivo effects of FSH on proliferation and apoptosis during testis maturation. *J. Endocrinol.* 2005, 186, 429-446.

Meister, A. and M. E. Anderson. Glutathione. *Annu. Rev. Biochem.* 1983, 52, 711-760.

Moreno, R. D. and C. P. Alvarado. The mammalian acrosome as a secretory lysosome: new and old evidence. *Mol. Reprod. Dev.* 2006, 73, 1430-1434.

Moreno, R. D.; C. Lizama; N. Urzua; S. P. Vergara and J. G. Reyes. Caspase activation throughout the first wave of spermatogenesis in the rat. *Cell Tissue Res.* 2006, 325, 533-540.

Mruk, D. D. and C. Y. Cheng. Sertoli-Sertoli and Sertoli-germ cell interactions and their significance in germ cell movement in the seminiferous epithelium during spermatogenesis. *Endocr. Rev.* 2004, 25, 747-806.

Murray-Zmijewski, F.; D. P. Lane and J. C. Bourdon. p53/p63/p73 isoforms: an orchestra of isoforms to harmonise cell differentiation and response to stress. *Cell Death Differ.* 2006, 13, 962-972.

Nakai, A.; M. Suzuki and M. Tanabe. Arrest of spermatogenesis in mice expressing an active heat shock transcription factor 1. *Embo J.* 2000, 19, 1545-1554.

Nikkanen, V.; K. O. Soderstrom and M. Parvinen. Identification of the spermatogenic stages in living seminiferous tubules of man. *J. Reprod. Fertil.* 1978, 53, 255-257.

Oakberg, E. F. A description of spermiogenesis in the mouse and its use in analysis of the cycle of the seminiferous epithelium and germ cell renewal. *Am. J. Anat.* 1956, 99, 391-413.

Oatley, J. M. and R. L. Brinster. Regulation of spermatogonial stem cell self-renewal in mammals. *Annu. Rev. Cell Dev. Biol.* 2008, 24, 263-286.

Ohta, H.; S. Aizawa and Y. Nishimune. Functional analysis of the p53 gene in apoptosis induced by heat stress or loss of stem cell factor signaling in mouse male germ cells. *Biol. Reprod.* 2003, 68, 2249-2254.

Ortiz, R. J.; C. Lizama; V. A. Codelia and R. D. Moreno. A molecular evaluation of germ cell death induced by etoposide in pubertal rat testes. *Mol. Hum. Reprod.* 2009, 15, 363-371.

Ott, M.; V. Gogvadze; S. Orrenius and B. Zhivotovsky. Mitochondria, oxidative stress and cell death. *Apoptosis.* 2007, 12, 913-922.

Ozen, O. A.; M. A. Kus; I. Kus; O. A. Alkoc and A. Songur. Protective effects of melatonin against formaldehyde-induced oxidative damage and apoptosis in rat testes: an immunohistochemical and biochemical study. *Syst. Biol. Reprod. Med.* 2008, 54, 169-176.

Pacher, P.; J. S. Beckman and L. Liaudet. Nitric oxide and peroxynitrite in health and disease. *Physiol. Rev.* 2007, 87, 315-424.

Paul, C.; D. W. Melton and P. T. Saunders. Do heat stress and deficits in DNA repair pathways have a negative impact on male fertility? *Mol. Hum. Reprod.* 2008, 14, 1-8.

Paul, C.; A. A. Murray; N. Spears and P. T. Saunders. A single, mild, transient scrotal heat stress causes DNA damage, subfertility and impairs formation of blastocysts in mice. *Reproduction.* 2008, 136, 73-84.

Pentikainen, V.; K. Erkkila; L. Suomalainen; M. Otala; M. O. Pentikainen; M. Parvinen and L. Dunkel. TNFalpha down-regulates the Fas ligand and inhibits germ cell apoptosis in the human testis. *J. Clin. Endocrinol. Metab.* 2001, 86, 4480-4488.

Perez-Crespo, M.; B. Pintado and A. Gutierrez-Adan. Scrotal heat stress effects on sperm viability, sperm DNA integrity, and the offspring sex ratio in mice. *Mol. Reprod. Dev.* 2008, 75, 40-47.

Rabani, R. Effect of Cannabinoids on Testicular ischemia-reperfusion injury in rats. *Acta Medica Iranica*. 2006, 44, 365-370.

Raha, S.; A. T. Myint; L. Johnstone and B. H. Robinson. Control of oxygen free radical formation from mitochondrial complex I: roles for protein kinase A and pyruvate dehydrogenase kinase. *Free Radic. Biol. Med.* 2002, 32, 421-430.

Raha, S. and B. H. Robinson. Mitochondria, oxygen free radicals, disease and ageing. *Trends Biochem. Sci.* 2000, 25, 502-508.

Riedl, S. J. and Y. Shi. Molecular mechanisms of caspase regulation during apoptosis. *Nat. Rev. Mol. Cell Biol.* 2004, 5, 897-907.

Rockett, J. C.; F. L. Mapp; J. B. Garges; J. C. Luft; C. Mori and D. J. Dix. Effects of hyperthermia on spermatogenesis, apoptosis, gene expression, and fertility in adult male mice. *Biol. Reprod.* 2001, 65, 229-239.

Rodriguez, I.; C. Ody; K. Araki; I. Garcia and P. Vassalli. An early and massive wave of germinal cell apoptosis is required for the development of functional spermatogenesis. *Embo J.* 1997, 16, 2262-2270.

Russell, L. B.; P. R. Hunsicker; M. Kerley; A. Pyle and A. M. Saxton. Etoposide exposure during male mouse pachytene has complex effects on crossing-over and causes nondisjunction. *Mutat. Res.* 2004, 565, 61-77.

Russell, L. D.; H. Chiarini-Garcia; S. J. Korsmeyer and C. M. Knudson. Bax-dependent spermatogonia apoptosis is required for testicular development and spermatogenesis. *Biol. Reprod.* 2002, 66, 950-958.

Saez, M. E.; J. L. Gonzalez-Sanchez; R. Ramirez-Lorca; M. T. Martinez-Larrad; C. Zabena; A. Gonzalez; F. J. Moron; A. Ruiz and M. Serrano-Rios. The CAPN10 gene is associated with insulin resistance phenotypes in the Spanish population. *PLoS One*. 2008, 3, e2953.

Saez, M. E.; R. Ramirez-Lorca; F. J. Moron and A. Ruiz. The therapeutic potential of the calpain family: new aspects. *Drug Discov. Today*. 2006, 11, 917-923.

Salmand, P. A.; T. Jungas; M. Fernandez; A. Conter and E. S. Christians. Mouse heat shock factor 1 (HSF1) is involved in testicular response to genotoxic stress induced by doxorubicin. *Biol. Reprod.* 2008, 79, 1092-1101.

Salvesen, G. S. Caspases: opening the boxes and interpreting the arrows. *Cell Death Differ.* 2002, 9, 3-5.

Sato, T.; T. Machida, et al. Fas-mediated apoptosome formation is dependent on reactive oxygen species derived from mitochondrial permeability transition in Jurkat cells. *J. Immunol.* 2004, 173, 285-296.

Scaffidi, C.; S. Fulda; A. Srinivasan; C. Friesen; F. Li; K. J. Tomaselli; K. M. Debatin; P. H. Krammer and M. E. Peter. Two CD95 (APO-1/Fas) signaling pathways. *Embo J.* 1998, 17, 1675-1687.

Scaffidi, C.; I. Schmitz; J. Zha; S. J. Korsmeyer; P. H. Krammer and M. E. Peter. Differential modulation of apoptosis sensitivity in CD95 type I and type II cells. *J. Biol. Chem.* 1999, 274, 22532-22538.

Scarabelli, L.; C. Lanza; I. Demori; R. Accomando; V. Giansanti; A. I. Scovassi and S. Palmero. Expression of antioxidant defense and poly (ADP-ribose) polymerase-1 in rat developing Sertoli cells. *Cell Biol. Int.* 2010.

Schultz, N.; F. K. Hamra and D. L. Garbers. A multitude of genes expressed solely in meiotic or postmeiotic spermatogenic cells offers a myriad of contraceptive targets. *Proc. Natl. Acad. Sci. U. S. A.* 2003, 100, 12201-12206.

Setchell, B. P. Spermatogenesis and spermatozoa. In: Austin, C. R. and R. V. Short (Eds), *Germ cells and Fertilization.* Cambridge: Cambridge University Press; 1993; 63-102.

Setchell, B. P.; G. Ekpe; J. L. Zupp and M. A. Surani. Transient retardation in embryo growth in normal female mice made pregnant by males whose testes had been heated. *Hum. Reprod.* 1998, 13, 342-347.

Sharpe, R. M.; C. McKinnell; C. Kivlin and J. S. Fisher. Proliferation and functional maturation of Sertoli cells, and their relevance to disorders of testis function in adulthood. *Reproduction.* 2003, 125, 769-784.

Shetty, J.; G. K. Marathe and R. R. Dighe. Specific immunoneutralization of FSH leads to apoptotic cell death of the pachytene spermatocytes and spermatogonial cells in the rat. *Endocrinology.* 1996, 137, 2179-2182.

Shi, Y. Apoptosome: the cellular engine for the activation of caspase-9. *Structure.* 2002, 10, 285-288.

Shi, Y. Mechanical aspects of apoptosome assembly. *Curr. Opin. Cell Biol.* 2006, 18, 677-684.

Shin, M. H.; Y. J. Moon; J. E. Seo; Y. Lee; K. H. Kim and J. H. Chung. Reactive oxygen species produced by NADPH oxidase, xanthine oxidase, and mitochondrial electron transport system mediate heat shock-induced MMP-1 and MMP-9 expression. *Free Radic Biol. Med.* 2008, 44, 635-645.

Shiraishi, K. and K. Naito. Nitric oxide produced in the testis is involved in dilatation of the internal spermatic vein that compromises spermatogenesis in infertile men with varicocele. *BJU Int.* 2007, 99, 1086-1090.

Shiraishi, K.; H. Takihara and H. Matsuyama. Elevated scrotal temperature, but not varicocele grade, reflects testicular oxidative stress-mediated apoptosis. *World J. Urol.* 2010, 28, 359-364.

Shiratsuchi, A.; M. Umeda; Y. Ohba and Y. Nakanishi. Recognition of phosphatidylserine on the surface of apoptotic spermatogenic cells and subsequent phagocytosis by Sertoli cells of the rat. *J. Biol. Chem.* 1997, 272, 2354-2358.

Sikka, S. C. Relative impact of oxidative stress on male reproductive function. *Curr Med Chem*, 2001, 8, 851-862.

Sinawat, S. The environmental impact on male fertility. *J. Med. Assoc. Thai.* 2000, 83, 880-885.

Skandhan, K. P. and A. Rajahariprasad. The process of spermatogenesis liberates significant heat and the scrotum has a role in body thermoregulation. *Med. Hypotheses.* 2007, 68, 303-307.

Skinner, M. K. Sertoli cell secreted regulatori factors. In: Skinner, M. K. a. G., M.D. (Eds), *Sertoli cell Biology.* New York: Elsevier; 2005; 107-121.

Socher, S. A.; Y. Yin; W. C. Dewolf and A. Morgentaler. Temperature-mediated germ cell loss in the testis is associated with altered expression of the cell-cycle regulator p53. *J. Urol.* 1997, 157, 1986-1989.

Somwaru, L.; S. Li; L. Doglio; E. Goldberg and B. R. Zirkin. Heat-induced apoptosis of mouse meiotic cells is suppressed by ectopic expression of testis-specific calpastatin. *J. Androl.* 2004, 25, 506-513.

Squier, M. K. and J. J. Cohen. Calpain and cell death. *Cell Death Differ.* 1996, 3, 275-283.

Sugimura, M.; T. Kobayashi; F. Shu; N. Kanayama and T. Terao. Annexin V inhibits phosphatidylserine-induced intrauterine growth restriction in mice. *Placenta.* 1999, 20, 555-560.

Tesarik, J.; F. Martinez; L. Rienzi; M. Iacobelli; F. Ubaldi; C. Mendoza and E. Greco. In-vitro effects of FSH and testosterone withdrawal on caspase activation and DNA fragmentation in different cell types of human seminiferous epithelium. *Hum. Reprod.* 2002, 17, 1811-1819.

Tramontano, F.; M. Malanga; B. Farina; R. Jones and P. Quesada. Heat stress reduces poly(ADPR)polymerase expression in rat testis. *Mol. Hum. Reprod.* 2000, 6, 575-581.

Tsounapi, P.; M. Saito; F. Dimitriadis; S. Shimizu; Y. Kinoshita; K. Shomori; I. Satoh and K. Satoh. Protective effect of sivelestat, a neutrophil elastase inhibitor, on ipsilateral and contralateral testes after unilateral testicular ischaemia-reperfusion injury in rats. *BJU Int.* 2011, 107, 329-336.

Turner, T. T.; H. J. Bang and J. J. Lysiak. Experimental testicular torsion: reperfusion blood flow and subsequent testicular venous plasma testosterone concentrations. *Urology.* 2005, 65, 390-394.

Turner, T. T.; H. J. Bang and J. L. Lysiak. The molecular pathology of experimental testicular torsion suggests adjunct therapy to surgical repair. *J. Urol.* 2004, 172, 2574-2578.

Tuteja, N.; P. Ahmad; B. B. Panda and R. Tuteja. Genotoxic stress in plants: shedding light on DNA damage, repair and DNA repair helicases. *Mutat. Res.* 2009, 681, 134-149.

Ueda, S.; H. Masutani; H. Nakamura; T. Tanaka; M. Ueno and J. Yodoi. Redox control of cell death. *Antioxid. Redox. Signal.* 2002, 4, 405-414.

Ugras, M. Y.; M. Kurus; B. Ates; H. Soylemez; A. Otlu and I. Yilmaz. Prunus armeniaca L (apricot) protects rat testes from detrimental effects of low-dose x-rays. *Nutr. Res.* 30, 200-208.

Vera, Y.; M. Diaz-Romcro; S. Rodriguez; Y. Lue; C. Wang; R. S. Swerdloff and A. P. Sinha Hikim. Mitochondria-dependent pathway is involved in heat-induced male germ cell death: lessons from mutant mice. *Biol. Reprod.* 2004, 70, 1534-1540.

Vera, Y.; S. Rodriguez; M. Castanares; Y. Lue; V. Atienza; C. Wang; R. S. Swerdloff and A. P. Sinha Hikim. Functional role of caspases in heat-induced testicular germ cell apoptosis. *Biol. Reprod.* 2005, 72, 516-522.

Vigueras-Villasenor, R. M.; I. Ojeda; O. Gutierrez-Perez; M. Chavez-Saldana; O. Cuevas; D. S. Maria and J. C. Rojas-Castaneda. Protective effect of alpha-tocopherol on damage to rat testes by experimental cryptorchidism. *Int. J. Exp. Pathol.* 2010, 92, 131-139.

Villunger, A.; E. M. Michalak; L. Coultas; F. Mullauer; G. Bock; M. J. Ausserlechner; J. M. Adams and A. Strasser. p53- and drug-induced apoptotic responses mediated by BH3-only proteins puma and noxa. *Science.* 2003, 302, 1036-1038.

Waites, G. M. H. and B. P. Setchell. Physiology of mammalian testis. In: Lamming, G. E. (Eds), *Marshall's Physiology of Reproduction.* New York: Churchill Livingstone; 2; 1990; 1-106.

Wang, L.; C. Beserra and D. L. Garbers. A novel aminophospholipid transporter exclusively expressed in spermatozoa is required for membrane lipid asymmetry and normal fertilization. *Dev. Biol.* 2004, 267, 203-215.

Wang, R. S.; S. Yeh; C. R. Tzeng and C. Chang. Androgen receptor roles in spermatogenesis and fertility: lessons from testicular cell-specific androgen receptor knockout mice. *Endocr. Rev.* 2009, 30, 119-132.

Wang, X.; H. Li, et al. p28GANK knockdown-derived reactive oxygen species induces apoptosis through mitochondrial dysfunction mediated by p38 in HepG2 cells. *Int. J. Oncol.* 2008, 33, 743-750.

Wang, Y.; H. Zhao; X. Sheng; P. E. Gambino; B. Costello and K. Bojanowski. Protective effect of Fructus Lycii polysaccharides against time and hyperthermia-induced damage in cultured seminiferous epithelium. *J. Ethnopharmacol.* 2002, 82, 169-175.

Weikert, S.; M. Schrader; M. Muller; H. Krause and K. Miller. Expression of the apoptosis inhibitor survivin in testicular tissue of infertile patients. *Int. J. Androl.* 2004, 27, 161-165.

Werdelin, L. and A. Nilsonne. The evolution of the scrotum and testicular descent in mammals: a phylogenetic view. *J. Theor. Biol.* 1999, 196, 61-72.

Westphal, D.; G. Dewson; P. E. Czabotar and R. M. Kluck. Molecular biology of Bax and Bak activation and action. *Biochim. Biophys. Acta.* 2010, 1813, 521-531.

WHO. Examination and processing of human semen. Fifth Edition. Switzerland: World Health Organization, 2010.

Widlak, W. [The heat shock response and HSP70 gene expression in male germ cells]. *Postepy Biochem.* 2006, 52, 289-295.

Widlak, W.; K. Benedyk; N. Vydra; M. Glowala; D. Scieglinska; E. Malusecka; A. Nakai and Z. Krawczyk. Expression of a constitutively active mutant of heat shock factor 1 under the control of testis-specific hst70 gene promoter in transgenic mice induces degeneration of seminiferous epithelium. *Acta Biochim. Pol.* 2003, 50, 535-541.

Widlak, W.; M. Markkula; Z. Krawczyk and I. Huhtaniemi. Functional analysis of spermatocyte-specific hst70 gene promoter in transgenic mice. *Acta Biochim. Pol.* 1994, 41, 103-105.

Wong, P. Y.; C. L. Au and J. M. Bedford. Biology of the scrotum. II. Suppression by abdominal temperature of transepithelial ion and water transport in the cauda epididymidis. *Biol. Reprod.* 1982, 26, 683-689.

Yamamoto, C. M.; A. P. Hikim, et al. Impairment of spermatogenesis in transgenic mice with selective overexpression of Bcl-2 in the somatic cells of the testis. *J. Androl.* 2001, 22, 981-991.

Yan, H. H.; D. D. Mruk and C. Y. Cheng. Junction restructuring and spermatogenesis: the biology, regulation, and implication in male contraceptive development. *Curr. Top Dev Biol.* 2008, 80, 57-92.

Yan, W.; J. X. Huang; A. S. Lax; L. Pelliniemi; E. Salminen; M. Poutanen and J. Toppari. Overexpression of Bcl-W in the testis disrupts spermatogenesis: revelation of a role of BCL-W in male germ cell cycle control. *Mol. Endocrinol.* 2003, 17, 1868-1879.

Yan, W.; J. Suominen; M. Samson; B. Jegou and J. Toppari. Involvement of Bcl-2 family proteins in germ cell apoptosis during testicular development in the rat and pro-survival effect of stem cell factor on germ cells in vitro. *Mol. Cell Endocrinol.* 2000, 165, 115-129.

Yan, W.; J. Suominen and J. Toppari. Stem cell factor protects germ cells from apoptosis in vitro. *J. Cell Sci.* 2000, 113 (Pt 1), 161-168.

Yin, Y.; B. C. Stahl; W. C. DeWolf and A. Morgentaler. Heat-induced testicular apoptosis occurs independently of hormonal depletion. *Apoptosis*. 1998, 3, 281-287.

Yin, Y.; B. C. Stahl; W. C. DeWolf and A. Morgentaler. p53-mediated germ cell quality control in spermatogenesis. *Dev. Biol.* 1998, 204, 165-171.

Yin, Y.; B. C. Stahl; W. C. DeWolf and A. Morgentaler. P53 and Fas are sequential mechanisms of testicular germ cell apoptosis. *J. Androl.* 2002, 23, 64-70.

Youle, R. J. and A. Strasser. The BCL-2 protein family: opposing activities that mediate cell death. *Nat. Rev. Mol. Cell Biol.* 2008, 9, 47-59.

Young, K. W.; L. G. Pinon; D. Dhiraj; D. Twiddy; M. Macfarlane; J. Hickman and P. Nicotera. Mitochondrial fragmentation and neuronal cell death in response to the Bcl-2/Bcl-x(L)/Bcl-w antagonist ABT-737. *Neuropharmacology*. 2010, 58, 1258-1267.

Zhai, D.; C. Jin; Z. Huang; A. C. Satterthwait and J. C. Reed. Differential regulation of Bax and Bak by anti-apoptotic Bcl-2 family proteins Bcl-B and Mcl-1. *J. Biol. Chem.* 2008, 283, 9580-9586.

Zhu, H.; Y. Cui, et al. Proteomic analysis of testis biopsies in men treated with transient scrotal hyperthermia reveals the potential targets for contraceptive development. *Proteomics*. 2010, 10, 3480-3493.

Zwirska-Korczala, K.; M. Adamczyk-Sowa, et al. Role of leptin, ghrelin, angiotensin II and orexins in 3T3 L1 preadipocyte cells proliferation and oxidative metabolism. *J. Physiol. Pharmacol.* 2007, 58 Suppl 1, 53-64.

In: Testis: Anatomy, Physiology and Pathology
Editors: Yoichi Nemoto and Norio Inaba
ISBN: 978-1-61942-739-6

Chapter 8

EFFECT OF PLASTICIZERS ON TESTIS WITH SPECIAL REFERENCE TO SERTOLI CELL FUNCTIONS*

***Oli Sarkar and P. P. Mathur*†**

Department of Biochemistry and Molecular Biology, School of Life Sciences, Pondicherry University, Pondicherry, India

ABSTRACT

Over the past five decades there have been reports of progressive decline in male reproductive health, which has been correlated with increase in the amount of chemical pollutants in the environment. Plastics are one of the major environmental pollutants today and have become an integral part of urban lifestyle. Polyvinyl chlorides (PVC) and polycarbonates (PC) make up most of household plasticware. During manufacture of PVC and PC, polymers are treated with phenolic additives called "plasticizers" that enhance their flexibility and toughness. Some of these phenolic compounds have estrogenic and anti-androgenic properties and are known to harm the male reproductive system in a time- (fetal, neonatal and adult), duration- and dose-dependent manner. The male reproductive system is responsible for the production of spermatozoa and enabling the male to be fertile. Testis is the site of spermatogenesis and is constituted by seminiferous tubules populated by Sertoli and germ cells. Sertoli cells are nurse cells that nourish developing germ cells to sustain spermatogenesis, which due to their non-regenerative nature are vulnerable to toxicants. In this review we discuss the effects of two commonly used plasticizer groups on Sertoli cell functions. The phthalate group of PVC additives that includes Bis- (2-ethylhexyl) phthalate (DEHP), its active metabolite Mono- (2-ethylhexyl) phthalate (MEHP) and dibutyl phthalate (DBP) has been shown to disrupt Sertoli cell cytoskeleton causing vacuolization. The inability of immature Sertoli cells to anchor germ cells resulted in an efflux of germ cells leaving behind Sertoli cell-only (SCO) tubules. DEHP has been shown to cause a decrease in testosterone synthesis

* A version of this chapter also appears in *Advances in Medicine and Biology. Volume 21*, edited by Leon V. Berhardt, published by Nova Science Publishers, Inc. It was submitted for appropriate modifications in an effort to encourage wider dissemination of research.

† Phone: 91 – 413 – 2655212; Fax: 91 – 413 – 2655211/2655265; E-mail: ppmathur@gmail.com.

resulting in delayed Sertoli cell maturation and to induce apoptosis of germ cells. The phenolic group of plasticizers that includes 4-(3’, 6’ dimethyl 3-heptylphenol) (Nonylphenol) and 4, 4'-dihydroxy-2, 2-diphenylpropane (Bisphenol A or BPA) has been shown to cause disassembly of Sertoli cell junctions by disrupting actin-binding proteins. Both Bisphenol A and Nonylphenol have been shown to hamper the activities of anti-oxidant enzymes and increase the levels of reactive oxygen species (ROS) leading to conditions of oxidative stress and induction of Fas/ FasL-mediated Sertoli cell apoptosis. Bisphenol A has been shown to cause sperm acrosomal abnormalities and inhibit spermatogenesis. Recent studies show that the use of plasticizers must be vigilantly monitored to avoid any adverse effects to male reproductive health.

INTRODUCTION

Accelerated urbanization and industrialization has lead to many lifestyle changes; some of them are harmful to the health of people. When these phenomena are taken in conjunction with the worldwide decline in male sperm counts and male fertilizing capability reported for the same period of time, it is clear that urbanization has caused a detrimental effect on male reproductive health. The progressive decline in male reproductive health and fertility has also been positively correlated with an increase in the levels of man-made chemicals in our environment [1]. These synthetic chemicals leach into ground water as a result of environmental pollution and are consumed by humans and animals through contaminated food and water. Among environmental pollutants biodegradable compounds are less toxic than non-biodegradable compounds. Plastics are the most common non-biodegradable pollutants and due to the widespread use of plasticware in urban households they are one of the major toxicants found in the environment. For example, plastic additives which are synthetic compounds and not found naturally in the environment, have been detected in the urine of 95% of people in the United States as per a study conducted by the Centers for Disease Control and Prevention (CDC) [2]. Plastics (from Latin *plasticus* or malleable) are polymers of carbon, hydrogen, oxygen, nitrogen, chlorine and/or sulfur. Since their manufacture in the nineteenth century plastics have undergone much development and today are an integral part of our day-to-day life. Plastics find widespread use in household, medical, industrial and military products ranging from toothbrushes to explosives. They come in different forms depending on their composition and manufacture: inclusion of different additives or “plasticizers” to the core polymer mix (composed of repeats of the basic monomer) is used to give the plastic specific properties like flexibility, toughness, opacity, thermo- and cryo-tolerance [3]. For example, introduction of phthalate derivatives into polyvinyl chloride (PVC) polymer chains increases the space between adjacent polymer chains and confers flexibility to the otherwise rigid plastic. This enables the use of PVC polymer in the manufacture of flexible objects. Most of the commonly used plasticizers are hydrophobic compounds that contain one or more phenol rings.

Among phenolic plasticizers, phthalates or phthalic acid esters are (or have been) the most extensively used. Like every industrial chemical, the use of plasticizers is closely monitored and *N*o *O*bserved *A*dverse *E*ffect *L*evels (NOAEL) have been assigned for each compound. The NOAEL doses for each toxicant is reviewed periodically in the light of findings from newer studies. Moreover, studies have shown that organs have independent toxicity thresholds, i.e., exposure to a particular toxicant may not cause adverse effects in a particular organ while being toxic to the other. Therefore, organ-specific NOAEL have also been assigned by the National Toxicity Panel (NTP) set up by the National Institutes of Health (NIH), USA. Phenolic compounds exert their physiological effects due to structural similarities with estrogen and have been known to bind estrogen receptor thereby causing estrogenic effects. Due to their hormone-like activities phenolic compounds disrupt endocrine regulation and are called "endocrine disruptors". The reproductive system is closely regulated by estrogens and androgens and thus is a vulnerable target of phenolic endocrine disruptors. In addition, the presence of endocrine disrupting plasticizers like Bis- (2-ethylhexyl) phthalate (DEHP), dibutyl phthalate (DBP), 4-(3', 6' dimethyl 3-heptylphenol) (NP) and 4, 4'-dihydroxy-2, 2-diphenylpropane (Bisphenol A or BPA) has been linked to the increasing incidence of testicular cancer and male infertility [1, 4, 5]. Male fertility is dependent on the successful production of sufficient number of viable spermatozoa. Endocrine disruptors have been shown to target the testis because the testis is the organ where stem cells begin their development to become spermatozoa via the process called "spermatogenesis" [6]. The survival of developing spermatozoa within the seminiferous tubule is completely dependent on nurse cells called Sertoli cells.

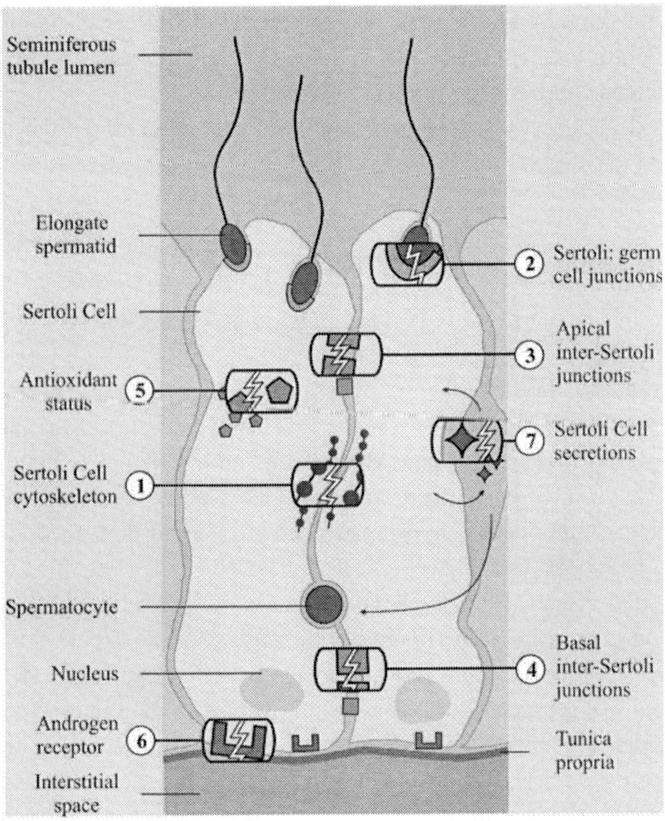

Figure 1. Sertoli cell processes targeted by plasticizers. Plasticizers disrupt the Sertoli cell cytoskeleton (6) resulting in a loss of Sertoli-germ (1) and Sertoli-Sertoli cell adhesion at the apical (2) and basal (4) regions of the seminiferous tubule. There is a concomitant alteration in pro/anti-oxidant balance that regulates Sertoli cell functions and junctions (7). Plasticizer-impaired testicular steroid production and transport affects androgen receptors present on the Sertoli cell (5). The secretory and endocrine

(autocrine and paracrine) functions of Sertoli cells (3) are affected by plasticizers like DEHP, DBP, NP and BPA, resulting in improper spermatogenesis and impaired male fertility.

Sertoli cells are flame-shaped columnar cells that line the interior of the seminiferous tubules of the testis. These types of cells are named after Enrico Sertoli who first described them in 1865 as "*cellule ramificate*" or branched cells [7]. The basal end of Sertoli cells resides along the lamina propria and their apical end extends into the center of the tubule. Sertoli cells undergo differentiation and proliferation only during fetal and pre-pubertal life [8]. These processes are inhibited by the presence of testosterone that is present from the onset of puberty. There are approximately 250-650 x 10^6 Sertoli cells/ testis at puberty. Sertoli cells anchor developing germ cells (in a ratio of 1:50) and provide them with essential nutrients. Sertoli cells adhere to each other to form a barrier called the blood-testis barrier (BTB) that separates the lumen of seminiferous tubule from systemic circulation [9]. Sertoli cells are both paracrine and autocrine cells: their functions are regulated by both germ cell and their own secretions [10, 11]. Sertoli cells are hormonally regulated by testosterone, FSH and estrogen. Therefore, they were considered to be potential targets of estrogen-mimickers or xenoestrogens. Plasticizers that share structural similarity with estrogen are known to possess estrogenic activity. In addition, the small size of estrogenic plasticizers enables them to pass through the blood-testis barrier and enter the seminiferous tubules directly. Thus, Sertoli cells are doubly susceptible to plasticizers (Figure 1). Recent studies have established the effects of various xenoestrogens on male reproductive system and have described the mechanism of their actions [12]. In this review we have summarized the effects of some of the most important plasticizers on the testis with special reference to Sertoli cells.

Effect of DEHP on Testicular and Sertoli Cell Functions

DEHP is included in the manufacture of plastic containers (kitchenware, shampoo, cream and other liquid product containers), toys and medical devices (intravenous tubes, catheters etc.). As a result of its extensive use and slow degradation phthalates, like DEHP, are widely distributed in the environment and find their way into water and food [13]. DEHP accounts for 50% of phthalates found in the environment and the United States alone produced close to two million tons of DEHP every year [14, 15]. The NOAEL dose for DEHP assigned for testis/ developmental effects is 3.7 mg/ kg body weight per day [16]. Once ingested from contaminated food and water, DEHP finds its way into the small intestine where it is hydrolyzed by lipases found therein into mono (2-ethyhexyl) phthalate (MEHP) units. Both residual DEHP and MEHP are absorbed and oxidatively degraded in the kidneys and excreted via urine [17]. Impaired renal clearance has been implicated in increased MEHP levels in the body and 'phthalate toxicity' [18, 19]. A NOAEL dose has not been assigned for MEHP probably because it is not used in its native form, and is present in an organism/ animal only as a result of exposure to DEHP. Despite being eliminated quickly, DEHP has been shown to affect the male reproductive system, impair male sexual behavior and possess anti-fertility actions in mice [20]. Following exposure to DEHP, rats showed decreased absolute and relative testis weights, testicular injury, cryptorchidism, hypospadia, decreased sperm counts [20, 21]. The condition of abnormal testicular descent is called cryptorchidism and is a common cause of infertility. During fetal life the testes are located in the abdominal region and descend to their external scrotal position by birth. This occurs because the mammalian body has a normal temperature of 37 ºC but cooler temperatures of 35 ºC are required for the production of viable sperm. The external location of testis allows it to be cooled by air circulation thereby facilitating normal spermatogenesis [22]. The development of external genitalia is critical to reproductive capacity and frequently there is improper seminal output due to penile defects. When the corpus spongiosum or penile foreskin is not properly regressed the penile urethra ends prematurely within the penis and sperm are ejaculated within the penis itself. This condition is called hypospadia and is a common cause of male infertility [23]. Following short-term exposure to DEHP, there is a loss of germ cells from seminiferous tubules accompanied by shrinkage of tubules [24]. Long-term exposure to DEHP retards spermatogenesis and causes spermatogenic arrest characterized by the presence of tubules that contain only Sertoli cell with a few spermatogonia and spermatocytes [20, 24]. DEHP affectes Leydig cell functions as evidenced by decreased insulin-like growth factor 3 (INSL3) and testosterone levels [25]. Decrease in testosterone levels has been implicated in testicular dysgenesis syndrome and germ cell apoptosis seen in DEHP-treated rats [26]. The term testicular dysgenesis syndrome loosely describes the combined appearance of cryptorchidism, hypospadia, germ cell cancer, sub-normal sperm production, abnormal development of Sertoli and Leydig cells, which are all risk factors for each other and for pregnancy [27]. A number of plasticizers are toxic to the testis, and many of them affect Sertoli cell physiology and functions [21]. Plasticizer-induced toxicity causes enlargement and vacuolization of Sertoli cells leading to dilation of seminiferous tubules. A large number of apoptotic germ cells are present and there is widespread efflux of germ cells from the tubules. In the absence of germ cells Sertoli cells lose their columnar shape and these de-structured Sertoli cells cause disassembly of testicular microtubules [28]. Interestingly, DEHP caused an up-regulation in the protein levels of N-cadherin, α-catenin, β-catenin and $p120^{ctn}$ at the basal region of seminiferous tubule. The catenin family of cytosolic proteins serves as adaptors that link the transmembrane cadherins to the actin cytoskeleton, and thereby enable cell adhesion (Sertoli-Sertoli and Sertoli germ cell) [29]. This suggests that DEHP could have an adverse effect on testicular junctions and similarly on Sertoli-germ or inter-Sertoli cell adhesion [24]. The effect of DEHP on Sertoli cell structure and functions has been shown to be dose-dependent. At low doses of 5 mg/ kg body weight/ day, DEHP does not alter Sertoli cell number, morphology (no vacuolization or atrophy) or ability to sustain spermatogenesis. But the same dose of DEHP, when administered in conditions of impaired detoxification (induced by folic acid administration), causes a decrease in testis weight, Sertoli cell vacuolization, seminiferous tubule atrophy and decreased sperm counts [19]. This signifies the critical role played by renal detoxification processes in the metabolism of toxicants. At a dose of 400 mg/ kg body weight/ day, severe vacuolization is seen in the cytoplasm of Sertoli cells and Sertoli-germ cell adhesion is affected leading to loss of germ cells from seminiferous tubules [16, 18]. DEHP causes a loss of germ cells from tubules by affecting Sertoli-germ cell adhesion and also induces germ cell apoptosis due to increased intra-testicular testosterone levels [30]. Testicular dysgenesis syndrome seen following DEHP exposure is considered a consequence of altered Sertoli cell functions [31-33]. Chronic doses of DEHP increase Leydig cell steroidogenesis resulting in elevated intra-testicular and circulatory levels of testosterone [34]. Apart from DEHP, Sertoli cells are targets of the mono-ester metabolite MEHP [15, 35]. During fetal life, Sertoli cell proliferation is regulated by FSH-stimulated cAMP production. MEHP caused inhibition of Sertoli cell proliferation but had no effect on FSH-cAMP pathway. It was rather shown that Sertoli cell proliferation was inhibited at a stage beyond FSH-stimulated cAMP production or via an FSH-independent pathway. But in pre-pubertal rat, MEHP decreases FSH-stimulated cAMP production but has no significant effects on Sertoli cell number [36]. This reiterates the fact that Sertoli cell proliferation is suppressed in an FSH-independent manner, probably by regulating testicular testosterone. In adult rat, MEHP exposure has been shown to affect the oxidation-reduction (redox) homeostasis and the mitochondrial anti-oxidant defense [37]. MEHP was also shown to disrupt the Sertoli cell cytoskeleton causing Sertoli cell vacuolization and germ cell apoptosis in a dose-dependent manner [38]. Interestingly, the number and size of Sertoli cell vacuoles increased progressively with the disappearance of cytoskeletal proteins (like vimentin) suggesting that Sertoli cell cytoskeleton is necessary to protect the cell against vacuolization and endocytosis [24]. Despite the fact that DEHP is more toxic to pre-pubertal rats than to adults, the fetus is the most vulnerable stage [39]. This could be because the fetus is minutely sensitive to variations in the hormonal, enzymatic or cytokine levels. Any imbalance in testosterone and estrogen levels of the mother alters organogenesis and cellular processes of the fetus. Therefore fetal or gestational exposure to xenoestrogens is an important hazard to fetus. Exposure to toxicants at levels that are non-toxic to adults have been shown to be toxic to fetuses. Rats exposed to low doses of DEHP during fetal life show numerous reproductive abnormalities during neonatal and adult life and gene-profiling studies have revealed that a host of genes are down regulated [3]. For example, down-regulation of the gene for Steroid Acute Regulatory (StAR) protein that is critical for incorporating cholesterol into testosterone during androgen synthesis, resulted in decreased cholesterol transport by Leydig cells. Similarly, down-regulation of genes encoding enzymes that regulate the steroidogenic pathway like the cytochrome family (Cyp11a1 and Cyp17a1) and 3-β hydroxy steroid dehydrogenase (Hsd3b1) cause decreased steroidogenesis in fetal Leydig cells [40]. During fetal life, testosterone is critical for the development of male phenotype and reproductive organs. Thus, male fetuses deprived of testosterone due to DEHP exposure during this critical phase result in offspring with abnormal external genitalia, underdeveloped or absent reproductive organs, decreased anogenital distance (AGD), female-like nipples, small testes, cryptorchidism and hypospadia [41-43]. Anogential distance, the distance between the anus and genitals, is used as a parameter to distinguish males and females at birth (with males having a larger anogenital distance than females). Reduction of anogenital distance at birth indicates impaired male reproductive organogenesis and has been correlated with endocrine disruption and decreased reproductive capability in adult life [44]. The testes of DEHP-treated rats are small with malformed seminiferous tubules containing multi-nucleated germ cells [43]. Even after they are sexually mature, rats have decreased daily sperm and spermatid production and associated low sperm counts [18, 43]. However, while testosterone deprivation hampers the development and functions of male reproductive system, lack of testosterone alone cannot be held responsible for all the abnormalities resulting from fetal exposure to low doses of DEHP. Other factors such as INSL3 that regulates testicular descent during fetal life have also been implicated in DEHP-induced toxicity [45]. In addition to hampering cholesterol synthesis and transport, low doses of DEHP cause fetal Leydig and germ cells to undergo apoptosis [18]. When fetal testicular sections were examined, large clusters of Leydig cells and germ cells were found in the interstitium and tubular lumen respectively. These cells underwent apoptosis as a result of up-regulation of the Caspase 3-

mediated signaling cascade. These Leydig cell clusters were retained even after birth and were also detected in neonatal offspring exposed to low doses of DEHP during fetal life [25].

It is interesting to note that DEHP, at low doses, is more toxic than at relatively higher doses. High dose exposures (5 mg/ kg body weight/ day) during fetal life did not have any significant effect on fertility, sexual behavior or on the weights of reproductive organs, though reduction in seminal vesicle sizes was observed in some animals [18]. Despite a reduction in sperm production, fetal exposure to high or low doses of DEHP had no significant effect on Sertoli cell number or their ability to support developing germ cells [18]. Moreover, DEHP was shown to hamper various Sertoli cell functions when adult males were exposed, but surprisingly did not have any toxic effect on fetal Sertoli cells. This apparent paradox may be due to the fact that DEHP has been shown to hamper certain Sertoli cells functions like junction formation [16, 24]. During fetal life Sertoli cells undergo proliferation and have no other known functions and therefore may be unaffected by DEHP. Taken together, these studies show that fetal exposure to DEHP did not significantly affect Sertoli cells, although numerous other repro-toxic effects were observed.

Effect of DBP on Testicular and Sertoli Cell Functions

The use of DEHP has been substituted in many products by DBP due to the low NOAEL and high toxicity of the former. DBP is used in the manufacture of food packaging, latex adhesives, fixatives for hair spray and solvents for perfumes and inks [46]. The reproductive NOAEL for DBP has been set at 50 mg/ kg body weight/ day [47]. The hydrophobic nature of DBP allows it to leach from plastic into water, soil and air. Once ingested, DBP is hydrolyzed to the mono-ester, monobutyl phthalate and cleared from the body of mammals within 48 hours [48]. In spite of having no bioaccumulation, DBP is considered a ubiquitous contaminant as it is found in almost all the animals and human population studied so far [49]. The effects of DBP on the testis occur in a systematic manner through a cascade involving several cell types. The first target of DBP is the interstitial cells (Leydig and peritubular myoid cells) since these cell types were the first to respond to DBP by alteration in their gene expression [50]. Peritubular myoid cells are responsible for the formation of seminiferous tubules and the peristaltic movements that propel the outflow of elongate spermatids at the end of testicular spermatogenesis [31, 51]. Abnormal myoid cell functions adversely affected Leydig cell functions and result in depleted testosterone in the testis. Lack of testosterone and the loss of peristaltic movements affect the Sertoli cells that constitute the seminiferous tubule and these cells are the second targets of DBP. This indicates that the toxicant could diffuse from interstitial space into tubular lumen. The presence of malformed tubules, loss of germ cells and decreased testosterone levels lead to a decrease in testis weights and hampered fertilizing capacity [50]. Phthalates have been implicated in low testosterone levels, underdeveloped reproductive organs, decreased anogenital distance, and poor sperm quality in humans [42, 52]. DBP, at a dose of 100 mg/ kg body weight/ day, has been shown to up-regulate gene expression of numerous transcription factors, signaling molecules, secreted proteins and transferrin receptor Tnfrsfl12a [50]. It is interesting to note that up-regulation of these factors preceded the down-regulation of Leydig cell mRNA levels of StAR protein and peripheral benzodiazepine receptor (PBR). Both StAR protein and PBR are responsible for the transport of cholesterol from the outer to inner mitochondrial membrane prior to androgen synthesis. Testicular androgen synthesis is regulated by P450scc and Cyp17a1, which were also shown to be downregulated by DBP. DBP decreased the gene expression of hormone receptors like thyroid hormone receptor–α1 (THRα1), estrogen receptor α (ERα) and androgen receptor (AR) [53, 54]. These results indicate that DBP affects testicular steroidogenesis and transport at the gene level without corresponding protein level changes [55]. At doses of 400 mg/ kg body weight/ day, DBP has been shown to decrease anogenital distance, caused malformed or absent epididymis and accessory glands, testicular atrophy, cryptorchidism, hypospadia, decreased sperm count and increased percentage of abnormal sperm, loss and abnormal clustering of germ cells, and Leydig cells hyperplasia [21, 31]. At a dose of 1000 mg/ kg body weight/ day, DBP has been shown to decrease testis weight concurrent with loss of germ cells from seminiferous epithelium. The tubules were devoid of virtually all types of germ cells except a few spermatogonia and spermatocytes resulting in a significant reduction in tubule diameter [56]. The effects of chronic doses of DBP on the testis were apparently restricted to the seminiferous tubules since neither androgen synthesis nor transport is affected as demonstrated by normal testosterone levels. These results indicate that high doses of DBP did not affect Leydig cell functions while low doses are toxic [56].

Sertoli cells are important targets of DBP in adults and a dose of 400 mg/ kg body weight/ day, has been shown to cause vacuolization of Sertoli cell cytoplasm [31, 57]. At a dose of 1000 mg/ kg body weight/ day, DBP produces tubules that contained Sertoli cells only [58]. Germ cells apoptosis resulting in tubules devoid of virtually all types of germ cells except a few spermatogonia and spermatocytes were observed in rats [59]. Without germ cells, the cytoskeleton of Sertoli cells is weakened and Sertoli cells lose their columnar shape, resulting in tubules that appeared shrunk or have reduced diameters. Following chronic exposure, testosterone levels were shown to be high due to increased androgen synthesis by Leydig cells [54]. The degradation of pyruvate to lactate by lactate dehydrogenase A (LDHA) present in Sertoli cells fulfills the energy requirements of developing spermatids. This phenomenon was shown to be down-regulated resulting in a marked decrease in sperm motility [55]. Following exposure to DBP, expression of the gene for sperm associated antigen 4 (spag4) was downregulated coinciding with germ cell depletion and loss of LDHA expression. Spag4 is a Sertoli cell secreted protein and is responsible for the temporal regulation of spermatogenesis [60]. *In vitro* studies have shown that phthalate exposure reduces Sertoli cell proliferation and down-regulates FSH receptor expression [61]. Thus, DBP-stimulated testosterone surge and decreased FSH receptor expression could together affect the ability of Sertoli cells to anchor developing germ cells resulting in germ cell efflux from tubules and hamperered spermatogenesis [56]. It is interesting to note that DBP causes a loss of vimentin cytoskeleton and a decrease in connexin43 and increased testin expression [40]. Connexin43 is a vital component of testicular gap junctions and any disruption in connexin43 invariably results in a loss of gap junction formation and arrested spermatogenesis (connexin43 null mice were shown to be sterile) [62]. Testin, a Sertoli cell secreted protein, is considered a marker of spermatocytes and a component of Sertoli-Sertoli and Sertoli-germ cell ectoplasmic specializations [63]. Taken together, these observations suggest that the blood-testis barrier (made up due to inter-Sertoli cell contacts) could be compromised, but no evidence is currently available to support this conjecture. Interestingly, following DBP exposure there appeared to be a “lag time” prior to changes in gene expression, i.e. gene expression changes are observed well after the maximal phthalate level. This suggests that the observed effects were not due to high levels of DBP present in the testis but due to the cumulative dose effect of DBP [50]. Exposure to DBP at doses that did not show any adverse effects on pregnant rats, caused a number of reproductive abnormalities in male offspring, like deformities in the vertebral column and cleft palate [4]. DBP has been shown to cause a decrease in testosterone levels resulting in abnormal development of testosterone-dependent reproductive organs like epididymis, vas deferens, seminal vesicles and prostate. Other reproductive abnormalities observed were retention of female-like nipples in male rats, decreased anogenital distance, cryptorchidism, hypospadia and testicular dysgenesis [31, 54, 64]. These abnormalities were shown to occur dose-dependently and are attributed to the decreased circulatory levels of testosterone seen in DBP-exposed offspring [31]. The seminiferous tubules appeared elongated, misshapen and cross-sections of testes showed fewer tubules per cross-section [65]. This may be due to the suppression of Sertoli cell maturation, and disorganization and vacuolization of Sertoli cell cytoplasm seen following DBP exposure in fetal testes [66]. The vimentin cytoskeleton, which along with actin cytoskeleton confers the columnar shape to Sertoli cells, was disrupted resulting in collapsed Sertoli cells with retracted apical evagination and convoluted plasma membrane. A loss in Sertoli-germ cell adhesive function was also observed due to loss in vimentin cytoskeletal disruption [65]. However, contrary to adult testes where a loss of vimentin cytoskeleton following exposure to heat has been shown to cause the death or apoptosis or germ cells, loss of vimentin cytoskeleton in the fetal testis does not cause germ cell apoptosis [57]. Exposure to DBP, caused signs of aberrant mitosis in fetal germ cells which appeared as multinucleated germ cell clusters at the basal region of seminiferous tubules [65]. The effects of DBP on fetal Sertoli cells are well documented but there are a few apparent contradictions on the effect of DBP on Leydig cells, especially on testosterone synthesis. The effects of DBP are biphasic: high dose (100 mg/ kg body weight/ day) exposure during fetal life caused decreased testosterone levels while low dose (38 mg/ kg body weight/ day) caused an increase in testosterone levels [25].

Effect of Nonylphenol on Testicular and Sertoli Cell Functions

Nonylphenol (NP), a lipophilic compound, is widely used as a nonionic surfactant. NP is used as an additive in detergents, paints, pesticides, leather processing, epoxy resins, photographic films, paper and textile manufacture and food packaging. Approximately 60% NP leached from contaminated products sediments into ground water and is orally ingested by humans and animals. NP is very stable with a high bioaccumulation rate: systemic NP levels have been shown to reach as high as 10-100 times more than environmental levels [67]. A reproductive NOAEL of 15 mg/ kg body weight/ day has been set for NP. Orally ingested NP finds its way via the gastrointestinal tract to the liver and intestine where it is conjugated to glucuronic acid by an Uridine diphosphate-glucuronosyl transferase (UGT2B1) into NP-glucuronide and *p*-nonyl-catechol glucuronide [68, 69]. Glucuronides are generally transported to various tissues by binding to multi-drug resistance-related protein-2 (MRP-2) [70]. But NP-glucuronide, is unable to bind MRP-2 possibly due to its long chain alkyl structure and/ or its hydrophobic nature. Both the NP metabolites are difficult to cleave and their stable nature allows them to be absorbed into serum and to be finally excreted in bile [68]. NP treatment leads to smaller testes and accessory organs, decreased sperm production and cryptorchidism in adult rats [71, 72]. The primary effects of NP on the male reproductive system are due to its ability to increase the levels of ROS in the epididymis and testis, especially in Sertoli cells, which are vulnerable targets of ROS [73-76]. Developing spermatozoa contain a very small amount of cytoplasm and thus the polyunsaturated fatty acids (PUFA) present in the sperm membrane are critical to sperm protection. Even a minute increase in the ROS level causes the peroxidation of sperm membrane PUFA and adversely affects sperm viability. To combat this ROS-induced toxicity, there are a number of enzymes that metabolize ROS and change them into harmless radicals. Superoxide dismutase breaks down superoxide radicals into hydrogen peroxide and molecular oxygen. Hydrogen peroxide is acted upon by catalase and glutathione peroxidase/ reductase system to form water and oxygen [12, 77]. Exposure to NP has been shown to hamper the activities of antioxidant enzymes (superoxide dismutase, catalase, glutathione peroxidase, and glutathione reductase) with a concomitant increase in hydrogen peroxide generation, peroxidation of sperm membrane lipids, loss of mitochondrial membrane potential and resulting in a state of oxidative stress [74-76]. When such a loss in sperm antioxidant defense was detected it was anticipated that there would be a reduction in sperm counts. This was shown to occur in a dose-dependent manner following NP exposure [74]. Conditions of oxidative stress in the testis have been shown to downregulate androgen synthesis and transport and decreased serum testosterone levels observed following NP-treatment could be due to increased ROS levels [78]. NP decreases the number of Sertoli cells and affected their morphology by causing a decrease in cytoplasmic volume and membrane integrity resulting in shrunk cells [76, 79]. *In vitro* experiments with Chinese hamster V79 cells (which are structurally similar to Sertoli cells and are often used to mimic Sertoli cell behavior *in vitro*) have shown that NP disrupts the cytosolic microtubule network [80]. However, these effects could not be duplicated *in vivo* suggesting the presence of other Sertoli cell factors that protect against NP toxicity. Apoptosis of germ cells occurs routinely to regulate the number of germ cells present in the seminiferous tubule. A significant increase in the number of apoptotic spermatocytes, but not of spermatids, is seen in NP-treated testes. Sertoli cell necrosis and apoptosis, via the Fas/ Fas ligand (FasL) pathway, were seen after exposure to NP [81, 82]. Sertoli cells possess the FasL, which, on interaction with the Fas protein present on germ cells, triggers germ cell apoptosis. This is a mechanism whereby excess germ cells are killed in order to maintain the optimum Sertoli-germ cell ratio, so critical to spermatogenesis [83]. Elevated ROS levels have been shown to affect Fas/ FasL signaling in addition to causing the peroxidation of mitochondrial inner membrane lipids, resulting in the dissociation of cytochrome c [81]. Once cytochrome c function is lost, the cell is committed to undergo apoptosis (via the caspase pathway) or necrosis, due to compromised cellular respiration resulting from elevated ROS levels [84]. Apoptotic pathways are seldom through a single signaling cascade, and NP has been shown to cause apoptosis in other cell types by inhibiting calcium pumps in endoplasmic reticulum or by stimulating a caspase-mediated signaling cascade [85, 86]. Whether these pathways are activated by NP in Sertoli cells still remains unclear. It is interesting to note that induction of oxidative stress has been correlated with germ cell depletion from seminiferous tubules due to loss of Sertoli-germ cell adherens junction functions [87]. ROS and reactive nitrogen species (like nitric oxide) are known to play a key role in the assembly/ disassembly of testicular junctions by regulating the levels and interactions of their constituent proteins [88, 89]. In addition to ROS, numerous signaling cascades act in tandem to regulate testicular junctions [90]. NP has been shown to downregulate connexin43 levels and to inhibit its phosphorylation, thereby compromising GJ functions in Sertoli cells [88]. Although NP has mild estrogenic properties, its effects on testicular junctions do not involve either the estrogen receptor pathway or the p38 mitogen-activated protein (p38MAP) kinase pathway [88]. Other compounds that affect testicular junctions have been shown to trigger the extracellular regulatory kinase (ERK) pathway and it is safe to speculate that NP-induced effects could be via the activation of this signaling cascade [91, 92]. The effect of fetal exposure of NP on the male reproductive system is dependent on dose and duration of exposure. There are some reports that show that rats exposed to NP during fetal life did not show any abnormalities in testis weight, morphology of seminiferous tubules or number of Sertoli cells [93, 94].

Other reports show that fetal exposure to NP causes decreased serum testosterone levels leading to feminization of male offspring at the level of hypothalamus and reproductive organs like epididymis [95-97]. Thus, these reports suggest that, in fetal rats, NP did not have significant effects within the seminiferous tubules while having adverse effects on the cells of interstitial space. These apparent discrepancies may be due to variations in the time and dose of exposure used in the respective experiments, i.e., short-term exposure during gestational day 11-18 in rats may not harm male reproductive functions whereas longer exposures from gestational day 7 to postnatal day 50 may be toxic. Although NP has no estrogenic effects on the fetus, gestational development is sensitive to the anti-androgenic properties of NP [96, 97]. Thus, the presence of NP at testosterone-dependent stages of development could be the reason for the observed effects of NP. Still the effects of fetal exposure to NP on male reproductive functions are not clearly understood and further studies are needed before precise conclusions may be drawn.

Effect of Bisphenol A on Testicular and Sertoli Cell Functions

Recently the use of another plasticizer, 4, 4'-dihydroxy-2, 2-diphenylpropane (BPA), has become a cause of controversy. BPA is used as an additive in the manufacture of polycarbonates to improve their opacity and non-stick properties. Due to its hydrophobic nature, BPA prevents food from sticking to the sides of (BPA-coated) containers and thus it is used to line disposable food containers, beverage cans and bottles. BPA is also found in epoxy and polystyrene resins, infant feeing bottles, microwave ovenware, refillable water containers, plastic utensils, infant toys and atmospheric dust. Due to its lipophilic nature, BPA leaches from contaminated plasticware into food and water and is ingested orally. BPA has been assigned a reproductive NOAEL of 50 mg/ kg body weight/ day. BPA is metabolized into BPA-glucuronide in the liver, excreted to the intestine as bile, and cleared rapidly via urine (with a half life of 6 hours). However, in rodents BPA-glucuronide is re-cleaved to BPA and glucuronide in the intestine and re-absorbed into the blood stream. Thus, oral bioavailability of BPA is relatively lower in humans than in rodents [98]. BPA has been shown to exert its estrogenic action by binding to estrogen receptor (ER)-α and -β (with higher binding affinity to ER-β) [99]. For long BPA was designated "weakly estrogenic" because it has 10, 000 times less affinity for ER than estradiol. However, recent studies have shown that BPA can act via other pathways and is as potent as estradiol and has numerous adverse effects on male reproductive system [100]. Rats, when treated with BPA, show retardation in spermatogenesis characterized by smaller reproductive organs (testis and epididymis) and accessory glands (prostate and seminal vesicle), under-developed seminiferous tubules, decreased daily sperm production and low sperm motility [101-103]. Estrogen advances the first wave of spermatogenesis at puberty, and the above-described effects would likely be the result of the estrogenic properties of BPA [101]. BPA has been shown to induce the generation of ROS with a concomitant decrease in the activities of antioxidant enzymes and thereby resulting in the peroxidation of membrane lipids [104]. The condition of oxidative stress in epididymis and testis is dose-dependent and impairs male fertilizing capacity [102, 103]. Exposure to BPA affects Sertoli cell viability and functions in a dose- and time-dependent manner [105, 106]. Sertoli cells are regulated by FSH and are the only cells (in the male) to contain FSH receptor. The binding of FSH to FSH-receptor which is regulated by cAMP was shown to be affected in BPA-treated testis [107]. BPA has been shown to increase the secretion of Inhibin B, which is a Sertoli cell secreted hormone that inhibits hypothalamic secretion of FSH [106]. Therefore, BPA suppresses FSH action by preventing FSH- to FSH-receptor binding and by inhibiting FSH secretion. BPA causes the downregulation of Sertoli cell genes associated with cell death, cell proliferation, cell cycle regulation, DNA replication and repair, and ER stress markers [108]. BPA-treated Sertoli cells showed signs of apoptosis like chromatin condensation, DNA fragmentation, membrane blebs, and cytoskeletal collapse. The trigger for BPA-induced Sertoli cell apoptosis was shown to be via the caspase-mediated signaling cascade [105]. As in the case of NP, BPA was shown to inhibit microtubule formation *in vitro* but these findings could not be replicated *in vivo* [80]. BPA does not have any significant effect on Leydig cells although elevations in testosterone levels been reported [66]. BPA treatment has a major impact on Sertoli cell junctions and causes incomplete apical ectoplasmic specialization resulting in detachment of elongate spermatids from Sertoli cells [109]. However, BPA does not affect either basal ES or the BTB [110]. The loss in apical ES may be due to BPA-induced decrease in the levels of cortactin, which is an actin-binding protein found in the apical ES. Cortactin binds to the integrin β1/ laminin and cadherin/ catenin complexes and anchors them to the actin cytoskeleton. Cortactin is considered a marker for spermiogenesis and is responsible for imparting proper shape to spermatid acrosome [111]. Decrease in cortactin levels may be the cause for the appearance of malformed spermatid acrosome and nuclei seen after BPA treatment [110]. BPA has been shown to decrease the level of N-cadherin, occludin and connexin43, but increase the level of ZO-1 in Sertoli cells [112]. Therefore, it would seem that BPA has an adverse effect on TJs (occludin and ZO-1), AJs (N-cadherin and ZO-1) and GJs (connexin43) present at the apical region of seminiferous tubules. These junctions are interspersed at Sertoli-Sertoli and Sertoli-germ cell contacts and are regulated by cyclic nucleotides and phosphodiesterases (PDE) [90, 113]. Guanylate cyclase catalyzes the conversion of GTP into cGMP and PDE the conversion of cGMP into GDP [90]. When the degradation of cGMP is prevented by PDE inhibitors there is de-localization of Sertoli cell junction proteins although there are no changes in their levels.

Upon removal of these inhibitors, i.e., when PDE functions are restored, Sertoli cell junction proteins have been shown to relocate to their native locales and junction adhesion is re-established. This would suggest that de-localization of junction proteins may be an early response to toxic threats such as the one posed by BPA [38]. Increased intracellular calcium levels are considered an indicator of cellular injury and the transient increase in intracellular calcium levels following BPA treatment shows that indeed BPA is cyto-toxic to Sertoli cells and significantly affects their viability [85]. Fetal exposure to BPA causes slow post-natal growth rates, premature puberty, increased prostate weight, reduced daily sperm count, and an increase in the number of Sertoli cells per testis [114-117]. BPA has been shown to accelerate embryonic development but when thyroid hormone action was blocked (by inhibiting the thyroid hormone receptor), this effect was negated suggesting that BPA has an adverse effect on developmental timing through a thyroid hormone pathway [118]. Fetal exposure to BPA causes a decrease in circulating testosterone levels of male offspring coinciding with abnormal socio-sexual and aggressive behavior [119, 120]. Embryos treated with as low a dose as 1nM of BPA show premature puberty and postnatal reproductive development while high doses of 100mM retard development [121]. It is interesting to note that pubertal body weight of pups exposed during gestation are decreased when compared to untreated controls although all animals had similar natal weight [121]. This may be due to retarded growth of pups exposed to BPA but no corroborative evidence has been put forth to support his claim.

EPILOGUE

In the past decade, the safety/ toxicity of plasticizers has been a controversial topic of debate between researchers, academia and industry. Past reports that plasticizers, especially BPA, at doses well below the NOAEL dose can cause numerous multi-generation repro-toxic effects in males [100, 122, 123].

Alarmed by the piling evidence showing the toxicity of BPA, the Association of Plastics Manufacturers (APM) created and funded a consortium that would undertake research to validate the safety of this plasticizer. The APM then hired Gradient Corporation to gather evidence on the non-toxicity of plastics primarily to fight litigation that alleges that plastics and plasticizers are a health hazard.

Not surprisingly, the findings from Gradient Corporation claim that "the weight of evidence to date does not support the hypothesis that low oral doses of BPA adversely affect human reproductive and developmental health" [124]. These findings do not sit well in academia primarily because from the 119 publications arising out of government-funded research on sub-NOAEL doses of BPA till 2004, 92% report that BPA causes health hazards. There were 11 industry-sponsored studies upto 2004, all of which report the safety of BPA [125]. To resolve this discrepancy, the NIH convened a National Toxicity Program that met in 2002 and 2004 to examine available literature and determine the safety of BPA. The National Toxicity Program in 2002 upheld the NOAEL dose and deemed BPA safe below NOAEL doses.

But in an about-turn (probably due to the spate of publications from different countries which show the toxicity of BPA), the NTP, in 2004, declared there were grounds for concern regarding the safety of BPA. Despite efforts by the APM, governments worldwide are taking notice of these growing concerns, and in 2008, the government of Canada issued a ban on BPA in all infant-care products citing toxicity concerns. Controversies such as the one surrounding BPA create awareness about the safety and toxicity of plasticizers which, by all accounts, are hazardous environmental pollutants.

CONCLUSION

We have summarized the effects and mechanisms of action of important plasticizers like DEHP, DBP, NP and BPA on the male reproductive system (Table 1). Studies performed over a span of two decades have very clearly demonstrated that the Sertoli cell is targeted by these plasticizers, both in adult and fetal life.

Table 1. A summary of phenolic plasticizers and their effects on the male reproductive system

Plasticizer	*Uses*	Effects on the reproductive system	References
DEHP or Di (2-ethylhexyl) phthalate 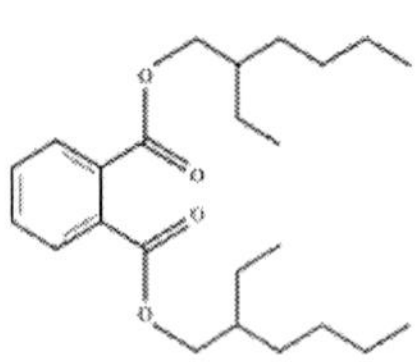	In the manu-facture of plas-tic containers (kitchen-ware, shampoo, cream and other liquid product con-tainers), toys, and medical devices (intra-venous tubes, catheters).	Decreased testis weights, testicular injury, cryptorchidism, hypospadia, decreased sperm counts, decreased AGD. Decreased INSL3 expression, de-creased T levels, induced capsase-3 mediated apoptosis in Leydig and germ cells. Vacuolization of Sertoli cells, atro-phy of seminiferous tubule, SCO. Disruption of AJs.	[16, 18-21, 24, 25, 42]
MEHP or Mono (2-ethyhexyl) phthalate 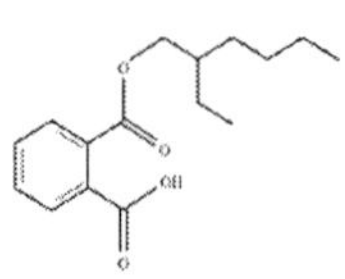	It is a degra-dation product of DEHP and is found in all DEHP- contain-ing plastics.	Affected redox homeostasis and mitochondrial anti-oxidant defence. Inhibited SC proliferation during fetal life. Disrupted SC cytoskeletal	[36, 37]

Plasticizer	Uses	Effects on the reproductive system	References
DBP or Dibutyl phthalate 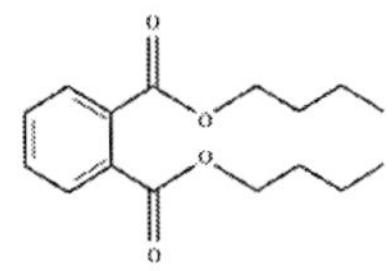	In the manu-facture of food packaging, latex adhesives, as fixatives for hair spray, and solvents for perfumes and inks.	Malformed or absent epididymis and accessory glands, decreased AGD, testicular atrophy, cryptorchidism, hypospadia, decreased sperm count, increased percentage of abnormal sperm, SCO. Downregulation of StAR, PBR, P450scc, ER-α, AR genes, germ cell loss, abnormal clusters of germ cells and Leydig cells hyperplasia. Vacuolization of Sertoli cell, loss in SC secretory functions De-structured vimentin cytoskeleton, disrupted GJ.	[31, 42, 46, 47, 50, 53-55, 60, 64]
NP or 4-nonylphenol 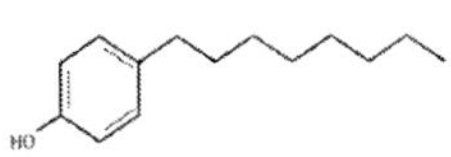	In the manu-facture of deter-gents, paints, pesticides, lea-ther processing, epoxy resins, photographic films, pa-per and textile ma-nufacture, and food packaging.	Decreased size of testes, epididymes, prostate and seminal vesicles, de-creased sperm production, crypt-orchidism, oxidative stress (in testis, epididymis and sperm). Decreased SC cytoplasmic volume and membrane integrity, SC necrosis and apoptosis via Fas/FasL pathway. Disrupted GJ.	[71, 74-76, 79, 81, 82, 88]
BPA or 4,4'-dihydroxy-2, 2-diphenylpropane 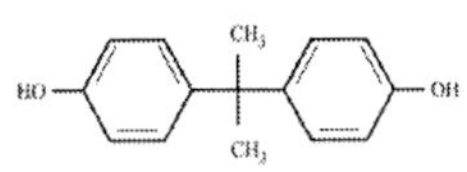	In the manu-facture of dis-posable food containers, be-verage cans, infant feeding bottles, micro-wave ovenware, refillable water containers and utensils.	Decreased size of testes, epididymes, prostate and seminal vesicles, under-developed seminiferous tubules, re-tardation in spermatogenesis, decrea-sed daily sperm production, decrea-sed sperm motility. Affected SC viability, induced SC apoptosis via caspase-mediated sig-naling. Caused incomplete apical ES for-mation, disrupted TJs, AJs and GJs.	[101-103, 105, 106, 109, 112, 114-117]

Abbreviations: AGD, anogenital distance; AJ, adherens junction; AR, androgen receptor; Cyp17a1, cytochrome 17; ES, ectoplasmic specialization; ER-□, estrogen receptor □□ FasL, Fas ligand; GC, germ cells; GJ, gap junction; LC, Leydig cells; NOAEL, No Observed Adverse Effect dose; P450scc, cytochrome p450 side chain cleavage; PBR, peripheral benzodiazepine receptor; SC, Sertoli cells; SCO, Sertoli cell only tubules; StAR, Steroid Acute Regulatory protein; T, testosterone and TJ, tight junction.

Due to its critical role in supporting spermatogenesis any threat to Sertoli cell function is intimately linked with a loss in male fertility. Therefore, the use of plasticizers must be vigilantly monitored to avoid any adverse effects to male reproductive health.

ACKNOWLEDGMENTS

P. P. Mathur acknowledges the receipt of financial support from the Department of Science and Technology, Government of India under the projects SP/ SO/ B-65/ 99 and DST-FIST to the Department, and the University Grants Commission, Government of India under the project 32-600/ 2006 (SR).

The authors wish to thank R. Jubendradass for help during preparation of the manuscript, and the staff of the Center for Bioinformatics, Pondicherry University for computational facilities.

REFERENCES

[1] Carlsen, E., Giwercman, A., Keiding, N. and Skakkebaek, N. E. (1992). Evidence for decreasing quality of semen during past 50 years. *Br. Med. J*, 305, 609-613.

[2] Calafat, A. M., Kuklenyik, Z., Reidy, J. A., Caudill, S. P., Ekong, J. and Needham, L. L. (2005). Urinary concentrations of bisphenol A and 4-nonylphenol in a human reference population. *Environ Health Perspect*, 113, 391-395.

[3] Latini, G., De Felice, C. and Verrotti, A. (2004). Plasticizers, infant nutrition and reproductive health. *Reprod. Toxicol*, 19, 27-33.

[4] Mylchreest, E., Cattley, R. C. and Foster, P. M. (1998). Male reproductive tract malformations in rats following gestational and lactational exposure to Di(*n*-butyl) phthalate: an antiandrogenic mechanism? *Toxicol. Sci*, 43, 47-60.

[5] Foster, P. M., Mylchreest, E., Gaido, K. W. and Sar, M. (2001). Effects of phthalate esters on the developing reproductive tract of male rats. *Hum. Reprod. Update*, 7, 231-235.

[6] Mathur, P. P., Saradha, B. and Vaithinathan, S. (2008). Impact of environmental toxicants on testicular function. *Immun. Endoc. Metab. Agents Med. Chem*, 8, 79-90.

[7] Hess, R. A. and França, L. R. (2005). History of the Sertoli cell discovery. In M. K. Skinner andM. D. Griswold (Eds.), *Sertoli cell Biology* pp. 3-14. San Diego: Elsevier Academic Press.

[8] Cupp, A. S. and Skinner, M. K. (2005). Embryonic Sertoli cell differentiation. In M. K. Skinner andM. D. Griswold (Eds.), *Sertoli cell Biology* pp. 43-70. San Diego: Elsevier Academic Press.

[9] Setchell, B. P. and Main, S. J. (1975). The blood - testis barrier and steroids. *Curr. Top Mol. Endocrinol*, 2, 223-233.

[10] Griswold, M. D. (1995). Interactions between germ cells and Sertoli cells in the testis. *Biol. Reprod*, 52, 211-216.

[11] Le Magueresse, B. and Jégou, B. (1988). Paracrine control of immature Sertoli cells by adult germ cells, in the rat (an *in vitro* study). Cell-cell interactions within the testis. *Mol. Cell Endocrinol*, 58, 65-72.

[12] Saradha, B. and Mathur, P. P. (2006). Effect of environmental contaminants on male reproduction. *Environ. Toxicol. Pharmacol*, 21, 34-41.

[13] Ministry of Agriculture, Fisheries and Food. (1998). Food surveillance information sheet no. 168: phthalates in infant formulae-follow-up survey.

[14] NTP-CERHR Expert Panel Report on Di(2-ethylhexyl) Phthalate. (2000). *Science International*, Inc. Alexandria, VA.

[15] Li, L. H. and Heindel, J. J. (1998). Sertoli cell toxicants. In K. Korach (Eds.), *Reproductive and Developmental Toxicology* pp. 657-693. New York: Marcel Dekker, Inc.

[16] Poon, R., Lecavalier, P., Mueller, R., Valli, V. E., Procter, B. G. and Chu, I. (1997). Subchronic oral toxicity of di-*n*-octyl phthalate and di(2-Ethylhexyl) phthalate in the rat. *Food Chem. Toxicol*, 35, 225-239.

[17] Toxicological profile for di(2-ethylhexyl) phthalate. (1993). Agency for Toxic Substances and Disease Registry. Atlanta.

[18] Andrade, A. J., Grande, S. W., Talsness, C. E., Gericke, C., Grote, K., Golombiewski, A., Sterner-Kock, A. and Chahoud, I. (2006). A dose response study following *in utero* and lactational exposure to di-(2-ethylhexyl) phthalate (DEHP): reproductive effects on adult male offspring rats. *Toxicology*, 228, 85-97.

[19] Nabae, K., Doi, Y., Takahashi, S., Ichihara, T., Toda, C., Ueda, K., Okamoto, Y., Kojima, N., Tamano, S. and Shirai, T. (2006). Toxicity of di(2-ethylhexyl)phthalate (DEHP) and di(2-ethylhexyl)adipate (DEHA) under conditions of renal dysfunction induced with folic acid in rats: enhancement of male reproductive toxicity of DEHP is associated with an increase of the mono-derivative. *Reprod. Toxicol*, 22, 411-417.

[20] Gangolli, S. D. (1982). Testicular effects of phthalate esters. *Environ. Health Perspect*, 45, 77-84.

[21] Gray, L. E., Jr., Ostby, J., Furr, J., Price, M., Veeramachaneni, D. N. and Parks, L. (2000). Perinatal exposure to the phthalates DEHP, BBP, and DINP, but not DEP, DMP, or DOTP, alters sexual differentiation of the male rat. *Toxicol. Sci*, 58, 350-365.

[22] Freeman, S. (1990). The evolution of the scrotum: a new hypothesis. *J. Theor. Biol*, 145, 429-445.

[23] Baskin, L. S. and Ebbers, M. B. (2006). Hypospadias: anatomy, etiology and technique. *J. Pediatric Surg*, 41, 1786-1791.

[24] Sobarzo, C. M., Lustig, L., Ponzio, R. and Denduchis, B. (2006). Effect of di-(2-ethylhexyl) phthalate on N-cadherin and catenin protein expression in rat testis. *Reprod. Toxicol*, 22, 77-86.

[25] Ge, R. S., Chen, G. R., Tanrikut, C. and Hardy, M. P. (2007). Phthalate ester toxicity in Leydig cells: developmental timing and dosage considerations. *Reprod. Toxicol*, 23, 366-373.

[26] Kim, J. M., Ghosh, S. R., Weil, A. C. and Zirkin, B. R. (2001). Caspase-3 and caspase activated deoxyribonuclease are associated with testicular germ cell apoptosis resulting from reduced intratesticular testosterone. *Endocrinology*, 142, 3809-3816.

[27] Skakkebaek, N. E., Rajpert-De Meyts, E. and Main, K. (2001). Testicular dysgenesis syndrome: an increasingly common developmental disorder with environmental aspects. *Hum. Reprod*, 16, 972-978.
[28] Sarkar, O., Mathur, P. P., Cheng, C. Y. and Mruk, D. D. (2008). Interleukin 1 alpha (IL1A) is a novel regulator of the blood-testis barrier in the rat. *Biol. Reprod*, 78, 445-454.
[29] Mruk, D. and Cheng, C. (2004). Sertoli-Sertoli and Sertoli-Germ Cell Interactions and Their Significance in Germ Cell Movement in the Seminiferous Epithelium during Spermatogenesis. *Endocr. Rev*, 25, 747-806.
[30] Park, J. D., Habeebu, S. S. and Klaassen, C. D. (2002). Testicular toxicity of di-(2-ethylhexyl)phthalate in young Sprague-Dawley rats. *Toxicology*, 171, 105-115.
[31] Fisher, J. S., Macpherson, S., Marchetti, N. and Sharpe, R. M. (2003). Human 'testicular dysgenesis syndrome': a possible model using *in-utero* exposure of the rat to dibutyl phthalate. *Hum. Reprod*, 18, 1383-1394.
[32] Foster, P. M. (2006). Disruption of reproductive development in male rat offspring following *in utero* exposure to phthalate esters. *Int. J. Androl*, 29, 140-147; discussion 181-145.
[33] Sharpe, R. M. (2001). Hormones and testis development and the possible adverse effects of environmental chemicals. *Toxicol Lett*, 120, 221-232.
[34] Akingbemi, B. T. and Hardy, M. P. (2001). Oestrogenic and antiandrogenic chemicals in the environment: effects on male reproductive health. *Ann Med*, 33, 391-403.
[35] Boekelheide, K., Lee, J. W., Hall, S. J., Rhind, N. R. and Zaret, K. S. (1993). A tumorigenic murine Sertoli cell line that is temperature-sensitive for differentiation. *Am. J. Pathol*, 143, 1159-1168.
[36] Grasso, P., Heindel, J. J., Powell, C. J. and Reichert, L. E. (1993). Effects of mono(2-ethylhexyl) phthalate, a testicular toxicant, on follicle-stimulating hormone binding to membranes from cultured rat Sertoli cells. *Biol. Reprod,* 48, 454-459.
[37] Onorato, T. M., Brown, P. W. and Morris, P. L. (2008). Mono-(2-ethylhexyl) phthalate increases spermatocyte mitochondrial peroxiredoxin 3 and cyclooxygenase 2. *J. Androl*, 29, 293-303.
[38] Boekelheide, K., Fleming, S. L., Johnson, K. J., Patel, S. R. and Schoenfeld, H. A. (2000). Role of Sertoli cells in injury-associated testicular germ cell apoptosis. *Proc. Soc. Exp. Biol. Med*, 225, 105-115.
[39] Sjoberg, P., Lindqvist, N. G. and Ploen, L. (1986). Age-dependent response of the rat testes to di(2-ethylhexyl) phthalate. *Environ. Health Perspect*, 65, 237-242.
[40] Liu, K., Lehmann, K. P., Sar, M., Young, S. S. and Gaido, K. W. (2005). Gene expression profiling following *in utero* exposure to phthalate esters reveals new gene targets in the etiology of testicular dysgenesis. Biol Reprod, 73, 180-192.
[41] Habert, R. and Brignaschi, P. (1991). Developmental changes in *in vitro* testosterone production by dispersed Leydig cells during fetal life in rats. *Arch. Androl*, 27, 65-71.
[42] Swan, S. H., Main, K. M., Liu, F., Stewart, S. L., Kruse, R. L., Calafat, A. M., Mao, C. S., Redmon, J. B., Ternand, C. L., Sullivan, S. and Teague, J. L. (2005). Decrease in anogenital distance among male infants with prenatal phthalate exposure. *Environ. Health Perspect*, 113, 1056-1061.
[43] Dostal, L. A., Chapin, R. E., Stefanski, S. A., Harris, M. W. and Schwetz, B. A. (1988). Testicular toxicity and reduced Sertoli cell numbers in neonatal rats by di(2-

ethylhexyl)phthalate and the recovery of fertility as adults. *Toxicol. Appl. Pharmacol*, 95, 104-121.

[44] Hsieh, M. H., Breyer, B. N., Eisenberg, M. L. and Baskin, L. S. (2008). Associations among hypospadias, cryptorchidism, anogenital distance, and endocrine disruption. *Curr. Urol. Rep*, 9, 137-142.

[45] Adham, I. M. and Agoulnik, A. I. (2004). Insulin-like 3 signalling in testicular descent. *Int. J. Androl*, 27, 257-265.

[46] McKee, R. H., Butala, J. H., David, R. M. and Gans, G. (2004). NTP center for the evaluation of risks to human reproduction reports on phthalates: addressing the data gaps. *Reprod. Toxicol*, 18, 1-22.

[47] Zhang, Y., Jiang, X. and Chen, B. (2004). Reproductive and developmental toxicity in F1 Sprague-Dawley male rats exposed to di- *n*-butyl phthalate *in utero* and during lactation and determination of its NOAEL. *Reprod. Toxicol*, 18, 669-676.

[48] Tanaka, A., Matsumoto, A. and Yamaha, T. (1978). Biochemical studies on phthalic esters. Metabolism of dibutyl phthalate (DBP) in animals. *Toxicology*, 9, 109-123.

[49] Kluwe, W. M., McConnell, E. E., Huff, J. E., Haseman, J. K., Douglas, J. F. and Hartwell, W. V. (1982). Carcinogenicity testing of phthalate esters and related compounds by the National Toxicology Program and the National Cancer Institute. *Environ. Health Perspect*, 45, 129-133.

[50] Johnson, K. J., Hensley, J. B., Kelso, M. D., Wallace, D. G. and Gaido, K. W. (2007). Mapping gene expression changes in the fetal rat testis following acute dibutyl phthalate exposure defines a complex temporal cascade of responding cell types. *Biol. Reprod*, 77, 978-989.

[51] Martineau, J., Nordqvist, K., Tilmann, C., Lovell-Badge, R. and Capel, B. (1997). Male-specific cell migration into the developing gonad. *Curr. Biol*, 7, 958-968.

[52] Pan, G., Hanaoka, T., Yoshimura, M., Zhang, S., Wang, P., Tsukino, H., Inoue, K., Nakazawa, H., Tsugane, S. and Takahashi, K. (2006). Decreased serum free testosterone in workers exposed to high levels of di-*n*-butyl phthalate (DBP) and di-2-ethylhexyl phthalate (DEHP): a cross-sectional study in China. *Environ. Health Perspect*, 114, 1643-1648.

[53] Rao, J. N., Liang, J. Y., Chakraborti, P. and Feng, P. (2003). Effect of thyroid hormone on the development and gene expression of hormone receptors in rat testes *in vivo*. *J. Endocrinol. Invest*, 26, 435-443.

[54] Lehmann, K. P., Phillips, S., Sar, M., Foster, P. M. and Gaido, K. W. (2004). Dose-dependent alterations in gene expression and testosterone synthesis in the fetal testes of male rats exposed to di (*n*-butyl) phthalate. *Toxicol. Sci*, 81, 60-68.

[55] Ryu, J. Y., Whang, J., Park, H., Im, J. Y., Kim, J., Ahn, M. Y., Lee, J., Kim, H. S., Lee, B. M., Yoo, S. D., Kwack, S. J., Oh, J. H., Park, K. L., Han, S. Y. and Kim, S. H. (2007). Di(2-ethylhexyl) phthalate induces apoptosis through peroxisome proliferators-activated receptor-gamma and ERK 1/2 activation in testis of Sprague-Dawley rats. *J Toxicol. Environ. Health A*, 70, 1296-1303.

[56] Cater, B. R., Cook, M. W., Gangolli, S. D. and Grasso, P. (1977). Studies on dibutyl phthalate-induced testicular atrophy in the rat: effect on zinc metabolism. *Toxicol. Appl. Pharmacol*, 41, 609-618.

[57] Boekelheide, K. (2004). Cracking the nut. *Toxicol. Sci*, 81, 1-2.

[58] Lee, S. K. and Veeramachaneni, D. N. (2005). Subchronic exposure to low concentrations of di-*n*-butyl phthalate disrupts spermatogenesis in Xenopus laevis frogs. *Toxicol. Sci*, 84, 394-407.

[59] Boekelheide, K., Johnson, K. J. and Richburg, J. H. (2005). Sertoli cell toxicants. In M. K. Skinner andM. D. Griswold (Eds.), *Sertoli cell Biology* pp. 345-382. San Diego: Elsevier Academic Press.

[60] Xing, X. W., Li, L. Y., Liu, G., Fu, J. J., Tan, X. J. and Lu, G. X. (2004). Identification of a novel gene SRG4 expressed at specific stages of mouse spermatogenesis. *Acta Biochim. Biophys. Sin.* (Shanghai), 36, 351-359.

[61] Lloyd, S. C. and Foster, P. M. (1988). Effect of mono-(2-ethylhexyl)phthalate on follicle-stimulating hormone responsiveness of cultured rat Sertoli cells. *Toxicol. Appl. Pharmacol*, 95, 484-489.

[62] Roscoe, W. A., Barr, K. J., Mhawi, A. A., Pomerantz, D. K. and Kidder, G. M. (2001). Failure of spermatogenesis in mice lacking connexin43. *Biol. Reprod*, 65, 829-838.

[63] Cheng, C. Y., Grima, J., Stahler, M. S., Lockshin, R. A. and Bardin, C. W. (1989). Testins are structurally related Sertoli cell proteins whose secretion is tightly coupled to the presence of germ cells. *J. Biol. Chem*, 264, 21386-21393.

[64] Mylchreest, E., Wallace, D. G., Cattley, R. C. and Foster, P. M. (2000). Dose-dependent alterations in androgen-regulated male reproductive development in rats exposed to Di(*n*-butyl) phthalate during late gestation. *Toxicol. Sci*, 55, 143-151.

[65] Kleymenova, E., Swanson, C., Boekelheide, K. and Gaido, K. W. (2005). Exposure *in utero* to di(*n*-butyl) phthalate alters the vimentin cytoskeleton of fetal rat Sertoli cells and disrupts Sertoli cell-gonocyte contact. *Biol. Reprod*, 73, 482-490.

[66] Sharpe, R. M. and Skakkebaek, N. E. (2003). Male reproductive disorders and the role of endocrine disruption: advances in understanding and identification of areas for future research. *Pure Appl. Chem*, 75, 2023-2038.

[67] Naylor, C. G., Mieure, J. P., Adam, W. J., Weeks, J. A., Castaldi, F. J., Ogle, L. D. and Romano, R. R. (1992). Alkylphenol ethoxylates in the environment. *J. Am. Oil Chem.* Soc, 69, 695-703.

[68] Daidoji, T., Inoue, H., Kato, S. and Yokota, H. (2003). Glucuronidation and excretion of nonylphenol in perfused rat liver. *Drug Metab. Dispos*, 31, 993-998.

[69] Daidoji, T., Ozawa, M., Sakamoto, H., Sako, T., Inoue, H., Kurihara, R., Hashimoto, S. and Yokota, H. (2006). Slow elimination of nonylphenol from rat intestine. *Drug Metab. Dispos*, 34, 184-190.

[70] Yamazaki, M., Suzuki, H. and Sugiyama, Y. (1996). Recent advances in carrier-mediated hepatic uptake and biliary excretion of xenobiotics. *Pharm. Res.* (NY), 13, 497-513.

[71] Lee, P. C. (1998). Disruption of male reproductive tract development by administration of the xenoestrogen, nonylphenol, to male newborn rats. *Endocrine*, 9, 105-111.

[72] de Jager, C., Bornman, M. S. and van der Horst, G. (1999). The effect of p-nonylphenol, an environmental toxicant with oestrogenic properties, on fertility potential in adult male rats. *Andrologia*, 31, 99-106.

[73] Zini, A. and Schlegel, P. N. (1997). Identification and characterization of antioxidant enzyme mRNAs in the rat epididymis. *Int. J. Androl*, 20, 86-91.

[74] Chitra, K. C., Latchoumycandane, C. and Mathur, P. P. (2002). Effect of nonylphenol on the antioxidant system in epididymal sperm of rats. *Arch. Toxicol*, 76, 545-551.

[75] Chitra, K. C. and Mathur, P. P. (2004). Vitamin E prevents nonylphenol-induced oxidative stress in testis of rats. *Indian J. Exp. Biol*, 42, 220-223.

[76] Gong, Y. and Han, X. D. (2006). Nonylphenol-induced oxidative stress and cytotoxicity in testicular Sertoli cells. *Reprod. Toxicol,* 22, 623-630.

[77] Sikka, S. C. (1996). Oxidative stress and role of antioxidants in normal and abnormal sperm function. *Front Biosci*, 1, e78-86.

[78] Saradha, B., Vaithinathan, S. and Mathur, P. P. (2008). Lindane alters the levels of HSP70 and clusterin in adult rat testis. *Toxicology*, 243, 116-123.

[79] Miles-Richardson, S. R., Pierens, S. L., Nichols, K. M., Kramer, V. J., Snyder, E. M., Snyder, S. A., Render, J. A., Fitzgerald, S. D. and Giesy, J. P. (1999). Effects of waterborne exposure to 4-nonylphenol and nonylphenol ethoxylate on secondary sex characteristics and gonads of fathead minnows (Pimephales promelas). *Environ. Res*, 80, S122-S137.

[80] Nakagomi, M., Suzuki, E., Usumi, K., Saitoh, Y., Yoshimura, S., Nagao, T. and Ono, H. (2001). Effects of endocrine disrupting chemicals on the microtubule network in Chinese hamster V79 cells in culture and in Sertoli cells in rats. *Teratog Carcinog Mutagen*, 21, 453-462.

[81] Han, X. D., Tu, Z. G., Gong, Y., Shen, S. N., Wang, X. Y., Kang, L. N., Hou, Y. Y. and Chen, J. X. (2004). The toxic effects of nonylphenol on the reproductive system of male rats. *Reprod. Toxicol*, 19, 215-221.

[82] Wang, X., Han, X., Hou, Y., Yao, G. and Wang, Y. (2003). Effect of nonylphenol on apoptosis of Sertoli cells *in vitro*. *Bull. Environ. Contam. Toxicol*, 70, 898-904.

[83] Richburg, J. H. (2000). The relevance of spontaneous- and chemically-induced alterations in testicular germ cell apoptosis to toxicology. *Toxicol. Lett*, 112-113, 79-86.

[84] Kroemer, G., Dallaporta, B. and Resche-Rigon, M. (1998). The mitochondrial death/life regulator in apoptosis and necrosis. *Annu. Rev. Physiol*, 60, 619-642.

[85] Hughes, P. J., McLellan, H., Lowes, D. A., Kahn, S. Z., Bilmen, J. G., Tovey, S. C., Godfrey, R. E., Michell, R. H., Kirk, C. J. and Michelangeli, F. (2000). Estrogenic alkylphenols induce cell death by inhibiting testis endoplasmic reticulum Ca(2+) pumps. *Biochem. Biophys. Res. Commun*, 277, 568-574.

[86] Kudo, C., Wada, K., Masuda, T., Yonemura, T., Shibuya, A., Fujimoto, Y., Nakajima, A., Niwa, H. and Kamisaki, Y. (2004). Nonylphenol induces the death of neural stem cells due to activation of the caspase cascade and regulation of the cell cycle. *J. Neurochem*, 88, 1416-1423.

[87] Sarkar, O. and Mathur, P. P. (2008). Adjudin-mediated germ cell depletion alters the anti-oxidant status of adult rat testis. *Mol. Reprod. Dev*, DOI 10.1002/mrd.20928.

[88] Aravindakshan, J. and Cyr, D. G. (2005). Nonylphenol alters connexin 43 levels and connexin 43 phosphorylation via an inhibition of the p38-mitogen-activated protein kinase pathway. *Biol. Reprod*, 72, 1232-1240.

[89] Sarkar, O., Xia, W. and Mruk, D. D. (2006). Adjudin-mediated junction restructuring in the seminiferous epithelium leads to displacement of soluble guanylate cyclase from adherens junctions. *J. Cell Phys*, 208, 175-187.

[90] Sarkar, O., Mathur, P. P. and Mruk, D. D. (2008). Nitric oxide-cGMP signaling: its role in cell junction dynamics during spermatogenesis. *Immun. Endoc. Metab. Agents Med. Chem*, 8, 28-35.

[91] Mograbi, B., Corcelle, E., Defamie, N., Samson, M., Nebout, M., Segretain, D., Fenichel, P. and Pointis, G. (2003). Aberrant Connexin 43 endocytosis by the carcinogen lindane involves activation of the ERK/ mitogen-activated protein kinase pathway. *Carcinogenesis*, 24, 1415-1423.
[92] Wong, C. H., Mruk, D. D., Siu, M. K. and Cheng, C. Y. (2005). Blood-testis barrier dynamics are regulated by {alpha}2-macroglobulin via the c-Jun N-terminal protein kinase pathway. *Endocrinology*, 146, 1893-1908.
[93] Dalgaard, M., Pilegaard, K. and Ladefoged, O. (2002). *In utero* exposure to diethylstilboestrol or 4-*n*-nonylphenol in rats: number of Sertoli cells, diameter and length of seminiferous tubules estimated by stereological methods. *Pharmacol. Toxicol*, 90, 59-65.
[94] Nagao, T., Wada, K., Marumo, H., Yoshimura, S. and Ono, H. (2001). Reproductive effects of nonylphenol in rats after gavage administration: a two-generation study. *Reprod. Toxicol*, 15, 293-315.
[95] Scallet, A. C., Bennett, C., Newbold, R., Delclos, K., Weis, C. and M., M. J. (1999). Decreased volume of the sexually dimorphic nucleus of the medial preoptic area (SDN-POA) in male rats after chronic nonylphenol exposure. *Soc. Neurosci. Abstr*, 25, 227.
[96] Hossaini, A., Dalgaard, M., Vinggaard, A. M., Frandsen, H. and Larsen, J. J. (2001). *In utero* reproductive study in rats exposed to nonylphenol. *Reprod. Toxicol*, 15, 537-543.
[97] Laurenzana, E. M., Weis, C. C., Bryant, C. W., Newbold, R. and Delclos, K. B. (2002). Effect of dietary administration of genistein, nonylphenol or ethinyl estradiol on hepatic testosterone metabolism, cytochrome P-450 enzymes, and estrogen receptor alpha expression. *Food Chem. Toxicol*, 40, 53-63.
[98] Opinion of the Scientific Panel on Food Additives, F., Processing Aids and Materials in Contact with Food on a request from the Commission related to 2, 2-bis (4-hydroxyphenyl) propane (Bisphenol A). (2006). *The EFSA Journal*, 428.
[99] Pennie, W. D., Aldridge, T. C. and Brooks, A. N. (1998). Differential activation by xenoestrogens of ER alpha and ER beta when linked to different response elements. *J. Endocrinol*, 158, R11-14.
[100] Welshons, W. V., Nagel, S. C. and vom Saal, F. S. (2006). Large effects from small exposures. III. Endocrine mechanisms mediating effects of bisphenol A at levels of human exposure. *Endocrinology*, 147, S56-69.
[101] Atanassova, N., McKinnell, C., Turner, K. J., Walker, M., Fisher, J. S., Morley, M., Millar, M. R., Groome, N. P. and Sharpe, R. M. (2000). Comparative effects of neonatal exposure of male rats to potent and weak (environmental) estrogens on spermatogenesis at puberty and the relationship to adult testis size and fertility: evidence for stimulatory effects of low estrogen levels. *Endocrinology*, 141, 3898-3907.
[102] Chitra, K. C., Latchoumycandane, C. and Mathur, P. P. (2003). Induction of oxidative stress by bisphenol A in the epididymal sperm of rats. *Toxicology*, 185, 119-127.
[103] Chitra, K. C. and Mathur, P. P. (2003). Induction of oxidative stress in epididymis of rats after short-term exposure to bisphenol A. *Arch. Med. Res*, 1, 1-16.
[104] Bindhumol, V., Chitra, K. C. and Mathur, P. P. (2003). Bisphenol A induces reactive oxygen species generation in the liver of male rats. *Toxicology*, 188, 117-124.
[105] Iida, H., Maehara, K., Doiguchi, M., Mori, T. and Yamada, F. (2003). Bisphenol A-induced apoptosis of cultured rat Sertoli cells. *Reprod. Toxicol*, 17, 457-464.

[106] Monsees, T. K., Franz, M., Gebhardt, S., Winterstein, U., Schill, W. B. and Hayatpour, J. (2000). Sertoli cells as a target for reproductive hazards. *Andrologia*, 32, 239-246.

[107] Bernard, L., Martinat, N., Lecureuil, C., Crepieux, P., Reiter, E., Tilloy-Ellul, A., Chevalier, S. and Guillou, F. (2007). Dichlorodiphenyltrichloroethane impairs follicle-stimulating hormone receptor-mediated signaling in rat Sertoli cells. *Reprod. Toxicol*, 23, 158-164.

[108] Tabuchi, Y., Takasaki, I. and Kondo, T. (2006). Identification of genetic networks involved in the cell injury accompanying endoplasmic reticulum stress induced by bisphenol A in testicular Sertoli cells. *Biochem. Biophys. Res. Commun*, 345, 1044-1050.

[109] Anahara, R., Yoshida, M., Toyama, Y., Maekawa, M., Kai, M., Ishino, F., Toshimori, K. and Mori, C. (2006). Estrogen agonists, 17□-estradiol, bisphenol A, and diethylstilbestrol, decrease cortactin expression in the mouse testis. *Arch. Histol. Cytol*, 69, 101-107.

[110] Toyama, Y., Suzuki-Toyota, F., Maekawa, M., Ito, C. and Toshimori, K. (2004). Adverse effects of bisphenol A to spermiogenesis in mice and rats. *Arch. Histol. Cytol*, 67, 373-381.

[111] Chapin, R. E., Wine, R. N., Harris, M. W., Borchers, C. H. and Haseman, J. K. (2001). Structure and control of a cell-cell adhesion complex associated with spermiation in rat seminiferous epithelium. *J. Androl*, 22, 1030-1052.

[112] Fiorini, C., Tilloy-Ellul, A., Chevalier, S., Charuel, C. and Pointis, G. (2004). Sertoli cell junctional proteins as early targets for different classes of reproductive toxicants. *Reprod. Toxicol*, 18, 413-421.

[113] Janecki, A., Jakubowiak, A. and Steinberger, A. (1991). Effects of cyclic AMP and phorbol ester on transepithelial electrical resistance of Sertoli cell monolayers in two-compartment culture. *Mol. Cell Endocrinol*, 82, 61-69.

[114] Nagel, S. C., vom Saal, F. S., Thayer, K. A., Dhar, M. G., Boechler, M. and Welshons, W. V. (1997). Relative binding affinity-serum modified access (RBA-SMA) assay predicts the relative *in vivo* bioactivity of the xenoestrogens bisphenol A and octylphenol. *Environ. Health Perspect*, 105, 70-76.

[115] vom Saal, F. S., Cooke, P. S., Buchanan, D. L., Palanza, P., Thayer, K. A., Nagel, S. C., Parmigiani, S. and Welshons, W. V. (1998). A physiologically based approach to the study of bisphenol A and other estrogenic chemicals on the size of reproductive organs, daily sperm production, and behavior. *Toxicol. Ind. Health*, 14, 239-260.

[116] Howdeshell, K. L., Hotchkiss, A. K., Thayer, K. A., Vandenbergh, J. G. and vom Saal, F. S. (1999). Exposure to bisphenol A advances puberty. *Nature*, 401, 763-764.

[117] Wistuba, J., Brinkworth, M. H., Schlatt, S., Chahoud, I. and Nieschlag, E. (2003). Intrauterine bisphenol A exposure leads to stimulatory effects on Sertoli cell number in rats. *Environ. Res*, 91, 95-103.

[118] Ramakrishnan, S. and Wayne, N. L. (2008). Impact of bisphenol-A on early embryonic development and reproductive maturation. *Reprod. Toxicol*, 25, 177-183.

[119] Dessi-Fulgheri, F., Porrini, S. and Farabollini, F. (2002). Effects of perinatal exposure to bisphenol A on play behavior of female and male juvenile rats. *Environ. Health Perspect*, 110 Suppl 3, 403-407.

[120] Kawai, K., Nozaki, T., Nishikata, H., Aou, S., Takii, M. and Kubo, C. (2003). Aggressive behavior and serum testosterone concentration during the maturation

process of male mice: the effects of fetal exposure to bisphenol A. *Environ. Health Perspect*, 111, 175-178.

[121] Takai, Y., Tsutsumi, O., Ikezuki, Y., Kamei, Y., Osuga, Y., Yano, T. and Taketan, Y. (2001). Preimplantation exposure to bisphenol A advances postnatal development. *Reprod. Toxicol*, 15, 71-74.

[122] Welshons, W. V., Thayer, K. A., Judy, B. M., Taylor, J. A., Curran, E. M. and vom Saal, F. S. (2003). Large effects from small exposures. I. Mechanisms for endocrine-disrupting chemicals with estrogenic activity. *Environ. Health Perspect*, 111, 994-1006.

[123] vom Saal, F. S. and Welshons, W. V. (2006). Large effects from small exposures. II. The importance of positive controls in low-dose research on bisphenol A. *Environ. Res*, 100, 50-76.

[124] Goodman, J. E., McConnell, E. E., Sipes, I. G., Witorsch, R. J., Slayton, T. M., Yu, C. J., Lewis, A. S. and Rhomberg, L. R. (2006). An updated weight of the evidence evaluation of reproductive and developmental effects of low doses of bisphenol A. *Crit. Rev. Toxicol*, 36, 387-457.

[125] vom Saal, F. S. (2005). Low-dose BPA: confirmed by extensive literature. *Chem. Indus*, 14 - 15.

INDEX

D

E

I

J

K

L

M

N

O

P

Q

R

S

T

U